This book is a comprehensive cyclopedia of reliable formulas intended to provide authentic, concise, and practical information for technical and non-technical people alike.

It presents hundreds of formulas which should fill many needs, not only of professional chemists, pharmacists, and others in related fields, but also of manufacturers, teachers, students, and laymen.

The author's vast and varied experience in industry and as a consultant has enabled him to compile these authoritative up-to-date formulas from many sources. Each formula here has been carefully selected, researched, tested, and proved. Instructions have been simplified, yet they are explicit enough to guide even a new experimenter to successful accomplishment.

Every section contains formulations that utilize the newest accepted materials for pharmaceuticals, natural and synthetic aromatics, preservatives, household and industrial products, etc. The comprehensive tables on the analysis of foods and the properties of gems are exceptional in a book of this type. The highly selective sections on cosmetics and on foods are especially well arranged for ready reference.

A good bibliography shows the broad background of the fields of science and technology from which this information has been assembled. And finally the list of suppliers at the end of the book will serve as a reliable buyer's guide to the chemicals needed for various formulations.

PRACTICAL and INDUSTRIAL FORMULARY

MITCHELL FREEMAN, Met.E.

Mitchell Laboratories

formerly with
The Standard Chemical Company
U. S. Metals Reduction Company
Pennsylvania Manufacturers and Extract Company
Duquesne Smelting Corporation

CHEMICAL PUBLISHING CO., INC.
212 Fifth Avenue · New York, N. Y.
1962

CHEMICAL PUBLISHING CO., INC.
New York N. Y.

Printed in the United States of America

Preface

This volume is a collection of new, modern, up-to-date formulae. The purpose of this work is to provide authentic, concise, and practical information of interest to all—laymen and technologists. It is a condensed, comprehensive, and reliable cyclopedia of formulas for the chemist, pharmacist, and those in allied professions. It is intended to fill a definite need of the manufacturer, teacher, student, and layman. Here, in one handy volume, is a wealth of new formulas and methods you can put right to work. No other book like it has been published. Most of the formulae may be varied to suit everybody's fancy.

This practical book offers you information equal to the services of a private staff of experts on many problems. The formulas in it are entirely practical—the kind you can put to use right away. Most of the formulas have been carefully selected, tested, and thoroughly researched by technical men.

To the thousands of professional workers for whom this book is intended, I extend my hope that it will prove to be a dependable and useful source of information. It is my sincere desire that this book will prove to be a significant contribution to the making of better things.

In keeping up with the times in this streamlined age, one is helped by various "digests" which one has come to require as first aids to one's knowledge. It is wise to know a little something about almost everything, hence one seizes upon the paper-covered things that give much in little.

I wish to acknowledge my indebtedness to the various government and scientific publications for much useful information.

Critical and constructive comments and suggestions from the users of this book will always be welcomed by the author.

This volume comprises a comprehensive Buyer's Guide, and it is hoped that this arrangement will enable users to find quickly an answer to their supply problems.

1962 Mitchell Freeman, Met.E.

Contents

Adhesives

Adhesive for Cellophane Films

	oz
Gum arabic, best grade	11.0
Glycerin	11.0
Glyceryl borate	9.0
Formalin	3.0

Mix the gum arabic with the glycerin and use gentle heat to effect complete solution. Finally, add the glyceryl borate, and formalin, and shake well.

Glue for Bookbinding

Skin gelatin	4.0 lb
Boiling water	3.0 lb
Glycerin	1.8 lb
Betanaphthol	10.0 oz
Alcosolve 2	10.0 oz

Dissolve the gelatin in the boiling water. Mix the betanaphthol with the glycerin and heat gently to effect solution. Mix the two solutions and shake well. Finally, stir in the Alcosolve 2.

Glue, Flexible

Skin glue, powdered, good quality	10.0 lb
Water	64.0 oz
Glycerin	2.5 lb
Sugar, granulated	2.3 lb
Betanaphthol	1.6 oz
Isopropyl alcohol, 88%	2.4 oz

Mix the first 4 ingredients, and beat until solution is complete. Allow it to cool and stir in the betanaphthol, previously dissolved in the alcohol. Put up in suitable containers. The resultant glue has extremely good tack and flexibility, it possesses excellent adhesive properties as well as flexibility.

Paste for Offices

White potato dextrin	5.0 lb
Boiling water	7.5 lb
Borax	6.8 oz
Glyceryl borate *	3.2 oz
Formalin	0.8 oz
Phenol	0.8 oz

Dissolve the dextrin in the boiling water. Stir in the borax and glyceryl borate. Finally, add the formalin and phenol, and shake well.

* Glyceryl Borate

	parts
Boric acid	12.4
Glycerin	36.8

Dissolve the boric acid in one half of the glycerin at 150°C. When solution is complete, add the other half of the glycerin and shake well.

Paste for Labeling Tin

	lb
White potato dextrin	1
Gum arabic solution, 20%	5
Boiling water	16½
Flake calcium chloride	1¾
Glycerite of starch *	1

Dissolve the dextrin in the boiling water. Add the calcium chloride and shake well. Finally, stir in the gum arabic solution and the glycerite of starch.

* Glycerite of Starch

Starch	1.27 oz
Distilled water	2.27 oz
Glycerin	11.30 oz

Make a slurry of the starch in the distilled water. Pour this slurry gradually with stirring into the glycerin at 140°C. When the frothing has subsided, keep the temperature at 135°C. and stir the gel until it becomes translucent.

Peel Paste

Mix suitable proportions of the following ingredients:

Methocel (methyl cellulose)
Glycerin
Water

The setting time of this adhesive can be adjusted by varying the amount of the glycerin. It is used in place of usual starch pastes in applying wallpaper to hard surfaces. This adhesive holds the paper in place for as long as required, and it can be stripped off easily when so desired.

Waterproof Cement

	oz
Lead monoxide, yellow, powdered	16
Glycerin	2⅓
Water	1

or

Lead monoxide	16
Glycerin	4
Water	1¾

Mix the glycerin with the water. Add the lead oxide, and mix thoroughly. The amount of water may be varied, depending on the rate of set desired. The resultant product yields a fast-setting, hard, waterproof cement which will adhere firmly to china, glass, iron, stone, wood and other materials.

Cleaning Preparations

For Aluminum

	oz
Trisodium orthophosphate	42.0
Sodium metasilicate, anhydrous	36.0
Soda ash	24.0
Alkyl aryl sodium sulfonate, 85% active	12.0
Tetrasodium pyrophosphate, anhydrous	6.0

Mix thoroughly and put in suitable containers. This product is satisfactory for precleaning metal specimens.

For Brass, Copper, and Bronze

	oz
Sodium dichromate	47.36
Sulfuric acid, 66°Bé	11.52
Water	69.12

Dissolve the dichromate in the water, add the sulfuric acid and shake well. Avoid contact of the substance with hands or any other part of the body, especially the eyes. This product will remove the superficial discoloration, thus restoring the original appearance and color of the metals.

For Cars (Paste)

	oz
Teepol (higher alkyd sulfate) *	75.0
Bentonite, white	30.0
Infusorial earth	45.0

* 30% active secondary fatty alcohol sulfate.

Heat the Teepol and stir in the powders. Continue to stir until a smooth paste is obtained. Put up in suitable containers. Rub the paste on the surface of the car, then rinse it off with water.

For Cars (Shampoo)

	oz
Dodecyl benzene sulfonate (40% active)	75
Sodium hexametaphosphate	22.5
Sodium sulfate, anhydrous	52.5

Mix the powders thoroughly and store in suitable containers. Make a 5% solution of this powdered compound in water, and apply to the body of the car with a rag or soft brush. Rinse the car with water from a hose.

For Dairy Pipe Lines

No. 1

	lb
Sodium tripolyphosphate, anhydrous	18
Trisodium phosphate, anhydrous	3.6
Soda ash	66
Sodium metasilicate, anhydrous	6
Sodium bicarbonate	14.4
Hyamine (germicide)	12

Have all the ingredients in a finely granulated form and mix thoroughly.

No. 2

	oz
Sodium hydroxide	4
Soda ash	14
Sodium metasilicate	100
Tripolyphosphate	70
Trisodium phosphate	12

Have all the ingredients in a finely granulated form and mix thoroughly. This now-sudsing mixture will minimize or prevent the formation of milk stone in glass pipe lines in dairies. The sodium hydroxide acts as a sanitizer; the trisodium phosphate as a water conditioner; and the metasilicate as a wetting and deflocculating agent. Do not handle the sodium hydroxide with bare hands.

Dishwashing Compounds

No. 1

	lb
Soda ash	48
Sodium metasilicate	54
Sodium tripolyphosphate	4.8
Trisodium phosphate	12
Wetting agent (Nekal BX)	1.2

Have all the ingredients in a finely granulated form and mix thoroughly.

No. 2

	lb
Sodium metasilicate	24
Sodium tripolyphosphate	18
Sodium carbonate	9
Trisodium phosphate	9

Have all the ingredients in a finely granulated form and mix thoroughly. The metasilicate acts as a suspending and dispersing agent, and also inhibits the corrosion of metals. As the tripolyphosphate has water-softening properties, it acts as a wetting and dispersing agent. The carbonate and trisodium phosphate augment the necessary alkalinity.

Dry-Wash for Hands

	oz
Stoddard Solvent *	64.00
Stearic acid	12.16
Triethanolamine	5.12
Hexalin	3.07
Lanolin	2.68
Water	40.97

* High flash point petroleum distillate.

Melt the stearic acid with the lanolin. Heat the triethanolamine and water to the same temperature, and pour slowly with constant stirring into the molten fats. When cool, stir in the Stoddard Solvent and Hexalin. Continue stirring until cold.

This preparation will remove oil, paint, grease, grime, tar and printer's ink from the hands.

Eyeglass Cleaner

Ammonium soap	6.40 oz
Glycerin	6.60 oz
Water, enough to make	1.00 gal
Fluorescein, soluble (D & C Yellow #7)	sufficient

Dissolve the soap in the water, add the glycerin and tint it with the fluorescein. Shake well. Place a few drops of this preparation on the eyeglass and wipe off clean with a soft cloth.

Glass Cleaner

	lb
Sodium sulfate	80
Sodium tripolyphosphate	33.34
Triton X-101	4
Trisodium phosphate	16

Have all the ingredients in powdered form and mix thoroughly.

Laundry Powder

	lb
Alkyl aryl sulfonate	30.00
Fatty alcohol ethylene oxide sulfate	10.00
Lauric ethanol	6.00
Sodium metasilicate	10.00
Sodium sulfate	30.00
Sodium tripolyphosphate	80.00
Tetrasodium pyrophosphate	14.00
Sodium carboxymethyl cellulose	1.00
Optical dye	0.06
Perfume and color	to suit

Have all the ingredients in a finely powdered form and mix thoroughly. The phosphates have detergent properties and act as dispersing and water-softening agents. The metasilicate inhibits the corrosion of metals. The sulfate is both a detergent and a diluent. The carboxymethylcellulose (CMC) assists in suspension of dirt.

Liquid for Floors and Walls

	oz
Coconut diethanolamide	49.00
Triethanolamine alkyl aryl sulfonate	28.00
Trisodium phosphate	14.00
Sodium tripolyphosphate	14.00
Water	4.65 gal

Mix all the ingredients and stir thoroughly until everything is dissolved.

Liquid Hand Soap

Coconut oil fatty acids	6¾ lb
Soya fatty acids	27 oz
Potassium hydroxide solution (50°Bé)	81 oz
Potassium chloride	9 oz
Distilled water	5⅜ gal
Perfume oil	to suit

Put the fatty acids in a jacketed kettle equipped with a stirring apparatus, and heat at 65°C. Make a mixture of the potassium hydroxide solution, potassium chloride, and water, and heat to the same temperature. Pour the alkaline solution into the fats with constant stirring. Continue to stir until saponification is complete. Stir in the perfume oil when the temperature is about 35°C. Use this soap in a dispenser in any public washroom. It may also be used for scrubbing floors. Use extreme care when handling potassium hydroxide (caustic potash).

Liquid Scrub Soap

Cottonseed fatty acid (sap. value 200)	4.95 lb
Pine oil	25.00 oz
o-phenylphenol	25.00 oz
Caustic potash 100%	15.84 oz
Water	4.00 gal

Mix the fatty acid, pine oil, *o*-phenylphenol, and heat at a low temperature. Dissolve the potash in the water and heat to the same temperature. Pour the potash solution into the fats with constant stirring. Continue to stir until saponification is complete. The pine oil increases the transparency of the finished product, and the *o*-phenylphenol imparts germicidal properties to it.

Metal Cleaner

	oz
Mineral spirits *	70.00
Triethanolamine	2.50
Oleic acid	5.00
Ethylene glycol monobutyl ether (Butyl Cellosolve)	1.25
Pine oil	19.50

* A petroleum product, intermediate between gasoline and kerosene.

Mix all ingredients thoroughly; add 10 or more volumes of water. Spray this mixture over the metal surface to be cleaned. An extremely thin protective coating remains which prevents rusting over a period of several weeks.

Pine Oil Cleaner

	oz
Pine oil	6.40
Sodium carboxymethyl cellulose	0.60
Renex 20 *	12.80
Water	108.20

* Polyoxyethylene ester of fatty and resin acids.

Heat the water and dissolve the Sodium CMC in it. Add the Renex 20 and stir thoroughly. Finally, stir in with mild agitation the pine oil. Use about 2 oz of this cleaner to a gallon of water for cleaning bathroom floors, linoleum, tile, etc.

For Rugs and Upholstery

	lb
Oleic acid	15.12
Isopropyl alcohol	1.89
Stoddard solvent (a clear, colorless petroleum distillate of a sweet odor and a flash point not lower than 100°F. It evaporates without leaving a stain)	19.50
Xylene	6.00
Potassium hydroxide solution (40°Bé)	1.95
Potassium carbonate (granular)	1.02

Mix the acid with the alcohol, xylene, and Stoddard solvent. Dissolve the potassium carbonate in the hydroxide solution and add this solution slowly, with constant stirring, to the oleic acid mixture. Continue to stir until saponification is complete.

Rust Remover

	oz
Sulfuric acid	2.17
o-Phosphoric acid	29.44
Oxalic acid	0.38
Water	96.01

Dissolve the oxalic acid in the water, add the phosphoric acid; finally, slowly add the sulfuric acid and shake well. Immerse items in this solution, using only a pottery, china, or glass vessel. Care should be exercised in handling this product.

For Steam Pipes

	lb
Soda ash	36
Sodium hydroxide	30
Sodium metasilicate (anhydrous)	38.4
Tetrasodium pyrophosphate (anhydrous)	12
Sodium dodecylbenzene sulfonate (40% active)	3.6

Have all the ingredients in a finely granulated form and mix thoroughly.

Waterless Hand Cleaners

No. 1

	oz
Glycerin	11.25
Veegum H.V.	3.75
Sucrose monostearate	11.25
Methyl *p*-hydroxybenzoate	0.30
Water	108.45
Kerosene, deodorized	15.00

Mix the Veegum H.V. with the glycerin. Dissolve the sucrose monostearate and the *p*-hydroxybenzoate in the water, and heat to 80°C. Stir the hot monostearate solution into the mixture of Veegum and glycerin. Continue the stirring until a smooth product is obtained. When the temperature reaches 50°C., stir in the kerosene and homogenize all. Package this soft paste in tubes.

No. 2

	lb
Vanishing cream	25.0
Deodorized kerosene	5.0

Stir the kerosene at a low speed into the vanishing cream, and continue stirring until the mass is uniform.

No. 3

	oz
Kerosene, deodorized	51.00
Lanolin	4.00
Sorbitan monopalmitate	3.20
Polyoxyethylene sorbitan monopalmitate	9.60
Water	60.20
Methyl *p*-hydroxybenzoate (preservative)	0.26

Mix the kerosene and lanolin with the two monopalmitates and heat to about 60°C. Dissolve the preservative in the water and heat to about

65°C. Pour the water solution into the kerosene mixture and stir continuously until cold. This lotion is excellent for cleaning grease and heavy dirt off the hands when working in garages, machine shops, etc. It should be wiped on the hands and then wiped off with a paper or cloth towel.

No. 4

	oz
Carbowax Compound 4000	25.00
Oleic acid	7.00
Anhydrous lanolin	3.50
Propylene glycol	25.00
Triethanolamine	4.00
Water	25.00
Sodium bisulfite	0.15
Mild abrasive, powdered	41.00
Terpineol	0.25

Heat the Carbowax, oleic acid, lanolin, and glycol to 45°C. Dissolve the triethanolamine and sodium bisulfite in a separate container and heat to the same temperature. Pour the water solution into the fats and keep on stirring until cool. Add the terpineol and stir in the abrasive slowly. Continue stirring until the mass is homogeneous and of proper consistency.

No. 5

Methylcellulose 4000 cps.	3.32 lb
Lanolin, anhydrous	1.77 oz
Glycerin	20.30 oz
Methyl *p*-hydroxybenzoate	0.70 oz
Alcohol, specially denatured	16.90 oz
Perfume oil	1.25 oz
Water	16.38 lb

Dissolve the methylcellulose in the water with heating. Add to this the lanolin, glycerin, and preservative. Finally, stir in the alcohol-perfume mixture, and continue to mix until cold.

Rub this paste on the skin and allow it to dry. Then rub again until dirt and grime roll off the skin, and wipe the hands with a towel. This paste is effective against resistant grime and soil and it leaves the skin clean and soft.

Cosmetics and Perfumes

Part I: Cosmetics

Acetylated Liquid Lanolin

This compound is soluble in alcohol. It is an excellent coupling agent. It has many potential uses in aerosols, emulsions, shampoos, nail polish removers, and powdered cosmetics.

Acid Cream

	oz by weight
Cetyl alcohol	19.20
Spermaceti	6.40
Sodium lauryl sulfate	2.56
Lactic acid, 85%	1.54
Water	91.90
Glycerin	6.40

Melt the cetyl alcohol and spermaceti at 50°C. and then add the lauryl sulfate. Stir until the mixture is uniform. Add 50 parts of the water at the same temperature and stir vigorously. Continue rapid stirring until the mixture becomes a uniform emulsion. Stir slowly until this begins to thicken and then add a warm mixture of the glycerin, lactic acid, and the remainder of the water. Continue stirring until cold.

Aerosol Antiperspirant

	oz
Specially denatured alcohol #40, 95%	1.70
Aluminum sulfocarbolate	1.13
Perfume oil	0.05
Propellent mixture *	2.86

* Propellent mixture: Freon 12, 5 parts; Freon 114, 20 parts.

Aerosol Cologne

	oz
Specially denatured alcohol 95%	1.80
Perfume oil	0.03
Propellent mixture *	4.20

* Propellent mixture: Freon 12, 5 parts; Freon 114, 20 parts.

Aerosol Hair Lacquer
No. 1

	oz
Specially denatured alcohol #40 anhydrous	2.260

Polyvinylpyrrolidone/ vinyl acetate (60:40%)	0.300
Ethoxylan	0.0063
Myristic alcohol	0.0063
Isopropyl myristate	0.0063
Perfume oil	0.0250
Propellent mixture *	10.16

* Propellent Mixture: Freon 11, 14 parts; Freon 12, 6 parts.

Dissolve the various components in the alcohol and shake well. Finally add the propellent mixture.

No. 2

	oz
Ethyl cellulose	3.20
Diethylene glycol oleate	1.92
Absolute alcohol	58.88
Freon 12	64.00

Dissolve the ethyl cellulose and glycol oleate in the alcohol. Finally add the Freon 12.

This preparation will dry on the hair in about 2 minutes, leaving a glossy film with good setting properties. It can be easily removed when required.

Aerosol Shaving Cream

	lb
Stearic acid	12.30
Polyoxyethylene sorbitan monostearate	9.00
Lanolin, anhydrous	0.75
Glycerin	3.00
Triethanolamine	5.55
Water, soft	119.40
Perfume oil	to suit

Melt the first three ingredients. Mix the triethanolamine, glycerin, and water, and heat to the same temperature. Stir the aqueous solution into the fatty mixture, and continue stirring until it is cold. Stir in the perfume oil at about 40°C. Use 90% by weight of the shaving cream to be pressurized and 10% by weight of the propellent (dichlorodifluoromethane).

Aerosol Suntan Cream

	oz
Stearic acid	2.55
Propylene glycol monostearate	5.10
Mineral oil, white	9.00
Filtrosol A (Schimmel)	12.00
Methyl *p*-hydroxybenzoate	0.15
Triethanolamine	1.20
Distilled water	120.00
Perfume oil	0.60

Mix the first five components and heat to 60°C. Dissolve the triethanolamine in the water, and heat to the same temperature. Pour the melted fats slowly into the aqueous solution with constant stirring. When a smooth mixture is obtained, stir in the perfume oil, and continue stirring at a slow speed until the mass is cold.

To 46 parts of this cream add 4 parts of

Propellent mixture: Freon 12, 17.1 parts; Freon 114, 12.9 parts.

After-Shampoo Rinse

	oz
Triton X-400	16.00
Diglycol laurate	1.28

Water	110.72
Perfume and color	to suit

Heat 52 oz of water to 150°F., add the Triton X-400 and diglycol laurate slowly, and stir slowly until a smooth uniform emulsion is obtained. Cool to room temperature. Cool the rest of the water to a temperature of about 40°F., and add this slowly to the other mixture. Stir slowly (rapid stirring tends to produce a thin and unstable dispersion) until the finished product is very smooth and homogeneous. Add the perfume oil and color while stirring in the cold water.

After-Shave Lotion

	oz
Aluminum chloride N.F.	1.28
Acetic acid U.S.P.	1.92
Sodium acetate U.S.P.	0.64
Lanolin, soluble	2.56
Glycerin	4.48
Witch hazel N.F.	25.60
Perfume oil	0.32
Alcohol	51.20
Water	40.00

Dissolve the perfume oil, lanolin, in the alcohols. Add the witch hazel and glycerin and shake well. Dissolve the aluminum chloride, acetic acid, and sodium acetate in the water. Stir the water solution into the alcoholic solution and shake well. Allow the mixture to stand at least 24 hours, and filter if necessary, using kieselguhr as a filtering medium.

Alcoholic Hair Dressing

	oz
Odorless castor oil	23.04
Deltyl extra (Givaudan)	8.96
Alcohol	96.00
Perfume	to suit

Dissolve the castor oil in the alcohol, add the Deltyl extra and the perfume, and shake well. Allow the mixture to stand at least 24 hours.

Allantoin

Allantoin is a derivative of uric acid, known as Glyoxyldiureide—the diureide of glyoxylic acid.

Allantoin is a healing agent which stimulates the formation of healthy tissue. It is stable, non-toxic, non-irritating, and soothing. When applied to ulcers, cuts, wounds, lacerations, etc., allantoin has the power to remove the objectionable necrotic (decayed) tissue, clear the area, and then follow through by causing the growth of healthy new tissue. Strong alkalies, such as sodium or potassium hydroxide, decompose allantoin; therefore, such alkalies must be neutralized before the allantoin is added to the formulation.

Add allantoin in a proportion of 0.05 per cent to 0.5 per cent in the various cosmetic preparations. Such an addition would enhance considerably the healing properties of those preparations.

Allantoin Hand Lotion

	oz by wt
Glyceryl monostearate, self emulsifying (Aldo 28)	4.48
Light mineral oil	0.64
Butyl *p*-hydroxybenzoate	0.26
Allantoin	0.26
Propylene glycol	2.56
Water	119.80
Perfume and color	q.s.

Heat the monostearate together with the oil and preservative to 75°C. Heat the water-glycol mixture to 75°C and dissolve the allantoin in it. Mix the two solutions while stirring, and continue to stir until the lotion has reached room temperature. Add some menthol and benzocaine to this lotion, and you have an effective sunburn preparation.

Allantoin After-Shave Lotion

	oz
Hexachlorophene	0.32
Allantoin	0.26
Propylene glycol	2.56
Specially denatured alcohol #40	76.80
Water	47.68
Perfume oil	0.38
Color, as desired	

Dissolve the hexachlorophene and perfume oil in the alcohol; color if desired. Mix the water with the glycol and dissolve the allantoin in it. Add the water solution slowly to the alcohol solution, and shake well. Allow the liquid to stand for at least a week, then filter.

Allantoin Night Cream

	oz
Triple-pressed stearic acid	12.80
White beeswax	12.80
Spermaceti	10.24
Sesame oil	71.68
Light mineral oil	79.36
Anhydrous lanolin	9.00
Butyl *p*-hydroxybenzoate	0.52
White oleic acid	2.56
Water	51.20
Allantoin	0.52
Triethanolamine	3.84
Perfume oil	1.02

Melt the first eight ingredients at 70–75°C. Dissolve the allantoin in a small portion of the water and heat it to 70°C.; then pour it into the molten fats. Add the triethanolamine to the rest of the water, and heat to 70–75°C. Mix the two phases, with rapid stirring. Allow the emulsion to cool. Add the perfume oil at 35°C., and continue stirring until it is cold.

Allantoin Lipstick

	oz
White beeswax	16.64
White ozokerite	2.56
Spermaceti	2.56
Carnauba Wax #1	3.84
Anhydrous lanolin	6.40

Castor oil (odorless, tasteless)	71.68
Light mineral oil	5.12
Butyl stearate	2.56
Bromo acid	2.56
Lake colors and white pigment	12.80
Allantoin, 200 mesh	0.07
Perfume oil	1.21

Melt the waxes, lanolin, and one half of the castor oil. Wet the bromo acid with the butyl stearate, then grind in the mineral oil and the rest of the castor oil, slowly adding the pigments and the allantoin. Add this ground pulp to the melted waxes and mix thoroughly. Finally add the perfume oil, and pour into suitable molds.

All-Purpose Cream

	oz
Acetylated lanolin alcohols (liquid fraction)	15.00
Diethyleneglycol monostearate C	3.00
Acetylated lanolin	3.00
Stearic acid	3.00
Cetyl alcohol	0.75
Triethanolamine	1.50
Water	123.75
Methyl *p*-hydroxybenzoate	0.30
Perfume oil	to suit

Place the fatty substances and the methyl *p*-hydroxybenzoate preservative in the mixing kettle and heat to 82°C., stirring constantly until all is completely melted. Place the triethanolamine and the water in a separate container and heat to 85°C. Pour the water solution into the molten fats, stirring at a medium rate. Add the perfume oil when the temperature drops to about 50°C., and continue to mix slowly until cool. Remix the following day. This cream is emollient and has a glossy appearance. It imparts a non-greasy film to the skin which may be washed off or left on.

Alum Sticks

Aluminum potassium sulfate, U.S.P.	7	lb
Glycerin	1.125	oz
Menthol	1.125	oz
Water	7	lb

Dissolve the first three ingredients in the water by means of a slow heat. Have the molds oiled with mineral oil, stir and pour the mixture into the molds and allow them to cool. Polish the finished stick with water.

Aluminum Methionate Astringent

Use aluminum methionate to improve antiperspirants. It is more effective for this purpose than other common astringent agents tested. It is harmless to fabrics, and it has the additional advantage of being very soluble, hygroscopic, and non-toxic. Because it is hygroscopic it will prevent creams containing it from drying out.

Anti-Dandruff Rinse

		oz
1	Water	108.00
	Glycerin	4.00
	Alkyldimethyl benzyl ammonium chloride	0.13
	Lauryl isoquinolinium bromide	0.13
	Color	to suit
2	Alcohol	16.00
	Perfume oil	to suit

Mix ingredients of (1) thoroughly until solution is complete. Dissolve the perfume oil in the alcohol (2), and pour this solution slowly into (1) with constant stirring. Allow to stand for 24 hours. Filter if necessary.

Antiperspirant Cream

		oz by wt
1	Stearic acid	21.0
	Beeswax, white	3.0
	Polyoxyethylene stearate (Myrj 52)	7.5
	Polyoxyethylene oxypropylene stearate (G2162)	7.5
	Mineral oil, white (65/75 viscosity)	1.5
2	Water	76.5
	Methyl *p*-hydroxybenzoatc	0.3
3	* Chlorhydrol	33.0
	Perfume oil	q.s.

* Chlorhydrol (sodium aluminum chlorhydroxy lactate complex) is an excellent astringent, which makes it effective as an anti-perspirant and deodorant.

Heat ingredients of (1) to 70°C. Heat (2) to the same temperature and stir it into (1). Cool, while stirring, to 40°C., then add (3), and continue to stir until it is dissolved. Finally, stir in the perfume oil and pack.

Antiperspirant Powder

Talcum powder	11 lb
Cornstarch, powdered	1.40 lb
Aluminum sodium sulfate, powdered	4.50 lb
Salicylic acid, powdered	11.25 oz
Boric acid, powdered	11.25 oz

Blend the powders thoroughly, and put the mixture through silk of at least 120 mesh. Use a modern mixing and sifting apparatus for this operation.

Antiperspirant Sticks (Cologne-Type)

	oz
Chlorhydrol,* 40% solution	35.28
Specially denatured alcohol	28.00
Glycerin	2.12
Sodium stearate	4.24
Perfume oil	to suit

* See note under Antiperspirant Cream.

Heat the chlorhydrol solution to 60–65°C. Stir in slowly the alcohol and glycerin and maintain the same temperature. Add the sodium stearate and continue stirring until the resultant soap dissolves. Finally stir in the perfume oil and, after thorough mixing, pour the solution into suitable molds.

The manufacture of alcohol gel sticks entails a fire hazard as well as the possibility of excessive loss of alcohol. These problems may be reduced to a minimum by using kettles with reflux condensers. It might be advisable to use a number of small containers instead of a single large one during the filling operation.

The 40% solution of chlorhydrol has a pH value of 8.5. This compound does not irritate the skin, and it does not injure or discolor standard fabrics.

Astringent Lotion

No. 1

		oz by wt
1	Mineral oil, white (65/75 viscosity)	15.0
	Polyoxyethylene cetyl alcohol (Texofor A6)	6.0
2	Aluminum sulfate N.F.	7.5
	Methyl *p*-hydroxybenzoate	0.3
	Water	120.0
	Perfume oil and color	q.s.

Heat (1) to 65°C. Heat (2) to the same temperature and add it to (1) with constant stirring. Allow mixture to cool, stir in the perfume and color at 40°C., and continue to stir at low speed until cold.

No. 2
(Mild)

	oz
Zinc sulfocarbolate, N.F	3.84
Propylene glycol	6.40
Camphor water	119.76

Mix all the ingredients and shake well. Allow mixture to stand overnight and filter if necessary.

Baby Lotion

	oz
White mineral oil (65/75 viscosity)	7.500
Silicone oil	1.125
Glyceryl monostearate S	1.500
Span 80 (Sorbitan monooleate)	0.450
Benzalkonium chloride	0.075
Glycerin	2.625
Water	61.500
Perfume oil	0.225

Heat the first five ingredients to 65°C. Dissolve the glycerin in the water and heat solution to the same temperature. Mix the two solutions, allowing the emulsion to cool. When the mass is at 35°C., stir in the perfume oil and continue stirring until cold.

Baby Oil

	oz
White mineral oil (65/75 viscosity)	105.00
Isopropyl myristate	3.50
Liquid lanolin	3.50
Ethyl stearate	4.50
Methyl *p*-hydroxybenzoate	0.20

Perfume oil	0.30

Mix all the ingredients, except the perfume oil, and heat slowly until the solution is clear. When somewhat cooler, stir in the perfume oil.

Barrier Cream

	oz
Stearic acid	2.56
Chlorothymol N.F.	0.30
Glycerin	7.68
Soap, powdered	15.36
Sodium chloride	1.28
Water	70.80
Kaolin, N.F.	25.70
Bentonite	4.00

Mix the stearic acid, chlorothymol, and glycerin, and heat to 70°C. Dissolve the powdered soap and sodium chloride in the water and heat to the same temperature. Mix the two solutions with rapid stirring, and keep on stirring until the mass is cold. Stir the kaolin-bentonite mixture into the finished cream.

This preparation will protect against cutting oils, industrial dirt and grime, lacquer, etc., and it can be easily removed by ordinary washing. It also acts as a barrier to harmful substances.

Bleaching Cream

Petrolatum U.S.P. white	18 lb
Zinc oxide U.S.P.	6 oz
Ammoniated mercury, U.S.P.	9 oz

Melt the petrolatum. Remove from the fire, stir in first the zinc oxide, then the ammoniated mercury. Continue to stir until mixture is cold.

Brilliantines

No. 1

	oz
Mineral oil (sp. gr. 0.88)	109.0
Sulfonated castor oil	19.0
Perfume and color	to suit

No. 2

Henna powder	2.5 oz
Olive oil	20.0 oz
Mineral oil, enough to make	1.0 gal
Perfume oil	to suit

Macerate the henna powder in the olive oil for about 3 days with frequent shaking, then filter and mix with the mineral oil and perfume. Filter the finished product before filling.

No. 3

	oz
Isopropyl myristate	7.04
Glycerin	6.40
Specially denatured alcohol	114.56
Perfume and color	to suit

Mix and shake well. This preparation is a very pleasant brilliantine of reduced greasiness and good fixative properties.

No. 4

	oz
Acetylated lanolin	6.40
Mineral oil (65/75 viscosity)	121.60

Mix the acetylated lanolin with the mineral oil and heat slightly until clear.

No. 5
(Solid)

	oz
Petroleum jelly	84.48
Mineral oil, sp. gr. 0.88	21.34
Paraffin wax	19.00
Rosin, U.S.P. XI	1.90
Perfume oil	1.28

Mix the petrolatum, oil, wax, and rosin, and heat at a low temperature. When melted, remove from the fire and stir well. Add the perfume oil, and keep on stirring while pouring into jars.

No. 6
(Solid)

Paraffin wax U.S.P.	4 lb
Mineral oil	6½ pt
Petroleum jelly	15 lb
Perfume and color	to suit

Melt the oil, wax and jelly together, stir, add the perfume and color, and pour into suitable containers.

No. 7
(With Oleyl Alcohol)

	oz
Refined oleyl alcohol *	19.20
White mineral oil (65/75 viscosity)	108.80
Perfume oil	q.s.

Mix and shake well. Allow to stand overnight.

* Oleyl alcohol is a light yellow, viscous oily liquid, with a fatty odor. It will darken slightly if exposed to light. It is soluble in alcohol, aromatic hydrocarbons, and esters; it will disperse homogeneously in mineral and vegetable oils. Oleyl alcohol is stable in the presence of acids and alkalies. It has good emollient properties. Oleyl alcohol can be used in hair lotions, indelible lipsticks, and mascara; as a solvent for essential oils; and as a superfatting agent in liquid soapless shampoos.

Brushless Shaving Cream

No. 1

	oz
Stearic acid	54.0
Propylene glycol monostearate	12.0
Anhydrous lanolin	9.0
Isopropyl palmitate	9.0
Cetyl alcohol, pure	6.0
Glycerin	6.0
Triethanolamine	3.0
Water	200.4
Perfume oil	0.6

Melt the first five components together in a suitable container, and heat to about 80°C. In a separate container heat the glycerin and water to the same temperature. Stir the triethanolamine into the hot water, and pour this hot mixture into the molten fats with constant stirring. Continue to stir until the cream begins to thicken. Allow it to cool, and when the temperature reaches about 40–45°C., stir in the perfume oil. Continue to stir intermittently until the cream is at room temperature. Allow it to set overnight, then stir it for about five minutes, and fill immediately.

No. 2

Stearic acid	8⅓	lb
Anhydrous lanolin	1	lb
Triethanolamine	4	oz
Borax	2⅔	lb
Glycerin	1	lb
Alcohol (S.D. 3A)	11	oz
Distilled water	23⅓	lb
Perfume oil	1½	oz

Melt the stearic acid and lanolin at 70°C. Dissolve the triethanolamine, borax, and glycerin in the water and heat to the same temperature. Pour the aqueous solution into the molten fats with vigorous stirring. Finally stir in the perfume oil, previously dissolved in the specially denatured alcohol, and continue to stir until cold.

No. 3

	oz
Diethylene glycol stearate	27.0
Mineral oil (65/75 viscosity)	1.0
Sodium lauryl sulfate	4.5
Glycerin	12.0
Methyl *p*-hydroxybenzoate	0.3
Water	106.0
Perfume oil	to suit

Mix the stearate with the mineral oil and heat to 65°C. Mix the sulfate, glycerin, preservative, and water, and heat to the same temperature. Stir the oily mixture into the aqueous solution, and continue mixing until cold. Stir in the perfume oil at 40°C.

No. 4

	oz
Stearic acid	37.0
Cetyl alcohol, pure	1.5
Mineral oil (65/75 viscosity)	1.5
Isopropanolamine	3.0
Glycerin	7.5
Methyl *p*-hydroxybenzoate	0.3
Water	100.5
Perfume oil	to suit

Mix the isopropanolamine, glycerin, preservative, and water and heat to 70°C. Mix the stearic acid, cetyl alcohol, and mineral oil in a separate container, and heat to the same temperature. Pour the oily mixture into the aqueous solution with rapid stirring. Reduce the stirring and cool to 40°C. Add the perfume oil, and continue mixing until cold.

Bubble Bath Powder

	oz
Powdered sodium lauryl sulfate	15.0
Powdered sodium sesquicarbonate	27.0
Powdered sodium alginate	1.0
Perfume and color	to suit

Mix the powders thoroughly.

Butylated Hydroxyanisole

Butylated hydroxyanisole is an excellent antioxidant for protecting vegetable oils from rancidity.

Use about 0.1 percent as an antioxidant in foods, drugs, and cosmetics.

Cake Mascara

Triethanolamine stearate	4½	lb
Carnauba wax	22½	oz
Beeswax, yellow	12	oz
Propylene glycol stearate	12	oz
Anhydrous lanolin	10½	oz
Ceresin, white	4½	oz
Isopropyl palmitate	7½	oz
Propyl *p*-hydroxybenzoate	164	gr
Earth pigment *	9	oz
Perfume oil	to suit	

* Only certified (mineral) colors may be used around the eyes.

Mix all ingredients except the perfume oil, heat gently, and stir until all have been completely melted. Continue to stir slowly till the mixture begins to thicken, then pass it through a heated roller mill several times. Remelt the mass, mix slowly to avoid air pockets, stir in the perfume oil, and pour into molds. Allow the molds to cool, then discharge. Imprint any name or design on the forms.

This cake mascara is non-irritating, water repellent, and is easily applied.

As aniline colors may not be used the following pigments must be employed to complete the shade range for these products (brown, blue, red, green, violet, tan, yellow):

Carbon black, carmine N.F., chromium oxide, titanium dioxide, ultramarine and mineral blues, zinc oxide, aluminum hydroxide, and iron oxides.

Finely powdered aluminum and bronze (low copper content), may be used to provide interesting iridescent color effects, especially in eye shadow.

Cera Emulsificans (B.P.)

Prepare this product by the following process:

	oz
Cetostearyl alcohol	64.0
Sodium lauryl sulfate	7.0
Distilled water	3.0

Heat the alcohol to 90°C. Add the sodium lauryl sulfate and mix thoroughly. Add the distilled water and heat to 115°C. Stir vigorously and continue the heating until frothing ceases and the product becomes translucent. Cool quickly.

Chamomile Extract

Make the extract by percolating 7 oz of the powdered flowers with 65 oz of 95% alcohol.

This extract has a soothing action on the skin and stimulates the hair roots. Use 1–5% in cosmetics.

Cleansing Cream

No. 1

	oz by wt
Paraffin oil, white	120
Stearic acid	36
Carbitol *	12
Ethanolamine	12
Water	120
Perfume oil	q.s.

* Carbitol (diethylene glycol monoethylether) enhances the stability of the emulsion and makes washing easier.

Melt the stearic acid together with the paraffin oil. Dissolve the carbitol and ethanolamine in the water and heat solution to the same temperature. Pour the oily mixture into the water solution slowly with constant stirring. Allow it to cool, add the perfume oil at 40°C., and continue stirring at low speed until the mass is cold.

No. 2

	oz
Beeswax	27.0
Paraffin wax	30.0
Cetyl alcohol	3.0
Water	102.0
Borax	1.8
Perfume oil	to suit

Melt the waxes and alcohol together and keep the mixture at 60°C. Dissolve the borax in the water and heat also to 60°C. With vigorous stirring, pour the borax solution slowly into the melted wax-alcohol mixture. When emulsification is complete keep stirring more slowly and allow the mass to cool. Stir in the perfume oil at 35–40°C. The cetyl alcohol promotes emulsification and prevents "weeping."

No. 3
(Cold Cream)

Paraffin wax	10¾	lb
Anhydrous lanolin	1¼	lb
Cetyl alcohol	8	oz
Olive oil	16	oz
Rose water	1 7/16	gal
Suitable perfume oil	⅖	oz

Heat the first four ingredients to 65°C. Heat the rose water, in a separate container, to the same temperature. Pour the hot rose water into the melted wax mixture with constant stirring. When cooling stir in the perfume oil. Continue stirring and pour into jars at 130–135°F.

No. 4
(Cold Cream)

	oz
Beeswax	27
Amerchol L-101 *	6
White mineral oil (65/75 viscosity)	66
Borax	1½
Water	49½
Perfume oil	to suit

* Amerchol L-101 contains cholesterol.

Heat the beeswax, mineral oil, and Amerchol to 65–70°C. Dissolve the borax in the water in a separate container, and heat to the same temperature. Pour the borax solution into the wax-oil mixture slowly with continuous stirring. Stir in the perfume oil at about 45–50°C., and continue the stirring until the cream is white and smooth. Excellent results are obtained by passing the cream through a colloid mill.

No. 5
(Cold Cream)

	oz
Acetylated lanolin	1.5
Beeswax	25.5
Mineral oil (65/75 viscosity)	67.5
Amerchol L-101	4.5
Methyl *p*-hydroxybenzoate	0.3
Borax	1.5
Water	49.5
Permume oil	to suit

Place the first five ingredients in the mixing kettle and heat to 82°C., stirring constantly until all is completely melted. Place the borax and the water in a separate container and heat to 85°C. Pour the water solution into the oily mixture, stirring at a medium rate. Allow the emulsion to cool and add the perfume oil when the temperature is about 50°C. Pour into jars at the same temperature.

This cream has a very smooth texture, and the consistency of whipped cream. Its spreading and cleansing properties are excellent, and its stability is good.

No. 6
(Cold Cream)

	oz by wt
Paraffin oil, white	66
Paraffin wax, U.S.P.	66
Stearic acid	42
Carbitol *	21
Ethanolamine	6
Water	99
Perfume oil	q.s.

* See note under No. 1.

Melt the oil, wax, and stearic acid together. Dissolve the Carbitol and ethanolamine in the water and heat to the same temperature. Pour the oily mixture into the water solution slowly with constant stirring. Add the perfume oil at 40°C., and continue stirring at low speed until the cream is cold.

Cleansing Lotion

	oz
Stearic acid	4.50
Bleached beeswax	18.00
Isopropyl myristate	4.50
Polyethylene glycol monostearate (400)	22.50
Anhydrous lanolin	9.00
Cetyl alcohol	2.25
White mineral oil (65/75 viscosity)	33.53
Sorbic acid (preservative)	0.45
Propylene glycol	11.25
Triethanolamine	2.25
Water	116.78
Perfume oil	to suit

Dissolve the triethanolamine in the water and heat to about 70°C. Heat the other components to the same temperature in another suitable container, and stir the aqueous solution into the molten fats, oils, and waxes with constant stirring. Continue the stirring until the cream cools to room temperature. Stir in the perfume oil at 40–45°C.

Cold Wave Lotion

		oz by wt
1	Polyoxyethylene cetyl alcohol (Texofor A6)	7.5
	Mineral oil, white, sp. gr. 0.83	3.0
2	Ammonia water	q.s. (3–4.5)
	Water	105.0
	Ammonium thioglycolate 35%	30.0

Heat (1) to 65°C. Heat (2) to the same temperature and add it to (1) with constant stirring. When the emulsion has cooled, stir in the thioglycolate, and continue stirring until it is cold.

Cream Hair Rinse

No. 1

Triton X-400 *	12.0 oz
Aldo 28 (glyceryl monostearate)	5.0 oz
Water	120.0 oz
Perfume oil	2.0 drams
French pink color	10.0 min

No. 2

Triton X-400 *	12.0 oz
Polyethylene glycol distearate (600)	5.00 oz
Water	120.0 oz
Perfume oil	2.0 drams
French pink color	10.0 min

* Alkyl dimethyl benzyl ammonium chloride with a higher alcohol.

Heat the water to 80°C. and disperse the Aldo 28 or 600 distearate in it. Place the Triton X-400 in a separate container, and when the dispersion cools to 65°C. add slowly 60 oz of this to the Triton. Stir slowly until the mixture is smooth and uniform. (Rapid stirring tends to produce a thin and unstable dispersion). Cool to room temperature, and add slowly the rest of the dispersion. Stir slowly until the finished product is very smooth and homogeneous. Add the perfume oil and color while stirring in the rest of the dispersion.

Cream hair rinse softens the hair, imparts luster, and facilitates combing. It is excellent after shampooing or cold waving. In use, mix 1 oz of cream hair rinse with 3 oz of warm water. Distribute mixture evenly and work well into the hair for 2 or 3 minutes, then rinse thoroughly.

No. 3

	oz by wt
Quaternary ammonium base (Pendit CA)	10.50

Poly-ethylene glycol distearate (400)	1.50
Water	136.50
Sodium chloride	0.45
Perfume oil and color	q.s.

Mix the quaternary base with the 400 distearate and heat, while stirring, until the mixture is a thick translucent gel. Stir this mixture into the water which has been heated to 72°C. Continue stirring for about 20 minutes. Allow the batch to cool slowly with moderate agitation. Add the sodium chloride and color at 60°C.; then add the perfume oil at 40°C., and continue stirring at low speed until the mass is cold. Fill into bottles.

Cream Mascara

Tegin	36	oz
Petrolatum, white	13½	oz
Isopropyl linoleate	4½	oz
Oleyl alcohol	3	oz
Methyl *p*-hydroxybenzoate	131	gr
Water	75	oz
Earth pigment *	15	oz
Veegum	3	oz
Perfume oil	to suit	

* Only mineral colors or lakes may be used around the eyes; see note under Cake Mascara.

Melt the first four components. Dissolve the preservative in the water and heat to the same temperature. Mix the two solutions with constant stirring. Add the Veegum and finely powdered pigment with continuous agitation and cooling. Stir in the perfume oil, and pass the resultant mass through a colloid mill.

This cream mascara is uniform in texture, it is easily applied, it dries readily, and it is somewhat water-resistant.

Cream Rinse for Hair

	oz
Triton X-400	16.0
Diglycol laurate	0.64
Acetic acid	0.64
Water	110.72
Perfume and color	to suit

Mix the acid with the water and heat to 65°C. Disperse the Triton X-400 together with the diglycol laurate in the acidulated water, with constant stirring. Stir in slowly the perfume and color and stir until cold.

Cream Lotion for Hair

	oz
Amerchol L-101 (lanolin derivative)	8.96
Modulan (lanolin derivative)	13.44
Isopropyl palmitate	19.20
Stearic acid	2.11
Glyceryl monostearate	0.64
Glycerin	4.48
Triethanolamine	0.45
Water	78.72
Perfume oil	to suit

Melt the first five ingredients at about 65°C. Dissolve the triethanolamine in the water, add the glycerin, and heat this solution to the same temperature. Pour the aqueous solution into the oily mixture slowly with constant stirring and continue to stir until the mass is cold.

Cream Rouge
(Anhydrous)

		oz
1	Petrolatum, white	82.50
	Isopropyl myristate	12.00
	Wecobee SS	10.50
	Carnauba wax	8.48
	Beeswax, white	3.00
	Cetyl alcohol	3.00
	Super Hartolan	0.75
	Methyl *p*-hydroxybenzoate	0.15
	Crystal O Castor oil	12.00
	Bromo acid (D & C Red 21)	0.38
	Pigments	11.25
	Albatex	6.00
	Perfume oil	0.75

Mix and melt (1). Heat the bromo acid and castor oil together, and stir them into (1), when a clear solution results. Premix the Albatex and pigments, and then blend it with the molten mixture. Continue to stir until cool, and then pass the resultant mass through a roller mill twice. Finally, remelt the mass, add the perfume oil, and pour into containers, avoiding excess of air.

Dandruff Remover and Scalp Stimulant

Absorption base (Falba)	3	oz
Pilocarpine hydrochloride	20	gr
Colloidal sulfur	132	gr
Water	½	oz

Melt the absorption base. Dissolve the pilocarpine hydrochloride in hot water, and pour it slowly, with constant stirring, into the molten base. Stir in the colloidal sulfur, and continue to stir until the mass is cold.

Deodorants (Liquid)
No. 1

	oz by wt
Aluminum chloride, N.F.	10.0
Urea	5.0
Perfume oil	0.8
Water	35.0
Specially denatured alcohol	49.2

Dissolve the aluminum chloride and the urea in the water, and shake well. Dissolve the perfume oil in the alcohol, and mix the two solutions. Allow mixture to stand overnight, and filter if necessary. You may use 15 parts of aluminum chloride instead of 10 parts, and 30 parts of water instead of 35 parts if desired.

No. 2

	oz
* Sodium zirconium lactate	19.20
Glycerin	6.40
Alcohol, specially denatured #40	25.60
Water	76.80
Perfume oil	q.s.

Dissolve the perfume oil in the alcohol, and add the glycerin. Dissolve the sodium zirconium lactate in the water. Mix the two solutions and shake well. Allow to stand overnight. Filter if necessary.

* Sodium zirconium lactate is an excellent deodorant. It is conceivable that the soluble zirconium salt has a direct affinity for the proteins of the skin. Hence its prolonged action as a deodorant. Check all perfume mixtures before using them, as some components may be inactivated by the zirconium compound.

No. 3
(Cologne)

	oz
Aluminum acetotartrate	10.24
Water	85.76
Glycerin	6.40
Eau de cologne	25.60

Dissolve the aluminum acetotartrate in the water; mix the glycerin with the eau de cologne, and pour it into the aqueous solution. Shake well and allow it to stand overnight. Filter if necessary.

Deodorant Cream

	oz
White petrolatum	32.00
Cetyl alcohol	7.00
Wool wax alcohol	1.00

Place the components in a suitable vessel and melt them. When somewhat cooler, stir in the following solution:

	oz
Urea	8.00
Aluminum chloride	16.00
Water	16.00

Continue stirring until mixture is cold.

Deodorant Powder

	oz
Sodium zirconium lactate, finely powdered	6.40
Talcum powder	64.00
Zinc stearate	6.40
Precipitated calcium carbonate	32.00
Colloidal kaolin	19.20
Perfume oil	q.s.

Rub the perfume oil into some of the calcium carbonate and screen in order to break all caked particles. Add the perfumed calcium carbonate to the rest of the powders and mix thoroughly for sometime until a good distribution is effected. Finally, sift the mixture through a 120 mesh silk screen.

Deodorant Stick

No. 1

	lb
Sodium zirconium lactate	1.10
Sodium stearate U.S.P.	1.71
Propylene glycol	1.10
Specially denatured alcohol #40	17.50
Perfume oil	q.s.

Melt the stearate together with the propylene glycol; remove it from the fire and allow it to cool. Dissolve the perfume oil and the sodium zirconium lactate in the alcohol, and stir this mixture into the molten fats. Continue to stir and pour into suitable molds. Allow the molded sticks to cool slowly in order to prevent the formation of air pockets. Wrap the cooled sticks in foil.

No. 2

	oz
Sodium stearate	16.00
Specially denatured alcohol	150.00
Glycerin	10.00
Hexachlorophene	0.51
Water	20.00
Perfume oil	3.50

Melt the sodium stearate together with the glycerin and water; remove it from the fire and allow it to cool. Dissolve the hexachlorophene, perfume oil, in the alcohol, and stir this mixture into the molten fat mixture. Continue to stir and pour into suitable molds. Allow the molded sticks to cool slowly in order to prevent the formation of air pockets. Wrap the cooled sticks in tin foil.

Deodorant Talcum Powder

Use antiseptics such as hexachlorophene, bithionol, benzoic acid, or *p*-chloro-meta-cresol. Add 8 oz of any one of these to 100 lb of talcum powder. Grind and mix thoroughly.

Emollient Oil

	oz
White mineral oil (65/75 viscosity)	57.6
Isopropyl palmitate	32.0
Lantrol	38.4
Perfume oil	to suit

Mix all the ingredients except the perfume oil, and heat slowly just until the solution is clear. As it cools stir in the perfume oil.

Emollient Vanishing Cream

	oz
Glyceryl monostearate	17.500
Lanolin, anhydrous	2.500
Glycerin, U.S.P.	5.000
Methyl *p*-hydroxybenzoate	0.125
Water	99.250
Perfume oil	0.625

Mix all the ingredients, except the perfume oil. Heat the mixture to about 80°C. Allow it to cool, stir in the perfume oil at 45–50°C., and continue stirring until it is cold.

Ethoxylan

Ethoxylan is an odorless, lanolin product, which forms crystal-clear solutions with water and dilute alcohol. It is a modified lanolin derivative with the full emollient properties of natural lanolin, but without its greasy and sticky effects. It is surface-active, whereas ordinary lanolin is not, and it therefore enhances the foaming qualities of other materials. Ethoxylan is an ideal compound for anti-perspirants, hair and shaving preparations, pharmaceutical ointments, and shampoos.

Eyebrow Pencil

	oz
Paraffin	57.0
Petrolatum, yellow	57.0
Ceresin	6.0
Hychol	3.0
Methyl *p*-hydroxybenzoate	0.3
Pigment *	27.0
Perfume oil	to suit

* See note on pigment under Cream Mascara.

Mix all ingredients except the perfume oil, heat gently until the mixture is fluid. Stir slowly till the mass is slightly thickened, then pass it through a heated roller mill several times. Remelt the mass, stir in the perfume oil, and pour into aluminum molds. Allow molds to cool, then discharge.

Eye Cream

Sesame oil, N.F.	80	oz
Lanogene	1⅓	oz
Beeswax, white, U.S.P.	20	oz
Wecobee R	32	oz
Methyl *p*-hydroxybenzoate	120	gr

Mix, heat gently and stir until melted. Continue the stirring until the mixture is cold. Fill into suitable containers.

This eye cream is valuable as an emollient for the delicate thin skin around the eyes.

Eye Lotion

Boric acid, U.S.P.	1.0	oz
Sodium borate, U.S.P.	74.0	gr
Antipyrine, U.S.P.	109.0	gr
Water, distilled, enough to make	100.0	oz

Bring the water to a boil, and dissolve the powdered ingredients in it.

Use extreme care and the most sanitary conditions in preparing the eye lotion. Fill only into sterilized bottles.

Eye Shadow (Pencil)

Petrolatum, white	1.50	lb
Beeswax, yellow, U.S.P.	15	oz
Carnauba wax	9	oz
Ceresin	7.50	oz
Cottonseed oil, hydrogenated	7.50	oz
Isopropyl palmitate	6	oz
Isopropylan	2.25	oz
Crodacol O deodorized	2.25	oz
Loramine OM 101	0.75	oz
Methyl *p*-hydroxybenzoate	131	gr
Pigments *	15	oz
Perfume oil	to suit	

* See note on pigments under Cream Mascara.

Mix all the ingredients, except the perfume oil, heat gently and stir until melted. Continue to stir slowly till the mixture is slightly thickened, then run it through a heated roller mill several times. Remelt the mass, stir in the perfume, and pour it into molds. Allow them to cool, then discharge.

The eye shadow in pencil form can be easily applied, thereby keeping the fingers and container clean.

Face and Hand Lotion

	oz
White mineral oil (65/75 viscosity)	45
Beeswax, white, U.S.P.	15
Spermaceti, U.S.P.	11¼
Liquid lanolin	12
Borax	¾
Water	66
Perfume oil	¼

Place the fatty substances in the mixing kettle and heat to 70°C., stirring constantly until all is completely melted. Place the borax and the water into a separate container and heat to 75°C. Pour the water solution into the molten fats, stirring at a medium rate. Stir in the perfume oil when the temperature drops to 40–35°C., and continue to stir until the mass is cold.

Face Powders

No. 1: Light Weight
(for dry skin)

Zinc oxide	8.0 lb
Zinc stearate	3.2 lb
Talcum powder	14.0 lb
Kaolin	2.4 lb
Magnesium carbonate	12.2 lb
* Perfume oil	3.2 oz
* Certified colors	q.s.

* See notes following No. 3.

No. 2: Medium Weight
(for normal or slightly oily skin)

Zinc oxide	8.0 lb
Zinc stearate	3.2 lb
Talcum powder	8.0
Kaolin	3.2
Magnesium carbonate	17.4 lb
* Perfume oil	3.2 oz
* Certified colors	q.s.

* See notes under No. 3.

No. 3: Heavy Weight
(for very oily skin)

Titanium dioxide	3.6 lb
Zinc stearate	2.4 lb
Talcum powder	25.8 lb
Kaolin	3.6 lb
Magnesium carbonate	4.0 lb
* Perfume oil	4.5 oz
* Certified colors	q.s.

* The basic colors in face powder are the earth pigments—ochre, umber, sienna, and cosmetic brown. Various tones may be produced by adding other certified colors. The lake colors must be chosen and used with caution as they are very powerful. It is best to dilute these colors with an absorbent inert powder, such as kaolin.

Pour the perfume oil into the magnesium carbonate, stir the mixture thoroughly, and allow it to stand overnight. Force the magnesium carbonate through a wide-meshed screen, place it in a suitable mixer together with the rest of the powders and mix thoroughly for about 45 minutes. Store the base for future use; or add the pigments directly to portions of it, and continue to mix for another 45 minutes. Finally pulverize the powder through a fine-mesh screen.

For suggestions on perfumes for face powders, see Part II.

Foam Wash Facial Cream

	oz
White petrolatum	112.00
Lanolin	2.56
Sodium lauryl sulfate	11.64
Water	1.80
Perfume	to suit

Melt and mix the first four ingredients thoroughly; then stir in the perfume, and pour into suitable jars.

This product is a combination of cold cream and soap. Apply it like cold cream, massage with wet finger tips to a light lather for a minute, then rinse it off with a face cloth.

Foundation Cream, Colored

	oz
Colored powder with preservative	22.5
Lanolin absorption base	22.5
Coconut fatty acids	9.0
Cetyl alcohol	6.0
White mineral oil (65/75 viscosity)	4.5
Triethanolamine	6.0
Soft water	79.5
Perfume oil	q.s.

Grind the colored powder with the lanolin in a triple roller mill. Add to this mixture the fatty acids, cetyl alcohol, and mineral oil, and heat to 70°C. with constant stirring. Dissolve the triethanolamine in the water and heat to the same temperature. Mix the two solutions with constant stirring. Allow the mass to cool, and when the temperature reaches about 35°C., stir in the perfume oil. This preparation may be packed in an aerosol dispenser.

A suitable colored powder may be composed of the following:

	oz
Titanium dioxide, powdered	15.0
Kaolin N.F., powdered	6.0
Burnt Sienna, powdered	1.2
Blue lake, powdered	0.3
Orange lake, powdered	0.6
Yellow lake, powdered	0.6

Mix thoroughly.

Germicides for Soap

Soap containing 1% of tetramethylthiuram disulfide, after one week of use, effected a reduction in transient and resident bacterial population of the hands. The germicidal activity persisted for at least 2 days after application was discontinued.

A soap containing 2% of hexachlorophene was less effective.

Greaseless Hand Cream or Lotion

The following greaseless preparation will leave the skin on the hands feeling soft, and it will aid in healing rough and chapped hands.

Stearic acid	11.52 oz
Cetyl alcohol	1.92 oz
Deltyl extra	11.52 oz
Triethanolamine	1.92 oz
Carbitol	19.20 oz
Glycerin	3.00 oz

Water	2.40 gal
Perfume oil	to suit

Melt the first three ingredients, and maintain the temperature at 75°C. Mix the triethanolamine, Carbitol, glycerin, and water in another container, and heat to 75°C. Pour the water solution into the melted fats, stirring at a medium rate of speed, and allow the mixture to cool. Add the perfume at 45°C., and continue to stir until the cream is cold. Allow it to stand over night and stir again before filling.

Hair Bleach

	oz
Hydrogen peroxide solution, 3% U.S.P.	124.29
Alkyl ethyl morpholinium ethosulfate	1.92
Adipic acid	1.03
Sodium stannate	0.76

Mix thoroughly until solution is complete. This acid bleach is good for partially decolorizing the hair. The *p*H value of this lotion is 4–4.5.

Hair Dressings

No. 1

	oz
White mineral oil (65/75 viscosity)	98.20
Isopropyl myristate, pure	4.40
Stearic acid	3.65
Stripped coconut fatty acids	1.21
Glycerin	4.05
Triethanolamine	6.48
Water	80.20
Silicone oil 96–100	0.81
Perfume oil	to suit

Mix the mineral oil and isopropyl myristate with the acids, and heat to 70°C. Dissolve the glycerin and triethanolamine in the water and heat to the same temperature. Stir the oily mixture into the aqueous solution with rapid stirring until emulsification is complete. Stir in the silicone oil and allow the mixture to cool to 40°C. Add the perfume oil, and continue stirring until it is cold.

No. 2

		oz by wt
1	Mineral oil, white (65/75 viscosity)	75.0
	Petrolatum, white	15.0
	Lanolin	6.0
	Beeswax, white	4.0
	Sorbitan sesqui-oleate (Arlacel 83)	6.0
	Zinc stearate, U.S.P.	2.0
2	Borax	1.0
	Methyl *p*-hydroxybenzoate	0.4
	Water	91.0
	Perfume oil	q.s.

Heat (1) to 75°C. Heat (2) to the same temperature and add it to (1) slowly with moderate but thorough agitation. Stir in the perfume oil at 40°C., and continue stirring at low speed until cold.

No. 3

(Liquid)

Glyceryl monostearate (Aldo 28)	5.12 oz
Isopropyl palmitate	12.80 oz
Lantrol	7.68 oz

Lanfrax	1.28 oz
Oleic acid U.S.P.	3.20 oz
Tegosept M	0.26 oz
Tegosept P	0.13 oz
Triethanolamine	1.54 oz
Water	6.00 pt
Perfume oil	to suit

Mix the first seven ingredients and heat slowly until a clear solution results. Dissolve the triethanolamine in the water, and heat to the same temperature. Then pour slowly the water solution into the melted fats with constant stirring. When cool, add the perfume oil and continue stirring until cold.

No. 4
(Cream)

	oz
Glycerin monostearate	24.0
Mineral oil, white	48.0
Cetyl alcohol	2.0
Isopropyl palmitate	2.0
Lanolin anhydrous	2.0
Triethanolamine lauryl sulfate	3.0
Water	119.0
Perfume oil	to suit

Melt the first five ingredients at 70°C. Mix the triethanolamine lauryl sulfate with the water and heat to 70°C. With the agitator running, pour the water solution slowly into the melted fats and allow the mixture to cool. When the temperature has dropped to 40°C., stir in the perfume oil, and continue to stir until cold.

Hair Lotions

No. 1

	oz
Butoxy-polyoxypropylene glycol	25.60
Monoester polyoxyethylene glycol with coconut fatty acids	2.56
Propylene glycol monolaurate	1.41
Cetyl-dimethyl benzyl ammonium chloride 50% solution	1.28
Capsicum tincture	0.66
Menthol	0.64
Specially denatured alcohol #40	65.60
Perfume oil	0.50
Water	29.75

Dissolve the organic compounds in the alcohol. Add the water with vigorous stirring.

No. 2

	oz
Specially denatured alcohol #40	64.0
Ethoxylan 100	9.6
Isopropyl palmitate	19.2
Water	35.2
Perfume oil	to suit

Dissolve the palmitate and ethoxylan in the alcohol. Add the perfume oil and shake well. Finally add the water with vigorous stirring. Allow solution to stand overnight, and filter if necessary

Hair Pomade
(for Negroes)

Petrolatum	18 lb
Lanolin, anhydrous	2 lb
Mineral oil (65/75 viscosity)	3½ pt
Bergamot perfume oil	3 dr
Drug and cosmetic color	to suit

Melt the fats and oil. Remove from the fire, and stir in first the color, then the perfume oil. Pour into glass jars.

Hair Rinses: Liquid
No. 1: Bronze Red

D & C Red #13	1.192 oz
D & C Brown #1	0.860 oz
D & C Black #1	0.150 oz
Citric acid	12.000 oz
Water, enough to make	1.000 gal

Dissolve the citric acid in the water, add the colors and shake well. Put up in 4 oz or 8 oz bottles.

No. 2: Jet Black

D & C Black #1	1½ oz + 27 gr
D & C Brown #1	½ oz + 82 gr
D & C Red #13	96 gr
Citric acid	11 oz
Water, enough to make	1 gal

Follow same procedure as for No. 1.

No. 3: Slate
(for silver gray hair)

Black #12186 (Leeben Chem. Co., Inc.)	3.5 oz + 5 gr
D & C Brown #1	25.5 gr
Citric acid	9 oz
Water, enough to make	1 gal

Follow same procedure as for No. 1.

Directions for Application

Shampoo hair thoroughly; rinse completely free of all soap and oil; dry with towel, leaving the hair slightly moist. Dissolve 16 drops of the Slate Hair Rinse in 4 oz of warm water (more or less, as desired). Apply the rinse with a brush until all coloring has been absorbed, and comb hair well to distribute the color evenly. Then dry the hair as usual. The bottle should bear the following label in some conspicuous place:

Caution: This product contains ingredients which may cause skin irritation on certain individuals, hence a preliminary test, according to accompanying directions, should first be made. This product must not be used for dyeing eye-lashes or eyebrows. To do so may cause blindness.

To test: Mix rinse to strength to be used. Apply behind ear or to skin in bend of elbow. Allow to dry and remain 24 hours. If no itching, swelling, or redness appears during test period, then rinse may be applied.

Hair Rinses: Powdered

No. 1: Jet Black

	oz
D & C Black #1	8.00
D & C Brown #1	2.25
D & C Red #13	1.10
Powdered citric acid U.S.P.	55.00

Mix the powders thoroughly and pack the dry mixture in glassine or similar water-resistant envelopes at the rate of 30 grains of mixture per envelope. Add the contents of each envelope to one gallon of water for use as a rinse.

No. 2: Jet Black

D & C Black No. 1	1. 20 oz
D & C Brown No. 1	0.36 oz
Ext. D & C Red No. 1	0.44 oz
Citric acid U.S.P., powdered	4.05 lb

Procedure as for No. 1.

No. 3: Platinum

D & C Violet No. 1	0.25 oz
Citric acid U.S.P., powdered	2.84 lb

Procedure as for No. 1.

Hand Creams

No. 1

	oz
Glyceryl monostearate S (Aldo 28)	18.0
Lanolin	3.0
White mineral oil (65/75 viscosity)	1.5
Methyl *p*-hydroxybenzoate	0.3
Glycerin	15.0
Water	111.6
Perfume oil	0.6

Heat the first four ingredients to 65°C. Dissolve the glycerin in the water and heat to the same temperature. Mix the two solutions and continue stirring until cold. Stir in the perfume oil when the mass is at 35°C.

No. 2

	parts by wt
Stearic acid	7.5
Isopropyl myristate, pure	1.5
Polyoxyethylene sorbitan monostearate	3.0
Sorbitan monostearate	3.6
Glycerin	7.5
Methyl *p*-hydroxybenzoate	0.3
Water	126.9
Perfume oil	q.s.

Melt the acid, myristate, monostearates, and bring to 75°C. Dissolve the glycerin and preservative in the water and heat to 80°C. Slowly pour the water solution into the melted fats with rapid stirring. Stir in the perfume oil at 40°C., and continue to mix at slow speed until cold.

Hand Lotions

No. 1

Stearic acid	12.00 oz
Mineral oil (65/75 viscosity	20.00 oz
Cetyl alcohol	4.00 oz
Glycerin	20.00 oz

Triethanolamine	6.00 oz
Water	19.25 pt
* Quince seed mucilage	14.00 oz
Specially denatured alcohol	20.00 oz
Perfume oil	to suit

Place the stearic acid, mineral oil, and cetyl alcohol in a separate container, and heat to 70°C. Dissolve the triethanolamine and glycerin in the water and heat to 80°C. Mix the two solutions and continue to stir until the dispersion is uniform, and then slowly until the temperature cools to about 50°C. At this point stir in the quince mucilage and then the alcohol, to which the perfume oil has been added. Continue to stir until the lotion has acquired room temperature.

* Quince Seed Mucilage

Clean quince seed	1 oz
Water	33 oz
Methyl *p*-hydroxybenzoate	30 gr

Dissolve the preservative in the water. Stir in the quince seed and allow it to stand overnight. Finally, strain the mucilage through a fine screen.

No. 2

	oz
Stearic acid	1.77
Anhydrous lanolin	1.77
Triethanolamine	0.64
Distilled water	31.04
Thymol	0.04
Perfume oil	0.04

No. 3

	oz
Change the lanolin to	3.53
and the water to	29.30

For both No. 2 and No. 3, melt the stearic acid together with the triethanolamine. Add the water and stir until a creamy soap is formed. Add the lanolin and continue the heating until it has melted. Continue the stirring until a creamy emulsion is formed. Stir intermittently until the mass has cooled to room temperature. Then add the thymol and perfume, previously dissolved in a small amount of alcohol, and put it through a hand-operated homogenizer. These lotions are very satisfactory, because very little is necessary to soften the skin of the hands and face.

No. 4

	oz
Glyceryl monostearate S (Aldo 28)	16.00
Lanolin	4.00
Cetyl alcohol N.F. extra	1.00
Glycerin and propylene glycol	4.00
Alcohol, specially denatured	4.00
Perfume oil	0.75
Chlorophyll color	to suit
Water	enough to make 1 gal

Melt the monostearate, lanolin, and cetyl alcohol. Heat the water to the same temperature and dissolve in it the glycerin and propylene glycol. Pour the water solution into the molten fats with constant stirring. Continue to stir until cool. Mix the perfume oil with the alcohol, and stir it into the finished product. Color it with chlorophyll.

No. 5

		parts by wt
1	Glyceryl monostearate	4.5
1	Isopropyl myristate pure	1.5
1	Anhydrous lanolin	1.5
1	Alkyl dimethyl benzonium chloride	1.5
	Glycerin	7.5
	Methyl-*p*-hydroxybenzoate	0.3
	Water	133.5
	Perfume oil	q.s.

Mix (1) and melt. Dissolve the glycerin and preservative in water and heat to the same temperature. Pour slowly the water solution into the melted fats with rapid stirring. Stir in the perfume oil at 40°C., and continue mixing at slow speed until cold.

No. 6: Creme

	oz
Diglycol stearate	2.56
Stearic acid	5.12
Olive oil	2.56
Propylene glycol	3.84
Triethanolamine	1.41
Lanolin	2.56
Stearyl alcohol	0.90
Butyl *p*-hydroxybenzoate	0.13
Water	109.05
Perfume	to suit

Place the stearate, stearic acid, olive oil, lanolin, stearyl alcohol, and butyl *p*-hydroxybenzoate together in a suitable container and heat to 80°C. Heat the water and glycol to the same temperature. Add the triethanolamine to the hot water and pour this mixture into the molten fats with constant stirring. Continue the agitation until the cream has cooled to 45°C., and stir in the perfume. This cream has a very pronounced pearly appearance. If the pearliness is to be enhanced, allow the cream to age for a week or two, and agitate it from time to time during the aging period.

No. 7: Aerosol

	oz
Polyethylene glycol (400) distearate	3
Isopropyl palmitate	6
Sodium lauryl sulfate paste	30
Glycerin	15
Water	96
Perfume oil	to suit

Mix all the ingredients, except the perfume oil, and heat to 160–180°F. to effect complete solution. Stir in the perfume oil while cooling, and continue to stir until cold. Mix about 90 parts of this lotion with about 10 parts of a propellent mixture.

Hollywood Face Mask

	oz
Gelatin, in small pieces	19.20
Powdered zinc oxide or calamine	19.20

Glycerin	44.80
Distilled water	44.80

Soak the gelatin in the water, till soft. Add the glycerin and heat on a water bath until the gelatin goes into solution. Stir in the zinc oxide, and fill warm in tubes. This tube must be warmed everytime in a water bath before use. Apply this paste to the face and leave it for about 20 minutes when it becomes like a piece of gum. It can be removed in one piece, with all the impurities of the skin adhering to it.

Lanette Wax

Prepare Lanette wax by melting and mixing the following ingredients:

	oz
Cetyl alcohol	90.0
Sodium lauryl sulfate	10.0

Lanolin Derivatives

Polyoxyethylene derivatives of acetylated lanolin are completely soluble in water, alcohol, many oils and solvents. These derivatives yield persistent, emollient films and have solubilizing properties desirable in cosmetics, pharmaceuticals, toiletries, and aerosol formulations. They are non-greasy clear liquids, designed to give a soft, non-tacky after-feeling when incorporated into water-alcohol preparations and emulsions.

The lanolin derivatives are produced in two forms: (1) Completely acetylated for use in preparations of high alcohol content; and (2) partially acetylated for use in aqueous and weak alcoholic preparations.

Lather Shaving Cream

Coconut oil	6.38 lb
Stearic acid	40.50 lb
Potassium hydroxide, 45°Bé	17.00 lb
Sodium hydroxide, 50%	3.37 lb
Lanolin	0.63 lb
Glycerin	19.75 lb
Neutral soap	0.25 lb
Water	29.50 lb
Perfume oil	7.00 oz

Heat the coconut oil, stearic acid, and lanolin together in a stainless steel container to a temperature of 180°F. Heat the water to the same temperature and add the soap, with stirring, until it is dissolved. When solution is complete add the glycerin, potassium hydroxide, and sodium hydroxide. Pour this soapy solution into the hot fats with slow mechanical agitation (8–10 rpm). Continue heating until the product starts to boil. Remove from fire, but keep stirring the cream until it has acquired room temperature. Stir in the perfume oil, and age for about two weeks in order to develop a pearl.

Leg Make-Up
(Liquid Stockings)

Colloidal China clay	10.22 oz
Powdered titanium dioxide	1.30 oz
Talcum powder	6.40 oz
Lake color	5.12 oz
Polyvinyl alcohol (medium molecular weight)	3.84 oz
Sulfonated lauryl alcohol, liquid	3.84 oz
Glycerin	12.80 oz
Water, enough to make	1.00 gal

Mix the powders with the lake color, add the alcohols and glycerin; stir in the water and shake well.

Light-Screening Cream

	oz
Glyceryl tristearate	50.0
Cocoa butter	2.0
Cetyl alcohol	1.0
Glycerin	20.0
Triethanolamine	2.0
Distilled water	125.0
Perfume	to suit

Melt the tristearate, cocoa butter, and cetyl alcohol at about 55°C. Mix the triethanolamine, glycerin, and water, and heat to the same temperature. Pour the aqueous solution into the oily mixture, stirring constantly until an emulsion forms. Add the perfume oil and stir until cold.

Lipstick
No. 1

	oz
Castor oil, very high grade	53.25
Isopropyl myristate	13.50
Glyceryl monostearate	60.75
Petrolatum	6.00
Carnauba wax	6.00
Bromo Acid	3.00
* Color lakes	7.50
Raspberry or strawberry flavor	to suit

* See suggestions following No. 2.

Mix the castor oil with the isopropyl myristate and heat on a steam bath to 160°F., with moderate agitation. Dissolve the bromo acid in this mixture. Weigh out the pigments into a small mixer, and agitate the mass until the color is uniform.

Place the petrolatum, carnauba wax, and glyceryl monostearate into a separate container and heat until the mixture is completely melted. Stir the lake colors into the molten mass, and mill it to ensure uniform dispersion of the colors. Add this milled mixture to the bromo acid solution and stir until it is homogeneous. Evacuate any air that might have been trapped in the material during mixing. When the temperature has dropped to about ten degrees above the solidification of the mass, pour it into molds to form sticks, and chill quickly by passing the molds through a refrigerating unit. Remove the sticks and pass a flame over them to make the surface glossy. The sticks are now ready for packaging and storage.

No. 2

	oz
Ceresin	13.50
Lanolin anhydrous, U.S.P.	7.50
Cocoa butter, U.S.P.	4.12
Beeswax, white, U.S.P.	3.38
Carnauba wax	3.15
Glyceryl mono-oleate	5.25
Mineral oil (white, high viscosity)	21.98
Olive oil fatty acid monoethanolamide	15.00
Tetrabromofluorescein	1.68
Insoluble lakes	7.32
Perfume oil	1.50

Mill the insoluble lakes with the mineral oil and glyceryl monooleate in a triple roller mill. Melt the fatty acid monoethanolamide and dissolve the tetrabromofluorescein in it. Melt the other waxes and fats at 650°C. and stir into it the hot solution of the tetrabromofluorescein, pouring it through a fine metal strainer in order to remove insoluble impurities. Finally stir in the milled insoluble lakes, add the perfume oil, and pour into lipstick molds. You may replace some of the olive oil fatty acid monoethanolamide with some castor oil. Olive oil fatty acid monoethanolamide is a pale yellow wax with a pleasant odor and bland taste. It is a better dye solvent than castor oil, and it is not hygroscopic.

Lipstick Colors

Red: Bromo

	oz
D and C Orange No. 5	1.5
D and C Red No. 21	1.5

Red: Color Lakes

	oz
D and C Red No. 11 Ca Lake	2.0
D and C Red No. 31 Ca Lake	2.5
D and C Red No. 19 Al Lake	3.0
D and C Red No. 9 Ba Lake	2.5

Pink: Bromo

	oz
D and C Orange No. 5	3.0

Color, not Lakes

	oz
D and C Red No. 19	6.0
D and C Red No. 37	2.8
D and C Red No. 13	1.0
D and C Red No. 11	0.2

Liquid Make-Up

Isopropyl myristate	51.00 oz
Liquid lanolin	9.00 oz
Stearic acid, triple-pressed	4.50 oz
Methyl *p*-hydroxybenzoate	60.00 gr
Triethanolamine lauryl alcohol sulfate	1.50 oz
Distilled water	83.52 oz
Perfume oil	0.50 oz

Heat the first four ingredients to 70°C. Dissolve the triethanolamine lauryl alcohol sulfate in the water and heat to the same temperature. Mix the two solutions and continue to stir until cold. Stir in the perfume oil at a temperature of 40–35°C.

Mineral Filler

Micro-Cel (Synthetic calcium silicate) will absorb six times its weight in water, and will remain a free-flowing powder even after absorbing twice its weight in liquids.

Because of its high absorbing power, Micro-Cel will prevent caking and will control deliquescent products. Because its particle size is only 0.02 micron (one millionth of a meter), Micro-Cel will ensure better suspension of heavy solids, and will provide even dispersion and blending. The physical properties of Micro-Cel suggest many uses in the manufacture of pharmaceutical and cosmetic products.

Moisture Cream

	oz
White mineral oil (65/75 viscosity)	25.60
Glyceryl monostearate (Aldo 28)	10.24
Polyoxyethylene lauryl ether (Brij 35)	10.24
Lantrol	6.40
Microcrystalline wax 155	6.40
Cetyl alcohol	2.56
Tegosept M	0.26
Tegosept P	0.13
Glycerin	3.84
Sodium lauryl sulfate paste	1.28
Water	61.06
Perfume oil	to suit

Melt together the first eight ingredients and keep at 70°C. Dissolve the glycerin and sodium lauryl sulfate paste in the water and heat to the same temperature. Add the water solution to the melted fats and stir vigorously. When emulsification is complete, stir more slowly until cold. Stir in the perfume oil at 40°C.

Nail Enamel

	oz
Dibutyl phthalate	20.25
D & C Red #19	0.15
D & C Red #31	0.30
Oil Pink	0.15
Nitrocellulose	17.10
Ethyl acetate	47.25
Butyl acetate	45.00
Tri-*o*-cresyl phosphate	12.45
Alcohol, anhydrous	7.35

Mix the colors in the dibutyl phthalate, and grind the mixture in a pebble or ball mill. Dissolve the nitrocellulose in the ethyl acetate, and add the butyl acetate to this mixture. Incorporate slowly the color dispersion in the nitrocellulose solution and mix with thorough stirring. Finally, stir in the rest of the ingredients, and continue to stir until the product is homogeneous. Add some perfume oil if so desired. For best results fill the enamel at once.

Nail Enamel

	oz
Acryloid B66	18
Arochlor 5460	13.20
Arochlor 1254	20.25
Ethyl acetate	47.25
Butyl acetate	45
Alcohol, anhydrous or Isopropyl alcohol (99%)	5.60
Dye	0.60
Perfume	to suit

Mix the dye with Arochlor 1254 and grind the mixture in a pebble or ball mill. Dissolve the resins in the butyl-ethyl acetate mixture. Incorporate slowly the color dispersion in the resin solution and mix thoroughly. Use a tumbling and rolling action for quick solution. When solution is complete, add the alcohol and the desired perfume. Continue to stir until the finished product is homogeneous.

Nail Polish Removers

No. 1: Creamy

	oz
Stearic acid	36
Castor oil	8
Butyl acetate	280
Triethanolamine	14
Water	60

Melt the stearic acid with the castor oil. Dissolve the triethanolamine in the water and heat to the same temperature. Pour the water solution into the melted fats and keep on stirring until the mass cools; then stir in the butyl acetate, and continue stirring until the mass is homogeneous.

This preparation leaves the nails shiny. It does not have such a strong defatting action as is the case with liquid removers, and the nails are not left so brittle.

No. 2

	oz
Acetic ether	54.40
Acetone	54.40
Specially denatured alcohol #40	12.80
Ethoxylan 100	1.28
Water	5.12

Dissolve the Ethoxylan 100 in the acetone-alcohol-ether mixture. Add the water slowly, with constant stirring.

Oleyl Oleate

Oleyl oleate is sold under the trade name of Cetiol-V. When purified, it has the properties of a thin oil with an interesting feeling. It is a colorless liquid mixture of unsaturated wax esters of animal origin. Its uses are manifold: as a superfatting agent for creams and ointments, and as a base for cosmetic oils.

It is manufactured in Germany, and distributed in the U.S.A.

Preservatives

Methyl *para*-hydroxybenzoate is a good preservative for cosmetics. Use one part of it to 500 parts of finished product (0.2%). Fifteen grains of methyl *p*-hydroxybenzoate dissolve in about 14 oz of water, 1.5 oz of warm oil, 2.5 oz of warm glycerin. It is freely soluble in alcohol.

The *alpha-glyceryl ether of p-chlorophenol* has good possibilities as a preservative for cosmetic emulsions. It is a colorless, almost odorless solid which is more soluble in water than are many phenolic preservatives. Its toxicity is rather low, and it does not act as a primary irritant.

Emulsified ointment bases when inoculated with cultures of *penicillium, aspergillus,* and dermatophytes were kept sterile by the addition of 0.3% of chlorophenyl glyceryl ether, whereas living molds were isolated from control samples.

Permanent Wave Solution

	oz
Triethanolamine	14.72
Sodium sulfite	1.92
Borax	5.12
Sodium carbonate	2.56
Water	103.68

Mix the triethanolamine with the water, add the powdered chemicals, and shake well until solution is complete. Perfume and color may be added if so desired.

Pine Bath Oils

	oz
Bornyl acetate	2.6
Sulfonated olive oil	125.4
or	
Sulfonated olive oil	108.8
Pine perfume compound	6.4
Distilled water	12.8

Dissolve the perfume compound in the olive oil, and add the water. Color and filter if desired.

Polyethylene Glycols

Substitute polyethylene glycols for castor oil in the compounding of hair dressings. The polyethylene glycols are of two types, namely, water-soluble and aqueous-alcohol-soluble. These compounds require about half as much alcohol as castor oil.

Powder Cream

	oz
Cetyl alcohol	5.12
Polyoxyethylene lauryl ether (Brij 35)	1.28
Zinc oxide powder	32.00
Talcum powder	12.80
Glycerin	15.36
Water	61.44
Color	to suit

Mix the powders and color thoroughly with the glycerin and half the water. Melt the cetyl alcohol and lauryl ether in the rest of the water; cool, and reheat to 70°C. with stirring. When this emulsion is cold again, stir it into the powder mixture. Finally pass through a colloid mill.

Preshave Lotion

	oz
Specially denatured alcohol #40	64.00

Glycerin	6.40
Lactic acid U.S.P.	2.56
Water	55.04
Perfume	to suit

Mix the perfume oil with the alcohol. Mix the water with glycerin and acid. Pour the water solution slowly into the alcohol mixture, and shake well. Allow to stand overnight, and filter if necessary. This preshave lotion is excellent for electric shavers; it helps to tauten the skin and stiffen the whiskers.

Pressing Oil—For Negroes

Petrolatum, white	28	lb
Mineral oil (65/75 viscosity)	3	pt
Lanolin, anhydrous	24	oz
Silicone fluid 555	7½	oz
Bergamot perfume oil	4	dr
Drug and cosmetic yellow	to suit	

Melt the fats and oil. Remove from the fire, and stir in the silicone fluid, then the color and perfume oil. Pour into glass jars.

Protective Hand Cream

		oz
1	Stearic acid	16.92
	Lanette wax	1.20
	Lanolin, anhydrous	3.39
	Zinc stearate	8.60
2	Triethanolamine	6.78
	Glycerin U.S.P.	16.92
	Sorbo	10.17
	Sodium benzoate	0.15
	Water, distilled	111.75
	Perfume oil	q.s.

Heat (1) to 80°C. Heat (2) to the same temperature. Pour (2) into (1) with steady agitation, and continue to stir until the temperature has dropped to 40°C. Stir in the perfume oil and homogenize it.

Rolling Massage Cream

	oz
Paraffin wax	1.28
Cetyl alcohol	7.68
Mineral oil	3.84
Glycerin	6.40
Distilled water	85.22
Borax	3.84
Corn starch	19.24
Perfume	0.50

Melt the wax, alcohol, and mineral oil together with the glycerin. Dissolve the borax in the water and heat to the same temperature. Pour the borax solution into the melted fats with constant stirring. Work the starch into the emulsion while it is still very warm and liquid. Add the perfume and keep on stirring until the mass cools.

Shampoo Base

	oz
Texapon BS (Sodium lauryl polyglycol ether sulfate)	64.00
Water	62.72
Sodium chloride	1.28

Mix thoroughly. Mix one part of this base with seven (7) parts of water.

Shampoo for Aerosols

Sodium lauryl sulfonate paste	53	oz

Isopropyl myristate	1½ oz
Polyethylene glycol (400) stearate	4½ oz
Water	92 oz
Perfume oil	4 dr

Mix the first four components and heat to 160–180°F. to effect complete solution. Allow to cool, and stir in the perfume oil. Continue to stir until cold. Mix 90 parts of this shampoo with 10 parts of a propellent mixture. (See suggestions under Aerosols.)

Cream Shampoos

No. 1

Sodium lauryl sulfate (30% active)	5.625 lb
Polyethylene glycol (400) distearate	8
Cetyl alcohol	1.500 oz
Water	3.125 pt
Perfume oil	to suit

Mix the first four ingredients and heat to 160–180°F. to effect complete solution. Allow to cool, and stir in the perfume oil. Continue the stirring until cold.

No. 2

	oz
Duponol WA paste	64.00
Polyethylene glycol (400) distearate	6.50
Water	54.48
Lanolin	1.28
Sodium polyphosphate	2.50
Perfume	to suit

Sodium polyphosphate is used in this formula as a foam builder. Heat to 85°C. with constant stirring until homogeneous. Add the perfume, and continue stirring until cold.

No. 3

	oz
Duponol WA paste	128.00
Polyethylene glycol (400) distearate	13.00
Lanolin anhydrous	2.56
Water	104.96
Perfume	to suit

Heat to approximately 85°C., stirring at a medium rate of speed. Allow the mixture to cool, add the perfume oil at 45°C., and continue stirring until the mass is cold. The resultant product is a thick white paste with a pearly appearance.

No. 4

Sodium lauryl sulfate paste	9¼ lb
Stearic acid	15 oz
Isopropyl myristate	3 oz
Sodium hydroxide	2¼ oz
Water	130 oz
Perfume oil	to suit

Mix the first three components and heat to 160–180°F. to effect complete solution. Dissolve the sodium hydroxide in the water and heat to the same temperature. Add the aqueous solution to the melted fats with thorough agitation. Continue the heating and stirring until saponification is complete. Stir in the perfume oil during cooling, and continue to stir until it is cold. Do not handle the sodium hydroxide with bare hands.

No. 5

Duponol WA paste	15¼ lb
Emcol MAS	2⅛ lb
Ninol AA 62 (foam stabilizer)	2⅛ lb
Coconut fatty acids	21 oz
Lantrol	14 oz
Triethanolamine	11⅕ oz
Sodium chloride	7 oz
Water	21 pt
Perfume oil	to suit

Mix all the ingredients, except the perfume oil, and heat to 160–180°F. to effect complete solution. Allow the mixture to cool, add the perfume oil, and continue to stir, using mild agitation, until the mass is cold.

No. 6

		oz
1	Coconut oil	25.00
	Coconut fatty acids	25.00
	Stearic acid	25.00
	Castor oil	10.00
	Triethanolamine lauryl sulfate	7.50
	Glyceryl monostearate (self-emulsifying)	5.00
	Stearyl alcohol pure	5.00
	Propylene glycol	5.00
2	Potassium hydroxide, 89% KOH	13.75
	Triethanolamine	5.00
	Sodium hydroxide, 98% NaOH	1.87
	Borax	1.25
	Alcohol, specially denatured	10.00
	Water	110.00
	Perfume oil	q.s.

Mix (1) and melt at the lowest possible temperature. Dissolve (2) in the water and heat to the same temperature. Pour (2) into (1) slowly, with constant stirring, and continue to stir until all is emulsified. Adjust the shampoo neutral to phenolphthalein (in neutral or acid solutions, it stays colorless) and only faintly alkaline to litmus (the red litmus paper is sensitive to 0.0005*N* NaOH). Stir in the alcohol, then the perfume oil, and continue stirring until the mixture is homogeneous. Tint it with D. & C. Naphthol Green if desired.

This shampoo lathers exceptionally well.

No. 7
(Liquid)

Sodium ethoxylated lauryl alcohol sulfate paste	3.5 lb
Magnesium stearate	2.56 oz
Polyvinyl alcohol (10% solution)	7.68 oz
Anhydrous lanolin	1.28 oz
Glyceryl monolaurate	2.56 oz
Cetyl alcohol	2.56 oz
Water, enough to make	1.00 gal
Perfume oil	to suit

Mix the first three ingredients with the water and heat to 168°F. Mix the lanolin, glyceryl monolaurate, and cetyl alcohol, and heat to the same temperature. Add the water solution to the melted fats with thorough agitation. Stir in the perfume oil, and continue stirring until cold.

No. 8
(Liquid)

Sodium lauryl sulfate, 86% active	4½	lb
Lauryl diethanolamide	33	oz
Ethylene glycol monostearate	15	oz
Phosphoric acid	3	oz
Water	178	oz
Perfume oil		q.s.

Dissolve the acid in the water. Mix the lauryl diethanolamide together with the ethylene glycol monostearate and melt at the lowest possible temperature. Heat the acidulated water to the same temperature, and gradually add it with constant stirring, then incorporate the sodium lauryl sulfate. Finally, add the perfume oil, and continue the stirring until cold. The resultant product is a pearly and viscous liquid cream shampoo.

Liquid Shampoos

No. 1

Sodium lauryl sulfate	2	lb
Miranol "MM" conc.	2	lb
Polyethylene glycol (400) distearate	4.25	oz
Polyterge 102	5	pt
Glycerin	24	oz
Borax	4	oz
Polyvinylpyrrolidone (PVP), type NP	8	oz
Perfume oil	3	oz
Color	6	oz
Distilled water	6.75	gal

Mix the perfume oil with the Polyterge 102, and add 3 pt of the distilled water. Shake well and allow to stand overnight. Now mix the sodium lauryl sulfate, Miranol, distearate, and borax, in about 4 gallons of the water and heat to 160°F. Remove the heat and stir the glycerin and PVP into about 1 gallon of the water. Continue to stir while adding the perfumed Polyterge 102. Stir in the rest of the water while adding the color.

No. 2

Sodium lauryl sulfate	2	lb
Miranol "MM" conc.	2	lb
Ultrapole S	4	pt
Glycerin	24	oz
Borax	4	oz
Perfume oil	3	oz
Color	6	oz
Water, distilled	6.75	gal

Mix the perfume oil with the Ultropole S, and add 4 pt of the distilled water. Shake well and allow to stand overnight. Now mix the sodium lauryl sulfate, Miranol, borax, and with about 4 gallons of the water heat to 160°F. Remove the heat, and stir in the glycerin with about 1 gallon of the water. Continue to stir while adding the perfumed Ultrapole S. Stir in the rest of the water while adding the color.

No. 3

Triethanolamine lauryl sulfate	76.80
Fatty alkylolamide	2.56
Water	48.00
Perfume oil	0.64

Dissolve the triethanolamine lauryl sulfate in the water, add the perfume oil to the fatty alkylolamide, and mix the solutions. Shake well, and allow to stand overnight.

No. 4

Triethanolamine lauryl sulfate	2.0 lb
Sodium alginate	3.2 oz
Glycerin	2.0 oz
Water, enough to make	1.0 gal
Perfume and color	to suit

Mix all the ingredients and heat to about 50°C. Keep on stirring until solution is complete. The resultant shampoo has good body and appearance. Use distilled water if necessary.

No. 5

Triethanolamine lauryl sulfate (40% active)	8.75 lb
Propylene glycol	6 oz
Oleic monoethanolamine	3 oz
Water (distilled) enough to make 26% active lauryl sulfate	
Perfume oil	to suit

Mix and stir until solution is complete.

No. 6

Sipon ES	17.500 lb
Ethoxylan 50	3.875 lb
Ninol AA62 (foam stabilizer)	3.500 lb
Polyethylene glycol (400) distearate	14.000 oz
Sodium chloride	7.000 oz
Versene Na_4	3.500 oz
Water	2.125 gal
Perfume oil	to suit

Mix all the ingredients, except the perfume oil, and heat to about 160°F. to effect complete solution. Allow it to cool, then stir in the perfume oil. Stir occasionally until cold.

No. 7

Sodium lauryl sulfate (28% active)	7.5 lb
Ethanolamide of coconut fatty acids	15 oz
Lanolin	3 oz
Ethylene glycol monostearate	4.5 oz
Water	10 pt
Hydroxyacetic acid (glycolic acid) q.s. for *p*H of 7.4	
Perfume oil	1.5 oz

Mix the first five components and heat to 160–180°F. to effect complete solution. Stir in enough of the acid in order to bring *p*H value to 7.4. Allow to cool, and stir in the perfume oil. Continue to stir until cold.

No. 8

	lb
Ammonium lauryl sulfate	20
Lauric diethanolamide (62% amide)	3–5
Water (soft)	75–77

Dissolve the sulfate in the water. Melt the amide, then add with stirring to the sulfate solution. Adjust the *p*H to 7.0 or 7.5 with a little citric acid. Stir in any desirable color and perfume, and add about 0.1% formalin U.S.P. to act as a preservative. Finally, adjust the *p*H of the finished shampoo to 7.2 in order to avoid the odor of ammonia.

Liquid Soap Shampoos

No. 1

	lb
Coconut oil	8.00
Castor oil, U.S.P.	0.50
Lauric acid	2.50
Oleic acid, U.S.P.	0.75
Water, distilled	5.00
Potassium hydroxide U.S.P., 88–90%	3.38
Sodium borate, U.S.P.	0.25
Triethanolamine	0.12
Sodium hexametaphosphate	0.15
Water, distilled	7.50
Alcohol, specially denatured	3.00
Perfume oil	0.45
Water, distilled	68.40

Melt the oils and acids together. Stir in the 5 lb of water cold, just before the alkaline mixture is added. This prevents frothing-over when the caustic solution is added. Dissolve the alkalies in the 7.50 lb of water, and when solution is complete, stir in the sodium hexametaphosphate. Now stir this caustic solution into the mixture of molten oils and acids. Introduce it in small portions, especially at the beginning, and stir constantly. When saponification has taken place, stir in some of the alcohol. Reserve some of the alcohol for dissolving the perfume oil. When the temperature has fallen sufficiently, and after the rest of the water has been thoroughly incorporated, stir in the perfume solution. Finally, filter the shampoo through a little talcum. If proper filtering equipment is not available, use brewers' bags.

No. 2: Pine Tar

Pine tar, U.S.P. (obtained from pine wood)	1.0 oz
Bornyl acetate	0.5 oz
Liquid soap shampoo No. 1	5.0 gal

Substitute the pine tar and bornyl acetate for the perfume oil, dissolve them in some alcohol, then mix the alcoholic solution thoroughly with the shampoo.

No. 3: Henna

A henna shampoo may be produced by stirring in a fraction of one per cent of synthetic Lawsonia (hydroxynaphthoquinone—the coloring matter of henna leaves).

Shampoo Thickener and Hair Conditioner

Use 1 to 5% of polyethylene glycol (400) distearate for the purpose of thickening both the cream and the liquid synthetic detergent shampoos. This compound definitely has "hair conditioning" properties. Polyethylene glycol 400 distearate is non-ionic and therefore its effect on reducing the lather is less than that of sodium stearate.

Shaving Creams

No. 1

	lb
Glyceryl tristearate	16.80
Myristic acid	8.40
Undecylic acid	4.80
Potassium hydroxide, U.S.P.	5.64
Sodium hydroxide, U.S.P.	0.27
Triethanolamine	0.81
Glycerin, U.S.P.	4.50
Eutanol G (saturated fatty alcohol)	1.50
Texapon CS (fatty alcohol sulfate)	2.25
Menthol, U.S.P.	0.15
Perfume oil	0.75
Water (soft) enough to make	84.00

Heat half of the glyceryl tristearate and myristic acid and all of the undecylic acid in a water-jacketed kettle to about 194°F. Dissolve the alkalies and triethanolamine in the water and heat to the same temperature. Stir in the hot alkaline mixture slowly into the molten fatty acids, and continue the stirring for about half an hour at about 165°F. Now stir in gradually the remaining glyceryl tristearate and myristic acid, previously melted. Cool the mixture to about 125°F., then stir in the glycerin, Eutanol, and Texapon.

Allow the cream to cool to about 85°F., then incorporate the menthol and perfume oil. Use some surplus water to make up for loss by evaporation. Stir the finished product again and then pass it through a suitable homogenizer. Repeat the operation after 24 hours. Finally, fill the finished cream in tubes.

No. 2

	lb
Stearic acid	30.0
Myristic acid	6.0
Coconut oil	12.0
Castor oil, U.S.P.	2.4
Potash (89–90%)	11.4
Borax	0.6
Water	6.0
Diethylene glycol stearate	2.4
Stearyl alcohol, U.S.P.	1.2
White mineral oil (65/75 viscosity)	1.8
Glycerin	6.0

Dissolve the potash and borax in the water in a stainless steel container. Add the fatty acids and oils to the alkaline solution; the heat from this reaction will start saponification. Heat this mixture on a water bath and stir it occasionally until saponification is complete. Add the remaining components, except the glycerin, and continue to stir the batch slowly. Cover it, allow it to stand on the bath for about one hour, and then stir in the glycerin.

Allow this shaving cream to age for some time. The resultant product has good stability and cutaneous properties.

Skin Bracer

Camphor, U.S.P.	93	gr
Menthol	31	gr
Specially denatured alcohol	46⅔	oz
Perfume oil	1	dr
Witch hazel extract	13⅓	oz
Glycerin	6	oz
Water	66	oz

Dissolve the camphor, menthol, and perfume oil, in the alcohol. Mix the witch hazel and glycerin, with the water. Finally mix the two solutions with vigorous shaking. Allow mixture to stand 48 hours, and if necessary filter it through kieselguhr.

Skin Freshner

	oz
Specially denatured alcohol #40	36.35
Propylene glycol	8.58
Zinc phenolsulfonate, N.F.	1.41
Boric acid, U.S.P.	2.75
Benzoic acid, U.S.P.	2.50
Menthol, U.S.P.	0.13
Perfume oil	0.89
Water	75.39

Mix the glycol with the water. Dissolve the zinc phenolsulfonate and the acids in the water-glycol solution, and stir until the solids are completely dissolved. Dissolve the perfume oil and the menthol in the alcohol, and stir this alcoholic solution into the water-glycol solution. Continue the stirring until the product is well mixed. Allow it to age for at least two weeks and then filter it through kieselguhr. Add color if desired.

Sodium Tripolyphosphate

This compound is a crystalline substance which can soften water without precipitation. Soap manufacturers using sodium tripolyphosphate find it superior to other phosphates for sequestering magnesium and iron. It is far more economical and better able to adjust and buffer the *p*H of solution. It is more soluble in water than some of the other complex phosphates; and more stable at higher temperatures in the presence of free alkalies.

Sunscreen Compounds

The ideal sunscreen compound has very slight or no absorption for the long ultraviolet rays beyond 3400 Angstroms which produce tanning without appreciable erythema (abnormal redness of the skin). Its decomposition products should be nontoxic and nonirritating.

The dialkyl-*p*-aminobenzoate esters meet all the requirements of the ideal sunscreen compound. They are neutral, relatively non-volatile, very soluble in the vehicle, slightly soluble in water, and have no absorption beyond 3500 Angstroms; they are nontoxic and nonirritating.

Ethyl-*p*-dimethyl aminobenzoate is a very effective sun screen. As little as 0.5 to 1% would be sufficient for the necessary filtering of harmful radiation.

p-Aminobenzoic acid, or especially its sodium salt, may also be used for filtering out the dangerous ultraviolet rays without preventing initial reddening or subsequent tanning of the skin. This substance will prevent or mitigate the undesirable and dangerous effects of sunburn.

The following compounds are approved for use in sunscreening preparations for preventing sunburn:

	%
Monoglyceryl *p*-aminobenzoate	3
Escalol 75 A	5
2-Ethylhexyl salicylate	5
Digalloyl trioleate	3
Menthyl salicylate	8
Dipropylene glycol salicylate	4

Propylene glycol salicylate may be used instead of menthyl salicylate as a screening agent in sunburn preventive preparations. Its cost per pound is less.

Sun Screen Evalution

Of five screening agents tested, tannic acid and *p*-aminobenzoic acid were the best; in 5% solutions, tannic acid was slightly the better of the two. The other three screening agents, namely, phenyl salicylate, glyceryl *p*-aminobenzoate, and menthyl anthranilate, showed no significant differences. The last-named compound was the poorest of the lot.

Sunscreen Indices Applying to 3080 Angstrom

Compound	*Sunscreen Index*
Ethyl *p*-dimethylamino-benzoate	14.80
Ethyl *p*-aminobenzoate	9.60
Isobutyl *p*-aminobenzoate	9.20
p-Aminobenzoic acid	7.40
Methyl umbelliferone	7.70
Umbelliferone acetic acid	6.00
Salicylic acid	4.30
Menthyl salicylate	4.00
Salicylamide	3.90
Sodium salicylate	2.40
Salicyl aldehyde	2.20
Digalloyl trioleate	2.30
Dipropylene glycol salicylate	1.90
p-Aminosalicylic acid	1.90
Ethyl gallate	1.40
Lauryl gallate	0.85

This table shows the relative absorption capacity of a number of sunscreens. The value of Ethyl *p*-dimethylaminobenzoate is clearly shown.

Sunburn Preventives

No. 1

	oz
Petrolatum U.S.P.	45.63
White mineral oil (65/75 viscosity)	19.00
Stearyl alcohol U.S.P.	4.38
Digalloyl trioleate	3.75
Sesame oil, N.F.	2.50
Calcium stearate	12.50
Kaolin, N.F.	37.50

Melt together the first five ingredients, and stir thoroughly until a clear solution results. Finally stir in the powdered ingredients, and continue the stirring until cold.

No. 2

	oz
Glycerin	1.18
Isobutyl-*p*-aminobenzoate	0.42
Tannic acid, U.S.P.	0.25
Specially denatured alcohol 70%	11.80

Dissolve the isobutyl-*p*-aminobenzoate in the alcohol. Add the glycerin, then the tannic acid, and shake well. Allow to stand overnight.

No. 3

	oz
β-Methyl umbelliferone	1.28
Propylene glycol	25.60
Alcohol	62.72
Water	38.40

Dissolve the umbelliferone in the alcohol, stir in the propylene glycol and then the water. Shake well.

No. 4

Stearic acid	8.06 oz
Triethanolamine	1.03 oz
Carbowax 1540	3.84 oz
Stearyl alcohol	5.76 oz
Benzocaine, U.S.P.	3.84 oz
Coumarin	26.30 gr
Titanium dioxide	1.28 oz
Calamine, prepared, N.F.	1.28 oz
Iron oxide, brown	83.13 gr
Methyl *p*-hydroxybenzoate	110.13 gr
Glycerin	12.80 oz
Water	89.50 oz

Melt the stearic acid together with the triethanolamine. Add the Carbowax and the stearyl alcohol and continue the heating until all are completely melted. Stir the benzocaine and coumarin into this mixture. Then stir in the finely powdered titanium dioxide, calamine and iron oxide, and keep on mixing with continued heating. Dissolve the preservative in the water-glycerin mixture, and heat to about 75°C. Slowly stir this hot water solution into the melted mixture with constant stirring. Remove from the fire and continue the stirring until the emulsion is cold and has an ointment-like consistency.

Suntan Creams

No. 1

	oz
Absorption base	44.80
Isopropyl myristate	6.20
Light-protective agent	3.84
Water	73.16
Perfume oil	to suit

Mix the fatty substances with the light-protective agent and heat to 55°C. Then stir in the water (previously heated to 55°C.), a small amount at a time, making sure that each portion added is thoroughly emulsified. Maintain the temperature at 55°C. until all the water has been added. Finally, stir in the perfume oil, and continue stirring until cold.

No. 2

	oz
Stearic acid	32.00
Cocoa butter	1.28
Cetyl alcohol	0.64
Triethanolamine	1.28
Glycerin	12.80
Distilled water	80.00
* Pyribenzamine	6.40

* Pyribenzamine is a synthetic drug, which can be obtained from Ciba Pharmaceutical Products, Inc., Summit, N. J.

Melt the first three ingredients at about 65°C. Dissolve the triethanolamine in the water, add the glycerin, and heat to the same temperature. Pour the oily mixture into the aqueous solution with constant but gentle stirring. Add the pyribenzamine, and continue to stir until cool. Package in air tight containers.

Suntan Lotions

No. 1

	oz
Methyl cellulose	0.64
Glycerin	2.56
Alcohol	13.44
Water	102.40
Menthyl salicylate	8.96

Wet the cellulose with the alcohol, add the glycerin and water, and stir until solution is complete. Add the menthyl salicylate and mix thoroughly.

No. 2

	oz
Isobutyl *p*-aminobenzoate	6.40
Alcohol	76.80
Glycerin	12.80
Water	32.00

Mix the alcohol with the glycerin and dissolve the amino-benzoate in the mixture; add the water and shake well. Add 2% of tannic acid; it will help in tanning the skin and it will also increase the sunburn-preventive action of the lotion.

No. 3

	oz
Specially denatured alcohol	76.80
Silicone (alcohol-soluble)	6.40
Light-protective agent	6.40
Glycerin	6.20
Water	32.20
Perfume oil	to suit

Dissolve the silicone, perfume oil, and light-protective agent in the alcohol; then stir in the water and glycerin a little at a time. Allow the mixture to stand overnight, and filter, if necessary, through kielselguhr.

No. 4

	oz
Propylene glycol ricinoleate	15.00
Glycerin	15.00
Glyceryl-*p*-aminobenzoate	4.50
Perfume oil	0.33
Specially denatured alcohol	97.50
Water	18.00
Color	to suit

Dissolve the first four components in the alcohol; add the water and color with rapid agitation.

No. 5

		oz
1	White mineral oil (65/75 viscosity)	26.24
	Sorbitan monostearate (Span 60)	5.12
	Polyoxyethylene sorbitan monostearate Tween 61)	7.68
2	Methyl *p*-hydroxybenzoate	0.26
	Water	78.72
3	Menthyl salicylate	10.24
	Perfume oil	to suit

Heat (1) to 55°C.; heat (2) to 60°C. Stir (2) into (1) with moderate agitation. When the temperature cools to 40°C. stir in (3) and keep stirring until cold. If desired, replace menthyl salicylate with 6.40 oz of Filtrosol and 30.08 oz of white mineral oil.

No. 6
(Water Repellent)

	oz
Dipropylene glycol salicylate	6.40
Alcohol-soluble silicone	6.40
Alcohol	115.20
Perfume	to suit

Dissolve the silicone and perfume in the alcohol, and stir in the salicylate. Allow it to stand overnight.

Suntan Oils

No. 1

	oz
Liquid lanolin	1.00
Petrolatum liquid, U.S.P.	10.00
Isopropyl myristate	8.60
Menthyl salicylate	2.00
Perfume oil	to suit

Mix and shake well.

No. 2

	oz
White mineral oil	70.40
Isopropyl myristate	26.00
Sperm oil	25.20
Light-protective agent	6.40
Perfume oil	to suit

Mix and shake well.

Tar Soap

	lb
Pine tar, U.S.P.	2.76
Sodium hydroxide, 38°Bé	2.04
Coconut oil	2.76

Place the pine tar in a kettle and liquefy it by means of heat. Add the sodium hydroxide and continue the heating until the mass becomes syrupy. Now stir in the coconut oil and the batch is ready to be poured into molds where the process of saponification is completed. Tar soaps are frequently used in the treatment of eczema, psoriasis, dandruff, and other chronic skin diseases.

Transparent Soap

	lb
Pressed tallow	21.61
Coconut oil	46.96
Castor oil, U.S.P.	25.35
Sodium hydroxide, 38°Bé	46.96
Specially denatured alcohol	32.41
Glycerin, 28°Bé	6.17
Sugar crystals, refined	26.90
Sodium chloride	0.44
Water	13.67
Perfume oil	1.50

Use a high grade of fats, clear lye, and thorough saponification in order to obtain a soap of good transparency. Mix the perfume oil with an equal amount of alcohol and add it to the soap at a temperature of 65°C. Run the soap into frames at a temperature of 63°C. in winter and about 55°C. in summer. Use shallow frames in order to speed solidification, because transparency is greatly improved by it.

Vanishing Creams

No. 1

1	Stearic acid	2.00 lb
	Glyceryl monostearate	6.00 oz
	Cetyl alcohol	2.00 oz
	Almond oil (sweet), U.S.P.	2.00 oz
	White mineral oil (65/75 viscosity)	2.00 oz
	Methyl *p*-hydroxybenzoate	0.20 oz
2	Propylene glycol	12.00 oz
	Water	8.94 pt
	Sodium hydroxide	0.32 oz
	Potassium hydroxide	0.40 oz
	Perfume oil	to suit

Heat (1) at 75°C. Heat (2) in another container to the same temperature. Pour (2) into (1) while the whole mass is briskly stirred. Keep stirring while cooling until a creamy product results; stir in the perfume oil at 45–50°C. Exercise great care in handling the hydroxide as it is very caustic.

No. 2

1	Stearic acid	2.00 lb
	Glyceryl monostearate	1.00 oz
	Cetyl alcohol	1.20 oz
	Sweet almond oil, U.S.P.	0.40 oz
	White mineral oil (65/75 viscosity)	2.00 oz
	Methyl *p*-hydroxybenzoate	0.20 oz

2	Water	8.75 pt
	Glycerin	1.00 pt
	Triethanolamine	1.20 oz
	Potassium carbonate, exsiccated	1.20 oz
	Borax	0.20 oz
	Perfume oil	to suit

Follow the same procedure as in Formula No. 1.

No. 3

	oz by wt
Stearic acid	66
Cetyl alcohol	2
Carbitol (diethylene glycol monoethylether)	30
Ethanolamine	3
Water	201
Perfume oil	q.s.

Melt the stearic acid with the cetyl alcohol. Dissolve the Carbitol and ethanolamine in the water and heat to the same temperature. Pour slowly the oily mixture into the water solution with constant stirring. Stir in the perfume oil at 40°C., and continue stirring at low speed until cold.

No. 4

	oz
Stearic acid	27.00
Cetyl alcohol	1.00
Isopropyl myristate	2.00
Methyl *p*-hydroxybenzoate	0.23
Potassium hydroxide, U.S.P.	0.75
Sodium borate, U.S.P.	1.05
Glycerin	5.25
Water	112.50
Rose oil	0.38

Heat the acid, cetyl alcohol, oil, and preservative at 170°F. Heat the potash, sodium borate, glycerin, and water at 175°F. and add it to the melted fats slowly while stirring rapidly for a few minutes until emulsification is complete. Allow the mixture to cool while stirring slowly. When the temperature has dropped to 130–125°F., stir in the perfume oil. Stir intermittently at low speed until cold. Pack this cream in air-tight jars.

No. 5
(Pearly)

		oz
1	Stearic acid	20.480
	Diethylene glycol stearate	4.480
	Almond oil	1.920
	White mineral oil (65/75 viscosity)	1.920
	Cetyl alcohol	1.280
	Propyl-*p*-hydroxybenzoate	0.260
2	Glycerin	9.600
	Potassium hydroxide	0.512
	Distilled water	87.550
	Perfume oil	to suit

Heat (1) at 170°F. Heat (2) at 175°F. Pour (2) into (1) while the whole is briskly stirred. Keep stirring while cooling until a creamy product results. When the temperature has dropped to 130°F., stir in the perfume oil. Exercise great care in handling the potassium hydroxide, as it is very caustic.

Part II: Perfumes

Aromatic Chemicals

BENZYL ACETATE: A colorless liquid with a fruity odor and a strongly marked jasmin character. It is found in many flower oils such as gardenia, hyacinth, jasmin (up to 65%), neroli, tuberose and ylang ylang. Benzyl acetate has a wide use in soap and cosmetic perfumes. It is especially suitable for floral bouquets such as gardenia, hyacinth, jasmin, lilac, mimosa, muguet and rose, and may be used in fruity flavors such as apple, plum and raspberry. This fragrant substance may be used to increase the top notes of floral compositions. When used in minute quantities, it helps to produce a harmonious blend of the many ingredients.

Benzyl acetate is an excellent pre-fixer, it adds mellowness and roundness to alcohol, thus covering its harsh, raw notes. Because of this fact it is widely used in such products as aftershave lotions and colognes. It is of paramount importance that benzyl acetate be free from chlorine, because its presence, even in trace amounts, may cause discoloration, or break down the composition of the perfume.

CEDRYL ACETATE: This is an ester with a woody undertone, which provides body to many florals and floral bouquets, and also acts as a blender and a binder. Cedryl acetate is stable in compositions designed for both cosmetics and soaps. Use it in concentrations of 2–5%.

CINNAMYL ESTERS: Cinnamyl acetate has a sweet flowery odor, with a spicy character. It has good fixative qualities for rose and hyacinth. Use this material only in small quantities.

Cinnamyl butyrate has a fruity odor, which blends well with hydroxy citronellal, cananga oil, and linaloöl. Use this product sparingly in floral perfumes.

Cinnamyl cinnamate has a sweet but powerful balsamic odor. Use it sparingly in oriental perfumes and heavy florals.

Cinnamyl formate has a sharp balsamic odor. Use this ester in heavy and oriental perfumes of the vetivert-santal type.

Cinnamyl propionate has a fruity grape odor. Use this product in floral narcissus, and in fruit flavors, particularly pear and grape.

Cinnamyl isovalerate has a pungent, spicy-fruity note. Use it in rose perfumes, and in flavors such as maple and walnut.

CYCLAMEN ALDEHYDE: This has an intensely floral note, and it is excellent for honeysuckle, lilac, lily-of-the-valley, linden, or cyclamen types and in all fancy floral bouquets. Because of its resistance to alkalies and the absence of skin irritating properties, it is most useful in association with hydroxycitronellal when used in perfume oils for cream and soap. Cyclamen Aldehyde Extra may be used as an extender or even as a substitute for hydroxycitronellal. It is a colorless to pale yellow oil and, like most other aldehydes; as it is not entirely stable, it must be properly stabilized. Use about 5% of it as a base for lily-of-the-valley and muguet. Use 0.25% to 5% as a floral modifier.

DIMETHYL ANTHRANILATE: This product is found naturally in some essential oils, and has a mandarin-grape-like odor. It can be used in such fancy floral compositions as gardenia, jasmin, neroli, orange flower and tuberose. Because of its stable and long lasting qualities it has become a valuable adjunct in colored soaps. Use it in perfumery at concentrations ranging from two to five per cent. It is widely used in peach, mandarin and grape flavors.

ETHYL AMYL KETONE: This product has a somewhat fruity, banana-like odor, and must be employed sparingly. It can be used advantageously in fougère, lavender and other fancy perfume compositions. Ethyl amyl ketone, when mixed with the less expensive lavandin oil, will convert it into a substitute for lavender oil.

ISOSAFROLE: This compound has a sweet sassafras-type odor. It may be used in the perfuming of disinfectants, detergents, insecticides, soaps, and many other products. Isosafrole has a stabilizing action in preventing the rancidification of certain types of oils and fats commonly used in the preparation of low cost products. Use isosafrole in very minute quantities to strengthen and modify chypre, fruity odors (root beer and sarsaparilla), oriental compounds, and spicy compositions.

METHYL HEPTINE CARBONATE: This compound is a colorless to pale yellow liquid, not found in nature. When it is used in minute quantities it develops the fine leafy fragrance of fresh violets. In this concentration, it has become very valuable in the compounding of perfumes. It is a desirable raw material for many floral compositions such as gardenia, honeysuckle, jasmin, and violet. When used in minute quantities, it is very useful in the blending of perfume compositions for soap. In low concentrations, methyl heptine carbonate blends well with ionones and methyl ionones. It is a good fixative, as it is stable and will not discolor. When used wisely, it can impart a pleasing freshness to lavender and rose fragrances.

n-OCTYLALDEHYDE (C_8): This aldehyde in concentrated form has a powerful, pungent odor, but when used in minute quantities, it imparts the odor of citrus peel to perfume compositions. It is widely used in colognes, as it fortifies such oils as bergamot, lemon, mandarin, and orange. In very minute quantities, it can be used in jasmin, lilac, neroli, and rose compositions for which it helps to round out the formulation. Dissolve 1% to 5% in alcohol and use this as a working solution.

n-NONYLALDEHYDE (C_9): This aldehyde has a warm, fatty, rose-type odor and it is widely used in floral compositions. In minute quantities, it may be used in colognes, and in blends for artificial jasmin and orris-type fragrances. It imparts power and top note to perfume oils for detergents and soaps. Dissolve 1% to 5% in alcohol and use this as a working solution.

n-DECYLALDEHYDE (C_{10}): This aldehyde has an orange-like, fatty odor, used as a bolsterer and intensifier for citrus oils. It is widely used in many classical perfumes. In minute quantities, it may be used in all types of floral compositions, especially in gardenia, jasmin, lilac, mimosa, and rose. Dissolve 1% to 5% in alcohol and use this as a working solution.

UNDECYLALDEHYDE (C_{11}): This aldehyde has a fatty, pungent odor, and because of its stability it is useful in perfume compositions for soap. In minute quantities, it may be used to round out blends for gardenia, jasmin, rose, and tuberose. This aldehyde gives the desired depth to these fragrances without its aldehydic top note. Dissolve 1% to 5% in alcohol and use this as a working solution.

LAURIC ALDEHYDE (C_{12}): This aldehyde has a powerful, sweet, fatty-like odor, useful in all types of floral compositions, especially in jasmin, lilac, muguet, and violet. It has a wide application in perfume compositions for soap. When this aldehyde is used together with Aldehyde C_{10} it yields one of the happiest combinations found in modern perfume compositions. Dissolve 1% to 10% in alcohol and use this as a working solution.

MYRISTALDEHYDE (C_{14}): This aldehyde has an orris-type, fatty odor and it can be used in blends that require ionone and orris notes, such as gardenia, jasmin, and violet. It has a wide application in extending orris absolute. This aldehyde, when used in perfume compositions, serves as a fixative effect for the other components. Dissolve 1% to 10% in alcohol and use this as a working solution.

SALICYLATES: Isoamyl salicylate has a powerful, persistent odor which is reminiscent of both orchids and clover. It is stable and has remarkable covering power. It is indispensable to perfumes of the types of orchid, clover, chypre, fougère and new mown hay. It imparts interesting tonal characters to cyclamen, carnation, camelia, and chrysanthemum types.

Isoamyl salicylate is offered on the market in two grades: prime and extra. The former is used in soap perfumes, and the latter, having a somewhat finer odor, is used in handkerchief perfumes.

Isobutyl salicylate is similar to isoamyl salicylate, but its odor is softer and more floral in character. It can be used either alone or in conjunction with the latter. Isobutyl salicylate is useful in blackberry and currant flavors.

Benzyl salicylate has a faint but sweet odor; it is used as solvent for the nitro musks, and as a fixative for carnation, lilac, lily, jasmine, and tuberose florals.

Phenylethyl salicylate with its soft balsamic-rose character is used as a modifier and fixative for such types as carnation, gardenia, honey-suckle, hyacinth, mimosa, tuberose, and ylang ylang. It is also used in flavors of the peach type. Great care must be exercised to keep all salicylates out of contact with iron salts in order to prevent the formation of color effects.

Aromatic Chemicals in White Soaps

ALPHA AMYL CINNAMIC ALDEHYDE: This compound has a strong jasmin odor; it can be used in white soaps without danger of discoloration.

CINNAMIC ALDEHYDE: This compound has a strong cinnamon odor, and should not be used in perfume compositions for use in white soaps since it tends to cause discoloration.

CITRAL: This compound has a citrus-lemon odor; it produces a yellow-brown color and a resin-like odor when used in soaps.

CITRONELLAL: This compound has an intense odor of lemon-citronella-rose, and it can be used in soaps without danger of discoloration.

JASMIN AND NEROLI: These compounds, because of the presence of indole and methyl anthranilate, tend to cause strong discoloration in soaps. Indole and methyl anthranilate should be omitted from synthetic jasmin and neroli oils which are intended for use in white soaps.

MUSK XYLENE: This musk—of all the nitro musks—tends to cause the least discoloration, and it imparts a persistent sweet freshness to the soaps. Benzyl salicylate, because of its ability to minimize the reactions of alkali on the nitro musks, is very often used as a solvent for the musks.

VANILLIN: This compound, being sensitive to light, darkens more rapidly in the presence of alkali, and it is also sensitive to traces of iron. A white soap will quickly turn brown if perfumed only with vanillin. As vanillin is a constituent of gum benzoin, balsam peru, balsam Tolu, Styrax, oakmoss, and oil of cloves, it is the source of the brownish discoloration which appears in white soaps containing these resins and this oil.

* Flash Points of Some Aromatic Chemicals

Acetone	2°F.
Amyl alcohol	105–115°F.
Ethyl acetate	31°F.
Ethyl alcohol	57°F.
Isoamyl acetate	77°F.
Isopropyl alcohol	56°F.
Methyl alcohol	57°F.

* The flash point of a volatile liquid is that temperature at which the liquid gives off vapor in sufficient quantity that, when mixed with air, it will flash, or ignite momentarily, on the application of a flame or spark.

The flash point of ethyl alcohol when mixed with water is as follows:

Ethyl alcohol	10%	120°F.
	20%	98°F.
	40%	80°F.
	60%	73°F.
	80%	66°F.
	100%	57°F.

Natural Aromatic Materials

GUMS, RESINS, AND BALSAMS not only impart to a perfume compound their pleasant sweetness, but also contribute in a very efficient manner, to its fixation, producing a film-like veil over the perfume.

Gums, resins, and balsams very often act as stabilizers as well as fixatives in good soap perfumes.

In labdanum and Mousse de Chene we have complementary and indispensable fixatives, especially for Orientals and Chypres. Styrax and labdanum are excellent fixatives, which will reinforce most types of odors in soaps.

RESINOIDS AND ABSOLUTE RESINS: Balsam Peru, Tolu, Styrax, benzoin gum, opoponax, myrrh, olibanum, fir balsam, mate, labdanum, orris root, costus, and oakmoss are resinoids of vegetable origin and are found in different parts of the plant. These crude resinoids contain foreign matter, such as bark, twigs, sand, and it is for the purpose of removing this foreign material that the crude resinoids are extracted with alcohol. The extract is then filtered and the volatile solvent is distilled off, thus leaving the so-called absolute resins.

Ambergris, castoreum, civet, and

musk are aromatics of animal origin, and are classified as resinoids. Ambergris is a pathological secretion of the sperm whale. It is the result of an intestinal irritant around which the ambergris is deposited. At times the whale is able to eliminate the solidified mass but sometimes the whale is killed by it. In either case the mass is finally washed ashore, where some lucky one finds it. It is very seldom that absolute resin of ambergris is offered on the market. The consumer prefers to prepare his own tincture or infusion directly from the crude resinoid.

The other three animal products are glandular secretions. Castoreum and civet are found in animals of both sexes, whereas musk is found in the male only. Castoreum is a product of the beaver of Canada and Siberia. Canadian castoreum is the more highly regarded. Civet is obtained from the Civet cat of Africa or Asia. Musk is a product of the musk deer of Tibet, Northern India and China. The scent glands of the caged animals are drawn off at regular intervals by hand. As with ambergris, the perfumer prefers to prepare his own tincture from the dried musk glands, called pods.

The absolute resins of vegetable origin have warm, balsamic odors, and are indispensable to the creator of oriental-type odors. These resins, when used in moderation, impart warmth to almost all floral odors. Labdanum and oakmoss are especially used in perfumes of the fougère and chypre type.

Ambergris has an earthy note; castoreum has an animal-like odor; civet has a fecal odor when concentrated, but in great dilution it acquires a floral character.

The absolute resins are mostly used as fixatives. Styrax and oakmoss are especially used as fixatives in soap perfumes. The animal resinoids are used in all high-quality perfumes; they impart a warmth, a tonal character, a oneness which cannot be accomplished in any other way.

Tincture of Oakmoss

Dry ground oakmoss	2.65 lb
Alcohol, 95%	4.23 pt

Macerate for ten days, with frequent shaking for some minutes everyday. Filter and press the residue. Macerate the residue again for 10 days in 4.23 pts of 95% alcohol. Wash the resulting residue with 2.12 pts of 95% alcohol. Mix the alcohol of the two macerations and the one washing, thus yielding about 10.56 pts of tincture of oakmoss.

Tragacanth Gum

Experiments have shown that the presence of gum tragacanth and other vegetable gums exerts a strong neutralizing effect on the bactericidal potency of chlorbutanol, *p*-hydroxybenzoate, benzalkonium chloride, and to a lesser extent on other bactericides. The reduction of the bactericidal potency is a function of the concentration of gum tragacanth, and it is found that jellies of this composition undergo a continuous loss of bactericidal potency on storage.

Perfumes for Cosmetics

For Brilliantine
(Rose Oil)

	oz
Palmarosa oil	3.00
Geraniol, palmarosa	2.25
Ginger grass oil	1.50
Bois de Rose oil	1.50
Clove oil, twice rectified	0.75
Phenylethyl alcohol, extra fine	1.50
Diphenylmethane	1.05
Musk ambrette	0.45
Terpineol, extra	3.00
Benzyl benzoate	1.50

Mix and allow to stand a week or more.

For Cleansing, Cold, and Vanishing Creams

	oz
Terpineol extra	3.37
Hydroxycitronellal extra	2.80
Geraniol pure	1.90
Sandalwood oil, Mysore	1.46
Bergamot oil	0.84
Benzyl acetate, F.F.C.	0.82
Linaloöl (from Bois de Rose)	0.74
Styrolyl acetate	0.74
Anisic aldehyde, C.P.	0.64
Rhodinol extra	0.63
Geranyl acetate pure	0.62
Alpha-amyl cinnamic aldehyde	0.42
Phenylethyl alcohol, extra fine	0.40
Amyl salicylate, extra	0.38
Linalyl acetate	0.33
Methyl ionone	0.32
Methyl anthranilate, extra	0.26
Cyclamen aldehyde, extra	0.40
Cinnamic alcohol (from Styrax)	0.24
Ylang-Ylang oil, Bourbon	0.24
Methyl isoeugenol	0.22
Isoeugenol	0.12
Geranium oil, Bourbon	0.08
Dimethylbenzylcarbinol	0.92
Musk ambrette	0.51
Heliotropine, recrystallized	0.33
Vanillin, 100%, U.S.P.	0.06
Coumarin, N.F.	0.19
Octyl aldehyde, 100%	0.014

For Cleansing, Cold, and Massage Creams

	oz
Citronellol, extra	4.00
Sophora 55 (Givaudan)	4.00
Phenylethyl alcohol, extra fine	2.60
Linalyl acetate, extra	2.00
Terpineol, extra	2.00
Lilial (Givaudan)	2.00
Geranyl acetate pure	1.00
Cinnamic alcohol pure	1.00
Ionone pure	1.00
Versalide (cyclic musk)	0.40

For Emollient Creams

	oz
Bergamot oil	3.00
Geraniol pure	2.90
Phenylethyl alcohol, extra fine	2.00
Sandalwood oil, Mysore	2.00
Geranium oil, Bourbon	1.00
Terpineol, extra	3.00
Linaloöl (from Bois de Rose)	1.00
Rhodinol, extra	0.60
Sage clary oil, extra	0.80
Palmarosa oil	0.40
Linalyl acetate, extra	0.40
Patchouli oil, Singapore	0.50
Petitgrain oil, Paraguay	0.50
Ylang-Ylang oil, Bourbon	0.40
Neroli oil, synthetic	0.20
Musk ketone	1.00
Veraroma Tolu (Stafford Allen & Sons)	0.30

For Vanishing Creams
No. 1

	oz
Cinnamic alcohol, pure	2.00
Citronellol, extra	2.00
Linaloöl (from Bois de Rose)	1.00
Linalyl acetate, extra	2.00
Phenylethyl alcohol, extra fine	5.00
Sophora 53 (Givaudan)	4.00
Vetiverol	1.00
Ylang-Ylang oil, Bourbon	0.40
Lilial (Givaudan)	0.20
Versalide (cyclic musk)	0.40
Isopropyl myristate, pure	2.00

Mix thoroughly, and allow all perfume oils to mature for one month before use. Dissolve the Versalide in the isopropyl myristate.

Use about 0.5% of perfume oil for cleansing, cold, and vanishing creams.

Use about 0.75% of perfume oil for emollient and lubricating creams. Incorporate the perfume after the temperature of the cream has dropped to about 50°C. Continue the stirring after the addition of the perfume for at least ½ hour.

No. 2

	oz
Lilac oil	16
Jasmine oil	2
Ylang-Ylang oil	2

Mix well and allow to stand a week or more. Use 2 oz of this oil to 50 lb of vanishing cream.

For Face Powder
No. 1

	oz
Musk ketone	0.50
Benzyl benzoate, F.F.C.	2.50
Benzoin gum, Sumatra, tincture (1:10 in alcohol)	10.20
Ylang-Ylang oil, Bourbon Premier	1.20
Jasmia A	1.00
Muguet fleur	0.80
Tuberose, extra fine	0.70
Sandalwood oil, Mysore	0.60
Rose otto (Fritzsche Bros)	0.56
Neroli (Fritzsche Bros.)	0.48
Vetivert oil (English)	0.40
Lavender oil (English)	0.16

Vanillin	0.80
Civettine (1:10 in alcohol)	0.06
Orris concrete	0.04

No. 2

	oz
Opoponax, L.G. (Givaudan)	4.40
Jasmia A	4.40
Lilas fleur	3.00
Fougère (Givaudan)	2.80
Rose Rouge (Givaudan)	1.00
Phenylacetaldehyde dimethylacetal	0.80
Bouvardiol (Givaudan)	0.40
Musk ketone	1.20
Coumarin	1.00
Aroma benzoin Siam	0.86
Ambreine	0.12
Exaltolide (1:10 in alcohol)	0.02

Mix all the ingredients in order named, and allow the mixture to mature one month before use. Do not use more than 1% of the perfume in the face powder, because larger amounts may cause the powder to become damp and lumpy. These two tested formulas will produce fine powder perfumes of high stability.

No. 3

Opoponax oil, extra	6.40 oz
Cyclamen aldehyde, extra	1.60 oz
Jasmine oil, artificial	1.60 oz
Phenylethyl alcohol, extra fine	1.60 oz
Bergamot oil	7.68 dr
Lilac oil, artificial	2.56 dr
Rhodinol, extra	3.84 dr
Nerol, extra	5.12 dr
Geranium oil, Algerian, extra	6.40 dr
Santalol	6.40 dr
Raldeine A (Givaudan)	3.84 dr
Aldehyde C_{11}	2.56 dr

Mix and allow to stand a week or more. This perfume oil has a spicy note.

No. 4

	oz
Rose Otto	0.75
Vetivert oil, extra	0.75
Jasmine absolute	0.30
Vanillin	0.30
Coumarin	0.40
Musk ambrette	0.50
Tincture of benzoin, 10%	7.50
Tincture of Tolu, 10%	4.50
Benzyl benzoate, U.S.P.	1.00

Mix well and allow to stand a week or more.

Perfuming of Face Powders

Mix the perfume compound with a part of the magnesium carbonate in any suitable vessel. Put the face powder ingredients, after a preliminary mixing in a powder mixing machine, through a micro-pulverizing apparatus. As this micropulverizer generates an appreciable amount of heat when in operation, it is best to micro-pulverize the perfume oil with a small portion of the pre-mixed face powder before the machine has become hot. Then, put the rest of the face powder through the micro-pulverizer, return it to the powder-mixing machine together with the perfumed portion, and mix for twenty minutes.

For Lipsticks

No. 1

	oz
Isopropyl myristate, pure	4.6
Phenylethyl alcohol coeur	4.0
Sophora 55 (Givaudan)	3.0
Aldehyde C_{20}	2.0
Cinnamic alcohol (from Styrax)	2.0
Methyl ionone, extra (D.&O.)	2.0
Alpha ionone	1.0
Rose rouge (Vidal-Charvet)	0.6
Vanillin, U.S.P. (from Eugenol)	0.6
Versalide (polycyclic musk)	0.2

No. 2

	oz
Citronellol, extra	6.0
Phenylethyl alcohol coeur	6.0
Geraniol (from palmarosa)	4.0
Rose rouge (Vidal-Charvet)	2.0
Methyl ionone gamma (D.&O.)	1.0
Vanillin, U.S.P. (from Eugenol)	0.4
Versalide (polycyclic musk)	0.4
Aldehyde C_{20}	0.2

Mix well and allow to stand a week or more with frequent shaking.

Use from 1 to 3% of this oil for perfuming purposes. Stir in the perfume oil after the lipstick mass has been freed from the air that was entrapped during milling and mixing, and just before the material is to be poured into the molds. These oils are non-irritating and stable, and will not discolor.

No. 3
Rose-Strawberry

	oz
Rhodinol, extra	5.0
Hydroxycitronellal dimethylacetal	4.0
Phenylethyl alcohol, extra fine	3.0
Aldehyde C-16, pure	2.0
Geranium oil, Algerian, extra	2.0
Methyl ionone gamma (D.&O.)	2.0
Alpha ionone	1.6
Isobutyl phenylacetate	1.6
Dimethyl phenylethyl carbinyl acetate	1.6
Phenyl acetic acid, pure	1.6
Dimethylbenzylcarbinyl acetate	2.0
Cinnamyl isovalerate	1.2
Hydrocinnamic alcohol	1.0
Musk ambrette	1.0
Musk ketone	1.0
Methyl cinnamate	1.0
Phenyl propyl acetate	1.0
Ethyl vanillin	0.8
Isoeugenol, extra	0.8
Terpineol, extra	0.6
Allyl cyclohexane propionate	0.2
Coumarin, N.F.	0.2
Ethyl benzoate	0.2

Mix well and allow to stand a

week or more with frequent shaking.

For Shampoos

	oz
Soap perfume oil	5.50
Alpha amyl cinnamic aldehyde (Buxine)	4.00
Phenylethyl alcohol, extra fine	4.50
Rose oil	0.50
Benzyl benzoate	1.50

Mix and shake well. Allow to stand a week or more.

For Soaps

No. 1

	oz
Musk xylol, 100%	1.25
Terpineol, extra	4
Ionone for soap	2.50
Geraniol for soap	4
Amyl cinnamic aldehyde	2.50
Methyl isoeugenol	0.50
Benzyl benzoate, F.F.C.	2.50

Mix well and allow to stand a week or more with frequent shaking.

No. 2
(Rose)

	oz
Diphenyl oxide	4.0
Diphenyl methane	2.0
Terpineol, extra	5.0
Phenylethyl alcohol	5.0
Geranyl acetate, pure	1.0
Methyl phenylacetaldehyde	0.8
Isoeugenol	0.4
Phenyl propyl alcohol	0.4
Ethyl vanillin	0.4
Benzyl acetate, F.F.C.	1.0

Mix thoroughly. Allow to stand a week or more with frequent shaking.

Soaps, Germicides, Fly Sprays

	oz
Terpineol	10.0
Lemongrass oil	2.0
Steam-distilled pine oil	1.0
Bornyl acetate	1.0
Ti-Tree oil	1.4
Terpinolene, soluble	1.0
Benzyl acetate	1.6
Citronella oil, Ceylon	2.0

Mix and allow to stand a week or more.

(Many additional perfumes for soaps are given under various individual odors in the next section.)

Compounding of Perfumes

Amber Oil

	oz
Methyl ionone	4
Labdanum absolute	2
Rose oil	2
Vanillin	2
Musk ambrette	1
Musk ketone	1
Benzyl salicylate	1

Mix well, and allow to stand a week or more with frequent shaking.

Bergamot Oil, Artificial

No. 1

Iso-bergamate	5.00 oz
Menthanyl acetate	3.00 oz
Orange oil, cold pressed	2.00 oz
Lemon oil, cold pressed	2.00 oz
Bois de Rose oil, Brazilian	2.25 dr
Petitgrain oil, Paraguay	3.20 dr
Citral, C.P.	1.28 dr
Aldehyde C_{10} *	28.80 min
Aldehyde C_9 *	9.60 min
Ethyl acetate *	20.00 min
Geranyl acetate	1.60 dr
Musk ketone	44.00 gr
Dextro-limonene	6.50 oz
Linalyl acetate 75%	1.75 dr

* Dissolve 1 oz in 10 oz diethyl phthalate.

Mix thoroughly and allow to stand a week or more.

No. 2

Iso-bergamate	8.0 oz
Lemon oil	3.0 oz
Orange oil, sweet	2.6 oz
Linaloöl (from Bois de Rose)	1.2 oz
Citral, pure	0.8 oz
Geranyl acetate, pure	0.2 oz
Aldehyde C-10, 10% in benzyl benzoate, U.S.P.	20.0 min
Dextro-limonene	4.2 oz

Mix thoroughly. Allow to stand a week or more with frequent shaking.

Bergamot Perfume Oil

Menthanyl acetate (Givaudan)	8.00 oz
Lemon oil, cold pressed	3.00 oz
Orange oil, cold pressed	1.00 oz
Bois de Rose oil, Brazilian	0.40 oz
Citral, pure	0.20 oz
Geranyl acetate, pure	0.20 oz
Ethyl acetate *	20.00 min
Aldehyde C-10 *	10.00 min
Musk ketone	35.00 gr
Deer's tongue (Vanilla plant) resinoid *	10.00 min
Dextro-limonene	6.75 oz

* 10% in benzyl benzoate, U.S.P.

Mix thoroughly. Allow to stand a week or more with frequent shaking.

Carnation Oil, Synthetic

	oz
Eugenol, U.S.P., extra	3.75
Eugenyl phenylacetate	2.25
Hydroxycitronellal dimethylacetal	2.25
Isoeugenol, extra	3.00
Cinnamic alcohol (*ex* styrax)	1.80
Citronellol, extra	1.80
Geranyl acetate, pure	1.50
Musk ketone	1.50
Phenylethyl alcohol (extra fine)	1.20

Terpineol, extra	1.20
Diethyl hydroquinone	0.90
Heliotropine, recrystallized	0.75
p-Cresyl caprylate	0.75
Benzyl acetate coeur	0.60
Anisic alcohol	0.60
Aubepine liquid	0.60
Ylang-Ylang oil, Bourbon Premier	0.60
Ethyl vanillin	0.45
Dimethyl octanyl acetate	0.45
Hydratropyl alcohol	0.45
Hydratropyl propionate	0.45
Amyl cinnamic aldehyde	0.30
Cumin ketone	0.30
Methyl ionone Gamma (D.&O.)	0.30
Musk xylol	0.30
Phenylethyl propionate	0.30
Rhodinol, extra	0.30
Bay leaves oil, redistilled, N.F.	0.15
Birch tar oil, rectified, N.F., 5% in dimethyl phthalate	0.15
Benzyl propionate	0.15
Citronellyl oxyacetaldehyde	0.15
Methyl isopropyl acetophenone, 10% in dimethyl phthalate	0.15

Mix well and allow to stand a week or more with frequent shaking.

Clover Flower Oil, Synthetic

	oz
Orchid oil, artificial	25.0
Coumarin, N.F.	1.6
Ylang-Ylang oil (Bourbon Premier)	1.5
Amyl salicylate, extra	1.0
Bergamot oil, extra, N.F.	0.7
Musk ketone	0.6
Heliotropine, recrystallized	0.5
Benzyl acetate coeur	0.3
Isobutyl phenylacetate	0.3
Dimethyl hydroquinone	0.3
Lavender oil, U.S.P., Barreme, 42%	0.3
Palatone, 5% in phenylethyl alcohol	0.3
Acetophenone	0.2
Oakmoss resin	0.2
Tuberyl acetate	0.2
Vanillin, U.S.P. (from Eugenol)	0.2
Benzyl alcohol, N.F.F.F.C.	1.3

Mix well and allow to stand a week or more with frequent shaking.

Crepe De Chine Perfume Oil

Bergamot oil, natural	2.00 oz
Oakmoss resinoid (Green)	2.00 oz
Linalyl acetate	2.40 oz
Hydroxycitronellal	1.00 oz
Lemon oil	1.00 oz
Rose otto type	1.00 oz
Linaloöl	0.80 oz
Sandalwood oil, natural	0.80 oz
Vetiverol	0.60 oz
Styrolyl acetate	0.48 oz
Musk ambrette	0.36 oz
Musk ketone	0.50 oz
Musk xylol	0.50 oz
Octadienol 1453	0.50 oz

Rhodinol extra	0.50	oz
Coumarin	0.36	oz
Ethyl Vanillin	0.24	oz
Petitgrain oil, extra	0.32	oz
Benzyl acetate, F.F.C.	0.30	oz
Aldehyde C_{11}, 10% solution	0.24	oz
Methyl nonyl acetaldehyde C_{12}, 10% solution	0.24	oz
Veronol aldehyde, 10% solution	0.12	oz
Civettiane	0.20	oz
Ylang-Ylang absolute	0.20	oz
Orange oil, bitter	0.20	oz
Phantolid	0.20	oz
Yara-Yara	0.18	oz
Amyl cinnamic aldehyde	0.16	oz
Methyl ionone	0.16	oz
Alpha ionone	0.12	oz
Citronellyl oxyacetaldehyde	0.12	oz
Eugenol, extra	0.12	oz
Isoeugenol	0.12	oz
Nutmeg oil, natural	0.12	oz
Cumin ketone	0.10	oz
Cardamom oil	40	min
Estragon oil, extra, French	20	min

Mix and shake well. Allow to stand a week or more with frequent shaking.

Cyclamen Flower Oil (Synthetic)

	oz
p-Isopropyl alpha-methyl hydrocinnamic aldehyde (Alpine Violet)	1.5
Hydroxycitronellol	3.0
Hydroxycitronellal dimethylacetal	1.0
Linaloöl, extra	1.5
Benzyl acetate coeur	1.0
Terpineol, extra	1.0
Rhodinol, extra	0.8
Lemon oil, Italian	0.6
Geranium oil, Algerian	0.5
Linalyl acetate, extra, 96–98%	0.5
Methyl ionone	0.5
Tolyl alcohol	0.5
Ylang-Ylang oil, Bourbon Premier	0.5
Musk ketone	0.4
Alpha ionone	0.4
Cinnamic alcohol, pure	0.4
Petitgrain oil, S.A.	0.4
Phenylacetaldehyde dimethylacetal	0.4
Hydratropyl alcohol	0.3
Cumin ketone	0.2
Amyl cinnamic aldehyde	0.2
Aldehyde C_{14}, 10% in dimethyl phthalate	0.1
Benzyl propionate	0.2
Coumarin, N.F.	0.1
Phenylethyl propionate	0.1
Benzyl alcohol, N.F.F.F.C.	1.4

Mix well and allow to stand a week or more with frequent shaking.

Eau de Cologne Oil

	oz
Bergamot oil, Melito (N.F. Sanderson's)	10.59
Lemon oil, U.S.P. (Sanderson's)	10.94

Neroli oil, Portugal	3.53
Rosemary oil, extra	3.53
Lavender oil, U.S.P., Barreme	2.82
Olibanum resin soluble	1.41
Pinus sylvestris oil, extra	1.41
Wintergreen oil, Northern, U.S.P.	0.71
Auranthiol, pure, 2% in alcohol	0.35

Mix well and allow to stand a week or more with frequent shaking.

Cologne Stick

	oz
Sodium stearate	10.24
Isopropyl myristate	12.80
Glycerin	3.84
Cologne perfume oil	3.84
Alcohol	97.28

Melt the stearate together with the myristate and glycerin; remove it from the fire and allow it to cool. Mix the alcohol with the perfume oil, and stir this mixture into the molten fats. Continue to stir and pour into suitable molds. Allow the molded sticks to cool slowly in order to prevent the formation of air pockets. Wrap the cooled sticks in tin foil. Glycerin helps to slow down the evaporation rate of the alcohol, and it also helps to enhance the translucent appearance of the finished stick.

Floral Sachets

	parts by weights
Dried orange flowers	74.4
Rose leaves	60.0
Orris root	45.6
Cassia flowers	6.0
Cloves	37.2
Coriander	16.8
Pimento	3.6
Ambrette seeds	7.2
Saint Lucia wood	7.2

Have the flowers, leaves, seeds, and spices ground together and pack weighed portions into envelopes of gauze or paper.

Fougère Oil

Bergamot oil	5	oz
Lavender oil	5	oz
Oakmoss absolute	1.33	oz
Coumarin	2.33	oz
Musk ambrette	75	gr
Patchouli oil	1	dr
Orange blossom oil	30	min
Benzyl benzoate	1	oz

Mix well, and allow to stand a week or more with frequent shaking.

Gardenia Flower Oil, Synthetic

	oz
Hydroxycitronellal dimethylacetal	3.0
p-Methylbenzyl propionate	2.6
Tolyl acetate	2.0
Civettiane	1.7
Rhodinol, extra	1.2
Geranium oil, Algerian, extra	1.0
Amyl cinnamic aldehyde	1.0
Phenylethyl dimethylcarbinol	0.8
Musk ketone	0.8
Linalyl acetate, 96–98%	0.8
Musk xylol	0.8

Ylang-Ylang absolute (Fritzsche)	0.8
Musk ambrette	0.3
Amyl salicylate, extra	0.6
Citronellyl acetate	0.5
Petitgrain oil, extra	0.5
Phenylacetic acid	0.5
Sandalwood oil, N.F.	0.5
Tuberyl acetate	0.5
Bay oil, N.F., extra	0.4
Citronellyl oxyacetaldehyde	0.4
Heliotropine, recrystallized	0.4
Mandarin oil, Italian	0.4
Methyl ionone	0.4
Palatone, 5% in phenylethyl alcohol	0.4
Phenylethyl dimethyl carbinyl acetate	0.4
Styrolyl propionate	0.4
Cumin ketone	0.2
Jasmine absolute	0.1
Rose otto	0.1
Astrotone, 100%	1.5

Mix well and allow to stand a week or more with frequent shaking.

Gardenia (For Soaps)

No. 1

Styrolyl acetate	1.50	oz
Heliotropin	2.50	oz
Nerolin	164.00	gr
Dimethyl hydroquinone	219.00	gr
Indole, extra pure (Givaudan)	54.00	gr
Bois de Rose oil	1.25	oz
Artificial bergamot oil	1.25	oz
Artificial ylang-ylang oil	0.75	oz
Petitgrain oil, Paraguay	1.75	oz
Benzyl acetate	2.00	oz
Amyl cinnamic aldehyde	1.12	oz
Isoeugenol	0.75	oz
Methyl *p*-cresol	2.00	dr
Methyl acetophenone	0.75	oz
Dimethyl benzyl carbinol	1.00	oz
Phenylethyl alcohol	2.00	oz
Diphenyl oxide	3.00	dr
Methyl anthranilate	0.75	oz
Styrax resinoid	1.25	oz
Bromstyrol	0.50	oz
Terpineol, extra	2.75	oz
Benzyl alcohol	1.50	oz
Benzyl benzoate	1.00	oz

Mix and shake well. Allow to stand a week or more, with frequent shaking.

No. 2

	oz
Terpineol, extra	4.0
Hydroxycitronellal	4.0
Benzyl acetate, F.F.C.	2.0
Benzyl phenylacetate	1.8
Geraniol	1.6
Cinnamic alcohol	1.0
Linaloöl	1.0
Styrolyl acetate	1.0
p-Methyl benzyl propionate	0.8
Heliotropine	0.8
Ionone, alpha and beta	0.4
Amyl salicylate	0.2
Methyl ionone	0.2
Aldehyde C_{14}, 10% in dimethyl phthalate	0.4
Dimethyl hydroquinone	0.4
Hydratropyl acetate	0.2
Phenylacetic acid	0.2

Mix well and allow to stand a week or more with frequent shaking.

Honey (Miel) (Synthetic)

	oz
Citronellol, extra	3.00
Hydroxycitronellal dimethyl-acetal	3.30
Phenylacetic acid, pure	2.70
Phenylethyl alcohol, extra fine	1.80
Dimethyl octanyl acetate	0.90
Benzophenone, C.P.	0.75
Ethyl phenylacetate	0.75
Methyl ionone	0.75
Rhodinyl phenylacetate	0.75
Terpineol, extra	0.75
Amyl cinnamic aldehyde	0.60
Benzyl propionate	0.60
Methyl acetophenone	0.60
Isoeugenol, extra	0.45
Musk ambrette	0.45
Alpha ionone	0.30
Benzyl acetate coeur	0.30
Isobutyl phenylacetate	0.30
Methyl phenylacetate	0.30
Veronol aldehyde, 10% in dimethyl phthalate	0.30
Benzyl salicylate	2.25

Mix well and allow to stand a week or more with frequent shaking.

Incense

	oz
Sandalwood, powdered	6.0
Cascarilla, powdered	3.0
Cardamom, powdered	0.8
Cubebs, powdered	0.7
Myrrh, powdered	0.2
Willow charcoal, powdered	2.4
Potassium nitrate, powdered	0.6
Benzoin Siam	3.0
Balsam Peru	0.6
Oleo-resin orris	0.2
Bergamot oil	0.6
Neroli oil	0.4
Cassia oil	0.3
Patchouli oil	0.2
Clove oil	0.1
Iso-butyl cinnamate	0.6
Methyl ionone	0.2
Musk grains	0.1

Mix the aromatic powders with the charcoal and potassium nitrate. Mix the oils with the gum resins, aromatic chemicals, and musk grains. Shake well and allow to stand until solution is complete.

Add the oils-gum resins mixture to the powders in such proportions that the finished powder is damp and adherent. Finally, press the finished powder into shapes of cones. Place each cone on an ash tray and light it.

Jasmin Absolute

Amyl cinnamic aldehyde	8.0 oz
Benzyl acetate, F.F.C., coeur	5.0 oz
Phenylethyl alcohol, extra fine	5.0 oz
Guaiac wood resin	10.0 oz
Indol extra, pure, 10% in dimethyl phthalate	4.0 oz
Ylang-Ylang absolute (Fritzsche)	5.0 oz
Linalyl acetate, extra, 96–98%	3.0 oz

Tolyl acetate	2.0 oz
Eugenol, extra, U.S.P.	1.0 oz
Benzyl alcohol, F.F.C., N.F.	2.0 oz
Hexyl cinnamic aldehyde	1.0 oz
Hydratropyl alcohol	1.0 oz
Lemon oil, Italian	4.0 dr
Linaloöl extra	4.0 dr
Orange flower absolute, 50% in dimethyl phthalate	4.0 dr
Tepyl acetate	4.0 dr
Celery seed oil, extra	45.0 min
Ethyl phenylacetate	45.0 min

Mix well and allow to stand a week or more with frequent shaking. This jasmin composition may serve as an extender for the natural absolute of jasmin flowers.

Jasmin, White

Benzyl acetate, F.F.C.	6.00 oz
Amyl cinnamic aldehyde	2.00 oz
Linaloöl (from Bois de Rose)	1.75 oz
Hydroxycitronellal dimethylacetal	2.50 oz
p-Methyl benzyl propionate	1.50 oz
Benzyl butyrate	6.00 dr
Indol, extra pure, 10% in dimethyl phthalate	6.00 dr
Tolyl acetate	4.00 dr
p-Cresyl phenyl acetate, 10% in dimethyl phthalate	4.00 dr
Ylang-Ylang oil, Bourbon Premier	4.00 dr
Ionone, alpha and beta, pure	2.75 dr
Cumin ketone	2.00 dr
Hexyl cinnamic aldehyde	2.00 dr
Hydratropyl alcohol	2.00 dr
Mandarin oil, Italian	2.00 dr
Orange oil, sweet	2.00 dr
Phenylethyl alcohol, extra fine	2.00 dr
Tepyl acetate	2.00 dr
Benzyl formate	1.00 dr
Myrrh oil, extra	45.00 min
Tarragon oil, extra	45.00 min
Aldehyde C_{14}, pure, 10% in dimethyl phthalate	45.00 min

Mix well and allow to stand a week or more with frequent shaking. Do not use this jasmin in soaps, because indole often causes discoloration.

Jasmin (for Soaps)

Benzyl acetate, F.F.C.	11.20 oz
Linaloöl (from Bois de Rose)	3.20 oz
Linalyl acetate	1.12 oz
Benzyl propionate	1.12 oz
Citronellol special	6.40 dr
Hydroxycitronellal	5.12 dr
p-Cresyl phenylacetate, 10% in dimethyl phthalate	5.12 dr
Ylang-Ylang oil, Bourbon Premier	1.60 dr
Benzyl isoeugenol	122.00 gr
Phenylacetic acid	140.00 gr
Dimethyl phthalate	4.00 dr

Mix well and allow to stand a

week or more with frequent shaking. This jasmin blends well with lilac and rose.

Jasmin Oil

No. 1

	oz
Benzyl acetate, F.F.C.	9.60
Linaloöl (from Bois de Rose)	3.00
Benzyl alcohol, F.F.C.	2.00
Linalyl acetate, extra	1.50
Buxine (Givaudan)	0.80
Benzoin resinoid, Siam	0.80
Ylang-Ylang oil, Bourbon Premier	0.60
Geraniol	0.50
Benzyl propionate	0.40
Methyl anthranilate	0.30
Terpineol, extra	0.20
Geranyl acetate	0.10
p-Cresyl phenylacetate	0.10
Indole, extra pure (Givaudan)	0.10

Mix and shake well. Allow to stand a month or more.

No. 2

Benzyl acetate, F.F.C	7.00 oz
Linaloöl, extra	4.00 oz
Linalyl acetate, extra	2.00 oz
Amyl cinnamic aldehyde, pure	3.26 oz
Phenylethyl alcohol, coeur	1.00 oz
Benzyl alcohol, N. F.	2.00 oz
Benzyl benzoate, U.S.P.	1.00 oz
Cinnamic alcohol, pure	0.60 oz
Musk ketone	35.00 gr
Methyl anthranilate	0.10 oz
p-Cresol	10.00 min
Indole, extra pure	10.00 min
Orange blossom oil	3.00 oz
Tuberose oil	2.00 oz
Bergamot oil	0.50 oz

Mix and shake well. Allow to stand a week or more, with frequent shaking.

No. 3

Benzyl acetate, F.F.C.	8 oz
Linaloöl (from Bois de Rose)	2 oz
Amyl cinnamic aldehyde	3 oz
Linalyl acetate, 97%	1 oz
Phenylethyl alcohol	1 oz
Musk ketone	70 gr
Orange blossom oil	2 oz
Indole, extra pure	40 min
Benzyl benzoate, U.S.P.	1 oz

Mix well, and allow to stand a week or more with frequent shaking.

No. 4

Benzyl acetate, F.F.C.	2.50 oz
Jasmin absolute	1.60 oz
Amyl cinnamic aldehyde	1.20 oz
Benzyl alcohol, N.F.F.F.C.	2.40 oz
Linaloöl, extra	1.30 oz
Phenylethyl alcohol	1.75 oz
Indole, extra pure	23 min
Alpha ionone	0.80 oz
Benzyl salicylate	0.80 oz
Dimethylbenzyl carbinyl acetate	0.64 oz

Methyl anthranilate	0.64 oz
Rhodinol	0.80 oz
Rose de Mai, essence (Schmoller & Bompard)	0.32 oz
p-Cresyl phenylacetate	0.32 oz
Isojasmone	0.20 oz
Rhodinyl isobutyrate	38 min
Benzoin Siam resinoid	0.58 oz

Mix well, and allow to stand a week or more. Filter if necessary.

Jasmin Oil (for Brilliantine)

	oz
Benzyl acetate, free from chlorine	3.00
Bois de Rose oil	3.75
Bergamot oil	0.75
Amyl cinnamic aldehyde	1.00
Cinnamic alcohol, pure	0.75
Orange oil, sweet	1.50
Hydroxycitronellal	0.90
Methyl anthranilate	1.05
Phenylethyl alcohol, extra fine	1.50
Ylang-Ylang oil, Bourbon	0.75
Undecalactone (Aldehyde C_{14})	0.15
Civet tincture (4 oz to 1 gal)	0.75
Benzyl benzoate	1.50

Mix and allow to stand a week or more.

Jonquille Flower Oil (Synthetic)

	oz
Hydroxycitronellal dimethyl-acetal	2.0
Tolyl acetate	2.2
p-Cresyl phenylacetate	1.5
Benzyl acetate, F.F.C., coeur	0.8
Eugenyl phenylacetate	0.8
Phenylethyl alcohol, extra fine	0.8
Amyl cinnamic aldehyde	1.2
Benzyl salicylate	1.2
Neroline crystals	1.0
Sandalwood oil, N.F.	1.0
Vanillin, U.S.P. (from Eugenol)	1.0
Rhodinol, extra	0.8
* Alpine Violet	0.6
Aubepine	0.6
Musk ketone	0.6
p-Cresyl caprylate	0.6
Phenylacetic acid, pure	0.6
Petitgrain oil, extra	0.6
p-Methyl hydratropic aldehyde	0.6
Ylang-Ylang, Bourbon Premier	0.6
Heliotropine, recrystallized	0.4
Phenylethyl acetate	0.2
Tarragon oil, extra	0.2

* Paraisopropyl alpha-methyl hydrocinnamic aldehyde.

Mix well and allow to stand a week or more with frequent shaking.

Lavender Oil (Artificial)

	oz
Iso-bergamate	2.00 oz
Menthanyl acetate	4.00 oz
Spike lavender oil, extra, Spanish	2.00 oz
Lavandin absolute	2.40 oz
Coumarin	1.20 oz
Moskene	175.00 gr

Bois de Rose oil, Brazilian	2.40 oz
Geraniol, pure	1.00 oz
Geranyl acetate	1.20 oz
Linalyl acetate, 75%	1.00 oz
Terpinyl propionate	2.00 oz

Mix thoroughly and allow to stand a week or more.

Lavender (For Soaps)

	oz
Lavender oil, French	6.0
Spike lavender oil, Spanish	2.0
Linalyl acetate	4.0
Isoamyl salicylate	1.0
Bornyl acetate, pure	1.0
Musk xylol	1.0
Geranium oil, Réunion	1.0
Patchouli oil, Sumatra	0.6
Galbanum resinoid	0.6
Oakmoss resinoid	0.4
Cedarwood oil	2.4

Mix thoroughly. Allow to stand a week or more with frequent shaking.

Lilac Oil

Terpineol, extra	4 oz
Hydroxycitronellal	1.5 oz
Phenylethyl alcohol	1.5 oz
Phenylacetaldehyde dimethylacetal	1 oz
Amyl cinnamic aldehyde	1 oz
Cinnamic alcohol, pure	1 oz
Linalyl acetate, extra	0.5 oz
Styrax resinoid	1 dr
Benzyl benzoate, U.S.P.	1.5 oz
Musk ambrette	0.5 oz

Mix thoroughly and allow to stand a week or more.

Lily of the Valley

No. 1

Hydroxycitronellal, extra	4.00 oz
Phenylethyl alcohol coeur	1.50 oz
Cinnamic alcohol, pure	1.00 oz
Terpineol, extra	1.00 oz
Rhodinol, extra	0.80 oz
Linaloöl, extra	0.50 oz
Heliotropine, recrystallized	175.00 gr
Musk ketone	20.00 gr
Amyl cinnamic aldehyde, pure	0.50 oz
Benzyl acetate, F.F.C.	0.10 oz
Ionone alpha	0.20 oz
Jasmine oil	2.25 oz
Orange flower oil	2.25 oz
Ylang-Ylang oil	1.50 oz
Cassie oil	1.50 oz

Mix and shake well. Allow to stand a week or more, with frequent shaking.

No. 2

	oz
Hydroxy citronellal	6
Linaloöl (from Bois de Rose)	3
Terpineol, extra	3
Rhodinol	2
Phenylacetaldehyde dimethylacetal, 10% solution	2
Benzyl benzoate	1

Mix well, and allow to stand a week or more.

No. 3 (Synthetic)

	oz
Hydroxycitronellal dimethyl acetal	6.0
Phenylethyl alcohol, extra fine	5.0
Rhodinol, extra	3.0
Linalyl acetate, extra, 96–98%	2.4
Heliotropine, recrystallized	2.0
Tolyl acetate	1.6
Benzyl acetate coeur	1.0
Hydratropyl alcohol	1.0
Linaloöl, extra	1.0
Terpineol, extra	0.6
Cumin ketone	0.4
Dimethyl octanyl acetate	0.4
Aubepine	0.2
Lemon oil, Italian	0.2
Ylang-Ylang absolute	0.2

Mix well and allow to stand a week or more with frequent shaking.

Magnolia Flower Oil (Synthetic)

	oz
Musk ketone	2.50
Hydroxycitronellal dimethyl-acetal	2.00
Methyl ionone, extra (D.&O.)	1.50
Phenylethyl alcohol, extra fine	1.50
Rhodinol, extra	1.50
Linalyl acetate, extra, 96–98%	1.25
Ylang-Ylang oil, Bourbon Premier	1.25
Auranthiol, 100%	1.00
* Alpine violet	1.00
Bergamot oil, extra, N.F.	0.90
Benzyl acetate coeur	0.75
Lemon oil, Italian	0.75
Vetiverol	0.75
Isoeugenol, extra	0.60
Amyl cinnamic aldehyde	0.50
Cinnamic alcohol, pure	0.50
Musk ambrette	0.50
Sandalwood oil, N.F., Mysore	0.50
Indole, extra pure, 10% in dimethyl phthalate	0.40
Aldehyde C_{14}, 10% in dimethyl phthalate	0.25
Dimethyl anthranilate	0.25
Ethyl vanillin	0.25
Phenylethyl propionate	0.25
Rose otto	0.20
Styrolyl propionate	0.20
Citronellyl oxyacetaldehyde	0.15
Aldehyde C_{12}, MNA, 10% in dimethyl phthalate	0.10
Oakmoss resin	0.05
Dimethyl phthalate	1.15

* *p*-Isopropyl alpha-methyl hydrocinnamic aldehyde.

Mix well and allow to stand a week or more with frequent shaking.

Narcissus Flower Oil (Synthetic)

No. 1

Hydroxycitronellal dimethyl acetal	6.0 oz
Sandalwood oil, N.F., East India	5.0 oz
Nerolin	5.0 oz
Musk ketone	4.0 oz

Petitgrain oil, S. France 4.0 oz
Phenylethyl alcohol, extra fine 4.0 oz
Amyl cinnamic aldehyde 2.0 oz
Benzyl acetate, F.F.C., coeur 2.0 oz
p-Cresyl caprylate 2.0 oz
p-Cresyl phenylacetate 2.0 oz
Rosacetol (Givaudan) 2.0 oz
Tolyl acetate 2.0 oz
Ylang-Ylang oil, Bourbon Premier 2.0 oz
Aubepine 1.6 oz
Amyl salicylate, extra 1.6 oz
Heliotropine, recrystallized 1.6 oz
Methyl ionone 1.6 oz
Musk xylol 1.6 oz
Cumin ketone 1.0 oz
Hydratropyl acetate 1.0 oz
Orange oil, bitter 1.0 oz
Labdanum oil, distilled, 10% in dimethyl phthalate 1.0 oz
Patchouli oil, Singapore 1.0 oz
Sage clary oil, extra 1.2 oz
Phenylacetic acid, pure 1.0 oz
Vetivert acetate 1.0 oz
Sweet basil oil, S. France 3.0 dr
Benzyl salicylate 2.4 oz

Mix well and allow to stand a week or more with frequent shaking.

No. 2

Terpineol, extra 4.80 oz
Benzyl acetate, F.F.C. 2.56 oz
p-Cresyl acetate 2.56 dr
Ethyl phenylacetate 5.12 dr
Bromstyrol 1.92 dr
Phenylacetaldehyde, 100% 5.12 dr
Pure linaloöl 5.76 dr
Oil Ylang-Ylang 1.92 dr
Oil petitgrain, French 5.12 dr
Indole, extra pure, 10% (Givaudan) 2.56 dr
Aldehyde C_{12}, 10% 2.56 dr
Isoeugenol 5.12 dr
Bezoin resinoid, Siam 5.12 dr
p-Cresyl phenylacetate 420.00 gr
Heliotropine, recrystallized 140.00 gr
Methyl naphthyl ketone 175.00 gr
Benzyl benzoate, U.S.P. 2.00 oz

Mix and allow to stand for one or two months.

Neroli Flower Oil (Synthetic)

Linalyl acetate, extra, 96–98% 4.0 oz
Petitgrain oil, extra 4.0 oz
Phenylethyl alcohol, extra fine 4.0 oz
Geranyl acetate, pure 2.0 oz
Ethyl decylate 6.0 oz
Hydratropyl alcohol 2.0 oz
Hydroxy citronellal dimethylacetal 2.0 oz
Linaloöl, extra 2.0 oz
Benzyl phenylacetate 1.50 oz
Methyl anthranilate, extra 1.0 oz
Coriander oil, U.S.P. 3.0 dr
Ethyl anthranilate 3.0 dr
Orange flower absolute 3.0 dr
Ylang-Ylang oil, Bourbon Premier 3.0 dr

Celery seed oil, extra	1.5	dr
Cuminic aldehyde	1.0	dr
Indol, extra pure	17.0	gr
Methylnonyl acetaldehyde, 10% in dimethyl phthalate	38.0	min
Citronellyl oxyacetaldehyde	20.0	min
Dimethyl phthalate	5.75	dr

Mix well and allow to stand a week or more with frequent shaking.

Neroli for Soaps

Limonene	10.0	oz
Geranyl acetate, special	4.0	oz
Bois de Rose oil	2.0	oz
Methyl anthranilate	2.0	oz
Amyl cinnamic aldehyde	1.2	oz
Benzyl acetate, F.F.C.	1.6	oz
Linalyl acetate	6.4	dr
Citral	1.5	dr
Nerolin	88.0	gr

Mix well and allow to stand a week or more with frequent shaking.

Orange Flower Oil (Synthetic)

	oz
Auranthiol, 100%	2.0
Petitgrain oil, extra	2.5
Rhodinyl acetate	2.0
Bergamot oil, N.F., extra	1.5
Phenylethyl dimethylcarbinyl acetate	1.5
Mandarin oil, Italian	1.0
Orange oil, bitter, N.F.	1.0
Rhodinol, extra	1.0
Rhodinyl butyrate	1.0
Benzyl phenylacetate	1.0
Cumin ketone	0.5
Linaloöl, extra	0.5
Methyl ionone, extra (D.&O.)	0.5
Musk ketone	0.5
Oranger crystals	0.5
Phenylethyl alcohol, coeur	1.0
Phenyl ethyl phenyl acetate	1.0
Ylang-Ylang, Bourbon Premier	0.3
Cinnamyl butyrate	0.2
Phenylacetic acid, pure	0.2
Amyl phenylacetate	0.1
Civettiane	0.1
Resin castoreum absolute, 10% in benzyl alcohol	0.1

Mix well and allow to stand a week or more with frequent shaking.

Orchid Flower Oil (Synthetic)

	oz
Amyl salicylate, extra	5.5
Isobutyl salicylate	4.0
Rhodinol, extra	3.0
Aubepine	2.5
Phenylethyl alcohol, extra fine	1.6
Linaloöl, extra	1.5
Heliotropine, recrystallized	1.0
Hydroxycitronellal dimethylacetal	1.0
Phenylacetaldehyde, 50% in benzyl alcohol	1.0
Acetophenone	0.5
Cumin ketone	0.5
Ylang-Ylang oil, Bourbon Premier	0.5

Coumarin, N.F.	0.4
Methylionone, extra (D.&O.)	0.4
Phenylacetic acid, pure	0.4
Citronellyl oxyacetaldehyde	0.2
Dimethyl hydroquinone	0.2
Palatone, 5% in phenylethyl alcohol	0.2
Vanillin, U.S.P., from Eugenol	0.2
Veronol aldehyde, 10% in dimethyl phthalate	0.2
Alpha ionone	0.1
Oakmoss resin	0.1
Dimethyl phthalate	0.6

Mix well and let stand a week or more.

Petitgrain Oil (Artificial)

Iso-bergamate	3.00 oz
Menthanyl acetate	4.00 oz
Petitgrain oil, French	3.00 oz
Bois de Rose oil, Brazilian	2.00 oz
Orange oil, sweet, distilled	1.00 oz
Indol, extra fine (1 oz in 10 oz diethyl phthalate)	1.60 dr
Methyl anthranilate, C.P.	1.20 oz
Linalyl acetate, 75%	2.00 oz
Geranyl acetate	1.20 oz
Oranger crystals (beta-naphthyl methyl ketone)	262.5 gr
Phenylethyl alcohol	1.8 oz

Mix well and allow to stand a week or more.

Rose Absolute (Synthetic)

	oz
Rhodinol, extra	7.50
Phenylethyl alcohol, extra fine	4.50
Geranium oil, extra, Algerian	1.50
Hydratropyl alcohol	1.50
Orange flower absolute, 10% in dimethyl phthalate	0.75
Citronellyl phenylacetate (D.&O.)	0.75
Guaiac wood acetate	0.75
Phenylacetic acid, pure	0.60
Benzyl propionate	0.45
Eugenyl phenylacetate	0.30
Geranyl benzoate	0.30
Mimosa absolute, 10% in dimethyl phthalate	0.30
Palatone, 2% in phenyl ethyl alcohol	0.30
Citronellyl oxyacetaldehyde	0.15
Ethyl pelargonate true (D.&O.), 10% in dimethyl phthalate	0.15
Eugenol, U.S.P., extra	0.15
Isobutyl phenylacetate	0.15
Labdanum absolute, 10% in dimethyl phthalate	0.15
Dimethyl phthalate	2.25

Mix well and allow to stand a week or more with frequent shaking.

Rose Garden Oil

	oz
Rhodinol, extra	5.00
Citronellol, extra	1.75
Phenylethyl alcohol, extra fine	2.00

Dimethyl octanol, pure	1.00
Octadienol 1473	1.25
Guaiac wood oil	1.00
Benzyl salicylate	1.50
Citronellyl acetate	0.80
Musk ketone	0.75
Musk xylol	0.40
Cinnamic alcohol, pure	0.50
Hydratropyl alcohol	0.50
Hydroxycitronellal dimethyl acetal	0.60
Phenylethyl phenylacetate	0.50
Tolyl alcohol	0.50
Dimethyl octanyl acetate	0.40
Isobutyl phenylacetate	0.40
Geranium oil, Bourbon	0.40
Phenylethyl propionate	0.30
Isoeugenol	0.30
Lemon oil	0.30
Ambergris tincture, 4 oz to gal	0.30
Civettiane	0.20
Methyl ionone	0.20
Bergamot oil	0.20
Galbanum oil, distilled, 10% solution	0.20
Rose oil natural	0.20
Tolyl acetate	0.20
Cumin ketone	0.10
Phenylacetaldehyde dimethyl-acetal	0.10
Ylang-Ylang, Bourbon, extra	0.10
Amyl salicylate, extra	0.10
Muguet aldehyde	0.10
Methylnonyl acetaldehyde (C_{12}), 10% solution	0.10
Mousse de Chene (Oak Moss Resinoid)	0.10
Methyl heptine carbonate, 10% solution	0.05
Hydratropyl acetate	0.10
Terpineol, extra	0.20

Mix well and allow to stand a week or more with frequent shaking.

Rose Oil, Basic

	oz
Citronellol	10.5
Phenylethyl alcohol, extra fine	4.8
Cinnamic alcohol, pure	1.5
Phenylethyl phenylacetate	0.9
Citronellyl acetate	0.6
Palatone, 5% in phenylethyl alcohol	0.6
Methyl ionone, gamma (D.&O.)	0.6
Isoeugenol, extra	0.6
Hydratropyl alcohol	0.45
Lemon oil, U.S.P., cold pressed	0.45
Benzyl propionate	0.30
Isobutyl phenylacetate	0.30
Phenyl acetic acid, pure	0.30

Mix well and allow to stand a week or more with frequent shaking.

Rose Otto (Synthetic)

	oz
Geraniol, from palmarosa	6.00
Rhodinol, extra	6.00
Geranium oil, terpeneless, Algerian	1.50
Phenylethyl alcohol, extra	1.50
fine	1.50
Geranyl acetate, pure	1.40
Alpha ionone	0.90

Hydratropyl alcohol 0.75
Dimethyl octanyl acetate 0.45
Hydroxycitronellal dimethyl-acetal 0.45
Aldehyde C-14 (Myristic), 10% in dimethyl phthalate 0.30
Aldehyde C-16, pure, 100% 0.15

Mix well and allow to stand a week or more with frequent shaking.

Rose Oil

No. 1

Geraniol, from palmarosa	3.70 oz
Citronellol, extra	2.50 oz
Phenylethyl alcohol, coeur	3.00 oz
Geranyl acetate, pure	0.10 oz
Ionone alpha	0.20 oz
Linaloöl, extra	0.40 oz
Aldehyde C_9	0.10 oz
Musk ketone	10.00 gr
Orange blossom oil	2.00 oz
Natural rose otto	1.50 oz

Mix and shake well. Allow to stand a week or more, with frequent shaking.

No. 2

Rhodinol, extra	1.0 oz
Geraniol, pure	6.0 oz
Citronellol, extra	2.0 oz
Phenylethyl alcohol, coeur	3.0 oz
Ethyl acetate	1.0 oz
Acetic acid	1.6 dr
Cinnamic alcohol, pure	3.2 dr
Bois de Rose oil	6.4 dr
Aldehyde C_{11}, 10%	1.6 dr
Geranyl acetate, pure	6.4 dr
Diphenyl oxide	4.3 dr
Lemon oil	1.5 dr
Benzophenone	1.0 oz
Benzyl acetate, F.F.C.	1.0 oz
Terpineol, extra	1.7 oz
Benzyl benzoate, U.S.P.	1.0 oz

Mix well and allow to stand a week or more. Add traces of clary sage oil in order to hasten the process of maturity.

No. 3

Musk ketone, 100%	¼ oz
Rosacetol	½ oz
Alcohol C_{12}	1 dr
Oil geranium rose, French	1 dr
Geraniol, pure	2 oz
Citronellol, extra	2 oz
Phenylethyl alcohol, extra fine	2 oz
Dihydrocitronellol (dimethyl octanol)	1 oz
Hydroxycitronellal	½ oz
Benzyl benzoate, F.F.C.	½ oz

Mix and shake well. Allow to stand a week or more.

No. 4

Geraniol, palmarosa	6 oz
Rhodinol	5 oz
Phenylethyl alcohol	5 oz
Linaloöl	1 oz
Orange blossom oil	1 oz
Musk ketone	80 gr
Rose oil, Bulgarian	1½ dr
Benzyl benzoate	1 oz

Mix well, and allow to stand a week or more with frequent shaking.

Tuberose Flower Oil (Synthetic)

Amyl cinnamic aldehyde	2.5 oz
Mimosa absolute (Fritzsche)	2.0 oz
Phenylethyl alcohol, extra fine	2.0 oz
Tolu oil, distilled	2.0 oz
Auranthiol, 100%	1.5 oz
Ylang-Ylang oil, Bourbon Premier	1.2 oz
Hydroxycitronellal dimethylacetal	1.0 oz
Methyl ionone	1.0 oz
Rhodinol, extra	1.0 oz
Civettiane	0.5 oz
Heliotropine, recrystallized	0.75 oz
Tuberyl acetate	4.75 dr
Hexyl cinnamic aldehyde	4.00 dr
Amyl salicylate, extra	3.00 dr
Tolyl acetate	3.00 dr
Glycidol	3.00 dr
Cinnamyl isobutyrate	3.00 dr
Celery seed oil, extra	1.50 dr
Cumin ketone	1.50 dr
Cuminic aldheyde, 10% in dimethyl phthalate	1.50 dr
Isoeugenol, pure	1.50 dr
Palatone, 5% in phenylethyl alcohol	1.50 dr
Phenylpropyl alcohol	1.50 dr
Phenylethyl isobutyrate	1.50 dr
Veronol aldehyde, 10% in dimethyl phthalate	1.50 dr
Aldehyde C_{14}, pure, 10% in dimethyl phthalate	45.00 min
Methylnonyl acetaldehyde (C_{12}), 10% in dimethyl phthalate	45.00 min

Mix well and allow to stand a week or more with frequent shaking.

Tearose Oil

	oz
Geraniol	5.0
Phenylethyl alcohol	15.00
Pelargol	7.00
Algerian Rose Geranium	7.00
Cinnamic alcohol	7.50
Diphenyl oxide	2.75
Geranyl formate	2.50
Guaiac wood oil	10.00
Guaiol acetate	1.00
Musk ambrette	1.25+

Violet Oil

Methyl ionone	6 oz
Alpha ionone	3 oz
Bergamot oil	2 oz
Ylang-Ylang oil	3 dr
Orris root resinoid	3 dr
Methyl heptine carbonate	48 min
Heliotropine recrystallized	350 gr
Benzyl benzoate	1 oz

Mix well, and allow to stand a week or more with frequent shaking.

Food Products

Agar-Agar Glaze for Cakes

Water	2	lb
Agar-Agar	2/3	oz
Corn syrup	1 1/3	lb
Sugar	1 1/3	lb
Water	1 1/3	lb
Citric acid, liquid	20	min

Soak the agar-agar in the water for 4 to 6 hours. Bring it to a boil to effect solution, then strain it through a fine sieve. In a separate enameled container bring to a boil the corn syrup, sugar, water, and the liquid citric acid, then stir in the strained agar-agar solution, and continue to simmer for about 4 minutes. Use the glaze while hot.

Allyl Cyclohexane Propionate

Usc this unexcelled ingredient in pineapple, strawberry and raspberry flavors. Strengthen lavender and other floral compositions by using 3–5% in such compounds. The fresh fruity pineapple odor of allyl cyclohexane-propionate does not predominate, but it adds fullness.

Almond Crescents

1	Almond paste	2 1/4	lb
	Egg whites	3/4	oz
2	Powdered sugar	1 1/2	lb
	Butter	2 3/4	lb
	Salt	82	gr
	Certified yellow color and flavor	to suit	
3	Egg whites (this can be varied)	2 1/4	oz
4	Cake flour	3 3/4	lb
	Baking powder	1 1/2	oz

Mix (1) to a smooth paste. Stir in (2) and cream it thoroughly. Add (3) and mix thoroughly. Mix (4) by sifting, add it to the other mixture, and mix only enough to accomplish a thorough incorporation.

Chill the finished dough, then roll it into strings, and cut it into slices weighing about one ounce. Roll into a thick thread-like form of about 3 inches long, tapering the ends slightly. Dip them into a heavy egg wash, roll them in grated almonds, then place them on paper-lined greased pans and shape them into crescent form.

Dry the crescents slightly by allowing them to stand for about an hour, then bake at 375°F.

Prepare the egg wash by mixing thoroughly the following ingredients:

Eggs	1¼ lb
Fresh milk	5 oz
Corn syrup or honey	2½ oz

Almond Paste

		lb
1	Blanched, broken almonds	48.0
	Granulated sugar	4.0
2	Granulated sugar	28.0
	Invert sugar	4.0
3	Water	9.6

Put some water in a steam-jacketed kettle and bring it to a boil. Now place the almonds of (1) into the kettle, and boil for about 2 minutes until they are fairly soft. Drain the water, and add the 4 lb of sugar, and run (1) several times through a peanut-butter mill. Grind the almonds to a fine particle size, and then add (2). Place the batch into a combination mixing-cooking kettle, equipped with double agitator, and add (3). Mix and cook the batch slowly until it becomes quite plastic (the paste will not stick to the back of the hand). Have the moisture content of the paste about 14%.

Do not use too much steam pressure during the mixing-and-cooking operation in order to avoid roasting the nuts. Try to maintain a pressure of about 30–40 pounds per square inch (psi). When the batch is cooked to the proper consistency, turn off the steam and mix for about 4 minutes. Empty the batch onto cooling slabs. When its temperature reaches 80°F., pack into suitable containers, and place a sheet of waxed paper over the paste before putting the lids into position.

It is expedient to brush the surface of the paste lightly with a thin film of glycerin or invert sugar at 130°F. You may substitute 5 lb of blanched bitter almonds if a slightly bitter-flavored paste is desired.

Almond Pastry

1	Egg whites	3¾ lb
	Sugar	1½ lb
	Salt	1¹⁄₁₆ oz
	Cream of tartar	3³⁄₁₆ oz
2	Almonds	4½ lb
	Sugar	4⅛ lb

Mix (1) and whip very lightly. Grind together (2) until the nutmeats are fine, add this to (1), and mix only enough to incorporate thoroughly. Mold the paste into any desired shape and place the patties on greased and flour-dusted baking sheets. Sprinkle thinly sliced almonds over the tops, then bake in moderate oven (325–350°F.). Remove from baking sheets, and cover the bottoms with a chocolate coating.

Almond Rings

Almond paste	1¼ lb
Butter	3¾ lb
Icing sugar	2½ lb
Eggs	15 oz
Cake flour	5 lb

Break up the almond paste, add a little of the butter to it and cream thoroughly. When the paste acquires the consistency of the butter, add the remainder of the butter and sugar, and cream thoroughly. While creaming, add gradually the eggs, and continue to mix until light. Finally, fold in the cake flour. Continue the mixing until the batter is smooth. Bag out into rings, crescents, or any desired shape. Bake at 350°F.

Alpha Furfuryl Mercaptan

This compound is an essential constituent of the aroma of roasted coffee. Use it in concentrations of 1:1,000,000.

Anise Drops

Sugar, powdered	5 lb
Eggs	42½ oz
Egg yolks	20 oz
Anise seed	2½ oz
Cake flour	2½ lb
Bread flour	2½ lb

Mix the eggs and egg yolks with the sugar and heat to 120°F. over a hot water bath, then beat until quite light and firm. Pulverize the anise seeds and mix them with the flours. Finally, fold the flour mixture into the whipped mass thoroughly, but carefully. Deposit on greased and dusted pans, and bake in a slow oven at 300–325°F.

Antioxidants in Foods

Confine the following to foods liable to oxidative rancidity, and add only to edible oils, fats, and essential oils:

Propyl, or octyl, or dodecyl gallate, or a mixture thereof in	
edible oils and fats	0.1 %
in essential oils	0.01%
Butylated hydroxyanisole in essential oils	0.1 %
Edible oils and fats	0.02%

Antioxidants for Essential Oils

Propyl gallate	0.01%
Butylated hydroxyanisole	0.02%

These two antioxidants give citrus oils in particular protection against becoming "terpeny."

These preservatives are approved for food use by the Food and Drug Administration.

Apple Crunch Cake

		oz
1	Sugar, fine granulated	27
	Shortening	9
	Baking soda	¾
	Salt	⅜
	Cinnamon	½
	Raisins, ground	6
2	Eggs	10½

Cream thoroughly (1), and add gradually, while creaming, (2). Finally add alternately the following:

	oz
Cake flour	34½
sifted together with the	
Baking powder	¾
Applesauce	33
Buttermilk	6

Continue the mixing until a smooth product is obtained. Weigh into heavily greased suitable molds lined with a liberal amount of the following crunch:

1	Coconut, long shred	13⅓	oz
	Sugar, powdered	6	oz
	Salt	40	gr
	Nutmeats, chopped fine	9	oz
	Eggs	3¾	oz
2	Lemon gratings	1½	oz

Mix together (1), then spread the mass evenly over a pan, and toast at 325°F. until dry—not too dark. When dry and not too hot, run it through a coarse food chopper and mix it together thoroughly with (2).

Apple Sauce Cake

1	Cake flour, high moisture	3¾	lb
	Baking powder	2¼	oz
	Baking soda	1⅛	oz
	Salt	⅛	oz
	Non-fat dry milk	3	oz
	Sugar, fine granulation	4⅞	lb
	Shortening, emulsifying type	30	oz
	Cinnamon	¼	oz
	Allspice	40	gr
	Cloves	40	gr
	Nutmeg	40	gr
2	Applesauce	2¼	lb
	Eggs	39	oz
	Applesauce	3¾	lb

Sift the flour, baking powder, and baking soda together, and mix (1) very thoroughly. Add at slow speed (2) and mix until smooth. Now mix together the eggs and applesauce, and add this in three separate portions, mixing until smooth after each addition.

Scrape the bottom and sides of the mixing bowl several times during the mixing operation. Finally, scale into loaf tins and bake at 365°F.

Apple Wine, Stabilization of

Add 0.15% of glucose oxidase and catalase to apple wine in order to prevent oxidation and the development of acetic acid.

The flavor of this stabilized wine is superior to the wine stabilized by the addition of sulfur dioxide, or by pasteurizing. Any discoloration that develops disappears with the aging of the wine.

Apricot Glaze

Water	2 lb
Agar-Agar	⅔ oz
Granulated sugar	3⅓ lb
Corn syrup	2 lb
Apricot pulp, strained	4⅓ lb

Soak the agar-agar in the water for 4 to 6 hours, then cook it slowly to effect solution, and strain through a fine sieve. Cook for 12 minutes the sugar, corn syrup, and strained apricot pulp, and then stir in the agar-agar solution. Use the glaze while hot.

Apricot Pie Filling

Dried apricots (washed)	5 lb
Water, hot	10 lb
Sugar	5 lb
Corn syrup	2½ lb
Salt	¾ oz
Starch	5 oz
Juice and water	12 oz

Wash the dried apricots twice and discard the water. Now soak the apricots in the hot water until they are soft and tender (about 20 hours). Drain the fruit and then, if necessary, add enough of the water to yield 5 lb. Retain 12 oz of the juice-water to suspend the starch. Place the rest of the juice-water in a cooking utensil, and stir into it the sugar, corn syrup, and salt, and bring all to a rolling boil. While stirring, add to this boiling mass the starch suspension, and continue to mix until thick and clear. Finally, add this thickened juice-water to the drained apricots and mix thoroughly—but gently—so as not to crush the apricots. Allow the mass to cool, then use as required.

Bagels

No. 1

High gluten flour (a wheat flour from which a large part of the starch has been removed)	7½ lb
Water (variable)	3⅜ pt
Sugar	9 oz
Yeast	1½ oz
Salt	1½ oz
Corn oil, refined	3¾ oz
Eggs	6 oz

Mix all the ingredients until the dough is smooth and pliable. Remove the dough from the mixer at approximately 80°F. Allow it to ferment for about 30 minutes. Shape into bagel form, and let them rest for 15 minutes, then place them in boiling water. As soon as the bagels appear on thc surface, remove them from the water, and bake at about 450°F.

No. 2
(With Eggs)

High gluten flour	4.00 lb
Water (variable)	27.00 oz
Yeast	0.80 oz

Salt	1.00 oz
Corn oil, refined	2.00 oz
Eggs	9.50 oz
Sugar	4.75 oz

Mix all the ingredients to a smooth dough of somewhat firm consistency. Remove the dough from the mixer at about 80°F. Allow it to ferment for about 30 minutes or longer, then shape the bagels. Let them lie for 15 to 20 minutes before placing them in boiling water. After properly conditioning the bagels in boiling water, remove them, drain, and then bake at about 450°F.

No. 3

High gluten flour	4.00 lb
Water	35.00 oz
Yeast	2.00 oz
Salt	1.00 oz
Corn oil, refined	1.20 oz
Barley malt	1.20 oz

Use the same procedure as for egg bagel.

No. 4
(With Onions)

High gluten flour	4.00 lb
Water (variable)	26.00 oz
Sugar	4.75 oz
Yeast	1.00 oz
Salt	1.00 oz
Eggs	3.00 oz
Corn oil, refined	1.60 oz
Onions, dehydrated	1.60 oz

Use the same procedure as for egg bagel. Add the onions to the dough several minutes before the mixing operation is completed.

No. 5
(Whole Wheat)

High gluten flour	2.00 lb
Whole wheat flour	2.00 lb
Water (variable)	2.00 lb
Eggs	6.50 oz
Sugar	4.75 oz
Yeast	0.80 oz
Salt	0.80 oz
Corn oil, refined	1.60 oz

Use the same procedure as for egg bagel.

Baking Powder Equivalents

No. 1

Cream of tartar (potassium bitartrate, U.S.P.)	2 oz
Baking soda (sodium bicarbonate, U.S.P.)	1 oz
is equivalent to	
Baking powder	4 oz

No. 2

Cream of tartar	3 oz
Baking soda	1½ oz
is equivalent to	
Baking powder	6 oz

No. 3

Cream of tartar	1 lb
Baking soda	8 oz
is equivalent to	
Baking powder	2 lb

Banana Cake

1	Sugar, granulated	5.7 lb
	Butter	1.5 lb
	Emulsifying shortening	1.5 lb
	Cinnamon	132.0 gr
	Salt	1.0 oz
	Honey	4.8 oz
	Bananas	6.0 lb
	Eggs	2.4 lb
	Cake flour	5.4 lb
	Baking powder	3.0 oz

Mix (1) and cream thoroughly. While creaming, add gradually the eggs. Now mix the cake flour with the baking powder and sift it, then add it to (1), and continue mixing until the batch is smooth. Scale, and bake at about 375°F. Nuts or coconut, or both, may be added if desired.

Banana Jam

Sugar	10 lb
Water	4 pt
Cream of tartar	262 gr
Lemon juice	1 pt
Ripe banana pulp	10 lb

Mix the sugar, water, and cream of tartar and cook to 230°F. Finally add the lemon juice and banana pulp, and boil to 224°F.

Barbecue Sauce

1	Starch (cold thickening)	1 oz
	Water	1 pt
2	Tomato paste (30% solids)	8 oz
	Sugar	6 oz
	White wine vinegar (5% acetic acid)	8 oz
	Salt	1 oz
	Water	2 pt
	Barbecue seasoning	1 oz

Mix (1) thoroughly until a slurry is formed. Now mix (2) thoroughly, and then apply some heat. While heating, stir in the starch-watery slurry and continue the heating until the starch develops. Finally stir in the barbecue seasoning. (See Barbecue Seasoning.)

Barbecue Sauce

Tomato juice	8 lb
Corn oil	1⅓ lb
Worcestershire sauce	1⅓ lb
Distilled vinegar	4 qt
Capsicum	⅔ oz
Mustard, dry	4 oz
Garlic, minced	⅔ oz
Onion, grated	2⅔ lb
Paprika	4 oz
Pepper, ground	4 oz
Salt	2 oz

Mix all the ingredients and shake well. Allow to stand overnight.

Barbecue Seasoning

	oz
Onion, grated	10⅔
Mustard, dry	1

Paprika	1
Pepper, ground	1
Salt	½
Garlic, minced	½
Capsicum	⅙

Mix well together, and pack in glass containers.

Basic Cream Icing

Icing sugar	12 lb
Butter	3 lb
Shortening, emulsifying type	2⅖ lb
Salt	33 gr
Condensed milk	33½ oz
Flavor	to suit

Cream thoroughly at medium speed the sugar, butter, shortening, and salt. Then add the condensed milk very slowly, at slow speed on a three-speed mixing machine. Finally stir in the flavor. Chocolate or cocoa, candied fruits, coconut, nutmeats, etc., may be added to this icing.

Basic Yellow Cake

1	Sugar, fine granulated	6 lb
	Shortening	1⅞ lb
	Butter	12 oz
	Corn starch	12 oz
	Salt	1 oz
	Vanilla	1½ oz
2	Egg yolks	1½ lb
	Eggs	1½ lb
	Milk	3¾ pt
	Cake flour	6¾ lb
	Baking powder (sift together with cake flour)	3¾ oz

Mix (1) and cream lightly, scraping the bowl very often. When the mixture is light, add (2) slowly while creaming. Then add the milk. Finally stir in the cake flour-baking powder, and continue mixing until smooth.

Use this formula for layers, sheet cakes, loaf, or wine cakes.

Bavarian Cheese Cake

1	Baker's special cheese	6.0 lb
	Granulated sugar, fine	2.4 lb
	Corn starch	3.6 oz
	Non-fat dry milk solids	1.2 oz
	Lemon juice, powdered	0.6 oz
	Salt	0.6 oz
	Shortening, emulsifying type	2.4 oz
	Eggs	28.8 oz
	Egg yolk	9.6 oz
	Vanilla and lemon flavor	to suit
	Warm water (120°F.)	12.0 oz

Mix (1) until it is very smooth. Add the shortening and mix thoroughly. Mix the eggs, egg yolk, vanilla and lemon flavor, and add this mixture in four portions to (1), mixing thoroughly after each addition. Scrape the sides and bottom of the mixing bowl at frequent intervals to ensure a smooth and lump-free batter. Finally, stir in slowly the warm water, and continue the mixing until the mass is smooth. Use spring forms. Line the pans (bottom and sides) with a cookie dough. Fill the tins to within one-half inch of the top. Bake for about 13 minutes at 485°F. in order to brown the dough, then bake at 225°F. until done.

Boiled Icing

		oz
1	Egg whites	21¼
	Salt	½
2	Icing sugar	21¼
3	Glucose	15
	Vanilla flavor	to suit

Whip (1) until light. Add (2) gradually while whipping and continue beating until the mass is stiff. Heat it to 180–200°F., and add (3) to it slowly, continuing to beat until the desired consistency is obtained.

Brazil Nut Fudge Kisses Fondant

	lb
Fine granulated sugar	45.00
Corn syrup	11.25
Invert sugar	5.63
Water	11.25

Place the ingredients in a suitable container and heat to 246°F. Cool the syrup to 125°F. and beat it into fondant (thick creamy paste). Heat 46.88 lb of the fondant to 125–130°F. in a warm mixing kettle, then add the following:

Long-shred, desiccated coconut	7.50 lb
Sliced Brazil nuts	3.75 lb
Salt	1.88 oz
Vanilla flavor	q.s.

Mix well.

Meanwhile, place in a separate container the following:

	lb
Fine granulated sugar	6.56
Corn syrup	4.69
Invert sugar	2.81
Sweetened, condensed milk	8.44
Hard coconut butter	1.50

Heat to 260°F., with constant stirring. Pour this batch into the mixture of fondant, coconut, and Brazil nuts and mix for about 10 minutes, or until the batch is firm enough to be spooned into kisses.

You can also spread this batch onto waxed paper, mark it, and cut it like fudge.

Bread Stuffing

Clean, lightly toasted bread crumbs	10.00 lb
Mono-sodium glutamate	0.20 oz
Mustard powder	0.15 oz
Celery salt	0.10 oz
Sage	0.10 oz
White pepper	0.10 oz

Mix thoroughly in order to obtain a uniform distribution of all the substances. The seasoning materials may be varied if so desired.

Buttercream Icing

1	Powdered sugar	7½ lb
	Butter	3⅜ lb
	Egg whites	3 oz
	Flavor and salt	to suit
2	Whipping cream	1$\frac{5}{16}$ lb
3	Powdered sugar	1½ lb
	Meringue powder (see Meringue Powder)	3 oz
	Water	1 pt

Cream (1) thoroughly at a slow speed. While creaming it add (2) very slowly and continue creaming at the same speed until the mixture is very light. Place (3) in another bowl and whip very light. Fold thoroughly and carefully the creamed mass into (3) and add a trace of certified aquamarine blue color in order to produce a whiter colored icing. Use the icing as required.

Buttercream Icing

1	Fondant	5 lb
	Emulsifying type shortening	1½ lb
	Butter	1¾ lb
	Salt (variable)	28 gr
	Vanilla	to suit
	Rum flavor	to suit
	Condensed milk	8 oz
	Water	3 oz
	Egg whites	8 oz

Cream the first 6 ingredients thoroughly. Mix the condensed milk with the water, and add slowly to the creamed mass. Finally, add gradually the egg whites, and continue to cream until the desired icing consistency is obtained.

Butter Cream Icing or Filling

		lb
1	Butter	2.00
	Emulsifying type shortening	1.17
	Icing sugar	4.00
	Salt and vanilla flavor	to suit
2	Whipping cream, about 36% butterfat	1.67
	Condensed milk	1.33
3	Finished marshmallow	1.17

Cream (1) thoroughly until fairly light. Mix (2) and add slowly to (1) while mixing at a slow speed. Finally fold (3) in thoroughly. Use this cream immediately or place it in the freezer and hold it for several hours to several days at 8–12°F. Remove from freezer as needed, and allow it to thaw at room temperature.

Butter Oil (Synthetic)

Diacetyl, very pure	6.0 oz
Methylacetylcarbinol	4.5 dr
Capryl butyric esters	3.0 dr
Acetyl isobutyryl	1.5 dr
Acetyl propionyl	1.5 dr
Acetal acetate	1.5 dr

Mix well and allow to stand overnight.

Butterscotch

Sorghum syrup	3 lb
Sugar	4 lb

Butter	1 lb
Vinegar	6 oz
Vanilla	to suit

Place the first 4 ingredients in a kettle and cook to 250°F. Remove the kettle from the fire and stir in the vanilla flavor. Pour the batch onto a greased slab, and score it into any desired shape and size. Pack in wax-lined boxes.

Buttermilk Custard

1	Buttermilk, liquid	42 oz
	Milk, fresh	42 oz
	Sugar	30 oz
	Corn syrup	6 oz
	Salt	55 gr
2	Eggs	18 oz
	Sugar	9 oz
	Milk	9 oz
	Corn starch, U.S.P.	7½ oz
	Vanilla flavor	q.s.

Bring (1) to a boil. Mix (2) and add it to (1). Continue to stir the mass until it thickens. Allow it to cool, then use it as required.

Butter Pecan Filling

Sugar, granulated	3 lb
Eggs	18 oz
Salt	75 gr
Cinnamon	¾ oz
Milk (variable)	42 oz
Cake crumbs	4½ oz
Pecans, finely chopped	24 oz

Mix the ingredients thoroughly. In case the filling does not spread readily, add enough egg whites to make spreading easier.

Butterscotch Icing

Sugar, granulated	2⅓ lb
Sugar, brown	2⅓ lb
Butter	20 oz
Condensed milk, sweetened	2⅓ lb
Water (variable)	17 oz
Fondant	4⅔ lb
Sugar, powdered	2 lb
Corn syrup	6⅔ oz

Mix the sugars with the butter and melt over heat until a medium caramel color is obtained. Mix the condensed milk with the water, then add it to the butter-sugar mixture. Allow it to cool slightly, then add the fondant, powdered sugar, and corn syrup, and continue mixing until the finished product is smooth. Use this icing at a temperature of 90°F. If necessary, thin it with simple syrup.

Butterscotch Topping
No. 1

1	Water	2.8 lb
	Sodium bicarbonate	175.0 gr
	Sodium citrate	175.0 gr
	Butter	19.2 oz
2	Brown sugar	3.2 lb
	Cane sugar	10.0 lb
3	Condensed skim milk, sweetened	12.8 oz
	Water	12.8 oz
4	Condensed skim milk, sweetened	2.4 lb
	Water	2.0 lb
5	Corn syrup	16.0 lb

6	Orange color	to suit
	Butter flavor	to suit
	Salt	2.0 oz

Place (1) in a steam-jacketed kettle and heat batch until the butter is melted. Now add (2). Mix (3) and introduce it into the kettle and heat to 240°F. Mix (4), slowly introduce it into the kettle, and bring the whole batch to a boil. Finally pour this hot mixture into (5)—previously heated to 170°F. At this point add (6), homogenize the whole at a pressure of 200 psi., and fill at 190°F.

No. 2

	lb
Brown sugar	25.0
Corn syrup, Stanley's	25.0
Water	16.5
Salt	0.5
Vanilla flavor	to suit

Place the first four ingredients in a steam jacketed kettle and cook rapidly to 228°F. Turn off the heat and stir in the flavor. Then fill hot into quart containers and seal. Use the product as is, or add 2 oz of melted butter to each quart of the topping, stirring thoroughly before serving.

Butter Sponge Cake

No. 1

Sugar	5.25 lb
Eggs	6.00 lb
Egg Yolk	1.50 lb
Corn syrup	12.00 oz
Water, warm (variable)	12.00 oz
Salt	1.00 oz
Flavor	to suit
Cake flour	4.50 lb
Baking powder	0.75 oz
Butter, melted	30.00 oz

Heat the first seven ingredients over a hot water bath to 110°F. Then whip this mixture until it is light and somewhat firm. Sift together the cake flour and the baking powder, and fold it into the whipped mixture. Finally, fold in the molten butter, thoroughly and carefully. Scale into pans and bake at a temperature of 390°F.

No. 2

Sugar	4⅞ lb
Eggs, mixed	7½ lb
Water	12 oz
Lemon oil	1 dr
Salt	¾ oz
Cake flour, high moisture type	4½ lb
Butter	1½ lb

Mix first five ingredients and heat to about 120°F., then beat until it is of a light and firm consistency. Sift the cake flour and fold it in by hand carefully (avoid overmixing). Finally, melt the butter and fold it in gradually. Scale into pans of any desired shape and size, and bake at about 400°F. Immediately upon removal from the oven, turn the cake out on dusted cloth to cool, with the pans inverted on cake for the purpose of retaining moisture.

Cake Filling

1	Fresh milk	3 lb
	Granulated sugar	12 oz
	Salt	39 gr
2	Fresh milk	6 oz
	Corn starch	7½ oz
	Granulated sugar	6 oz
	Whole eggs	10½ oz
3	Butter	1½ lb
	Granulated sugar	4½ oz
	Vanilla flavor	q.s.

Bring (1) to a boil and stir. Add (2), stirring constantly until the mass thickens. Cream it until very light, and cook it for several minutes. Cool the batch to 75°F., and add (3) after it has been well mixed. Use as required.

Cake Icing

No. 1

1	Meringue powder	2½ oz
	4X sugar	½ lb
	Cold water	½ pt
2	Glucose	¼ pt
	Glycerin	½ pt
	4X sugar	2¼ lb
	Liquid certified blue	as needed
	Flavor	as desired

Dissolve contents of (1) in mixing machine. Add sugar and liquid blue of (2) and mix together. Heat the glycerin and glucose of (2) together at 120°F., and when icing stands up clear and sharp, add it to the batch while mixing it. This icing will keep soft for a long time.

No. 2

Granulated sugar	7.5 lb
Corn syrup	12.0 oz
Cream of tartar	55.0 gr
Water	30.0 oz

Place in a clean kettle and cook to 222°F., then cool to 90°F. Add this sugar solution gradually to the following shortening mixture which has been creamed light at a medium speed:

Emulsifying type vegetable shortening	5.0 lb
Puff pastry margarine (high melting)	2.5 lb

Continue the creaming until the desired icing consistency is obtained.

Cake Topping

1	Granulated sugar	1½ lb
	Light brown sugar	12 oz
	Margarine or butter	1½ lb
	Corn Syrup	4½ oz
	Fresh milk	12 oz
2	Chopped almonds or pecans	2½ lb

Bring (1) to a boil. Remove from the fire, and add (2). Cool slightly, then use as required.

Calcium Cyclamate (Sweetening Agent)

Calcium cyclamate is an ideal sweetener for dietetic and diabetic products. It is very stable, and its sweetening properties are not affected by cooking, canning, baking, or freezing. It is safe and pure, free of salt, and it has no bitter off-taste or after-taste. All flavorings are compatible with it.

Caramels

No. 1

Sugar	6 lb
Corn syrup	4½ lb
Butter	6 oz
Sweet Cream 20%	6 pt

Mix and cook all the ingredients except the cream over a slow fire to 238°F.; add one half of the cream gradually and cook to 242°F.; add the rest of the cream and stir. Cook to 248°F. Pour the mass onto an oiled slab between bars. When cold, mark with a cutter and cut into the desired shapes.

You may use the above formula for making chocolate caramels by just adding 12 oz of chocolate liquor after all the cream has been added.

No. 2

Sorghum syrup	4½ lb
Brown sugar	1⅛ lb
Milk	18 oz
Chocolate	9 oz
Butter	4½ oz
Vanilla flavor	½ oz

Place the first 5 components into a kettle, and cook to 244°F. Remove kettle from fire, and stir in the flavor. Pour onto a greased slab, and cut into caramel size, while still warm. Wrap in waxed paper when cold.

Caramel Corn

1	Sugar	9.00 lb
	Corn syrup	4.50 lb
	Water	3.50 lb
2	Butter	2.25 lb
	Salt	to suit
	Popped corn	15 gal

Cook (1) in a steam-jacketed kettle to 285°F. While agitating the batch, stir in (2). Now stir in the popped corn.

Caramel Flavor

1	Coffee extract	12.000 oz
	Butter flavor	6.000 oz
2	Protovanol C	0.125 oz
	Palatone	0.100 oz
	Ethyl vanillin	0.125 oz
	Vanillidine acetone	0.125 oz
	Absolute resin vanilla	0.250 oz
	Absolute resin Tonka bean	0.125 oz
	Propylene glycol	3.000 pt
	Caramel	1.000 pt
	Water, enough to make	1.000 gal

Heat the propylene glycol to about 75°C. and stir in (2). When solution is complete, add (1), with constant stirring. Continue stirring while adding about 2 pts of water. Finally stir in the caramel and enough water to make one gallon.

Catsup

Ripe tomatoes, sliced	5 qt
Onions, chopped	1½ cups
Cinnamon (3-inch pieces)	2
Garlic clove, large, chopped	2
Whole clove	½ oz
Vinegar (5–6% acetic acid)	1 pt
Sugar	8 oz
Salt	½ oz
Paprika	½ oz
Capsicum powder	3–5 gr

Mix together the tomatoes with the onions and boil gently for about 30 minutes, then squeeze them through a sieve. Place the cinnamon sticks, cloves, and garlic in a clean, thin, white cloth, and tie the top tightly; add this spice mixture to the vinegar and boil gently for about 30 minutes, then remove it from the vinegar. Boil the strained tomato mixture rapidly until the original volume is reduced one-half. Keep on stirring to prevent sticking. Now stir the spiced vinegar, capsicum, salt, sugar and paprika into the tomato mixture and boil rapidly with constant stirring for about 10 minutes. Finally, pour into clean, hot, sterile bottles. Fill bottles to top and seal tightly.

Certified Food Colors

In preparing a solution of food colors, use distilled water and boil it. Then cool it to 180°F., and add 4 oz of the desired color per gallon, slowly with constant stirring. Continue to mix until solution is complete, then strain through cheesecloth. Use alcohol or glycerin as a preservative if desired. Use containers made of glass, enameled metal, Monel, or stainless steel.

The following coal tar dyes are no longer certified colors; therefore they can no longer be used in food products.

FD&C Orange No. 1 and 2.
FD&C Red No. 32.
FD&C Yellow Nos. 1, 2, 3 and 4.

Challis

(Jewish Egg Bread)

Strong bread flour	25 lb
Water (variable)	14 lb
Yeast	1 lb
Sugar	15 oz
Dry malt	15 oz
Salt	5 oz
Corn oil, refined	15 oz
Eggs (half yolk)	24 oz

Mix all the ingredients until the dough is smooth and pliable. Keep the dough at approximately 86°F., and allow it to ferment for about 2½ hours. Puncture and continue the fermentation for an additional hour before weighing the dough. Divide the dough into pieces, allowing 1¼ lb for each loaf. Shape into strands tapering a little at one end. Plait the strands as desired. Wash the loaves with egg wash, then besprinkle with sesame seeds. Allow them to proof 15 minutes or more before panning, then bake at about 425°F.

Cheese Buns

Baker's cheese	9	oz
Flour	21	oz
Eggs	27	oz
Sugar	2¼	lb
Salt	1	oz
Lemon juice	enough to flavor	

Carefully mix all the ingredients until the batch is of smooth consistency. Scale as required, then bake it at a temperature of 325° to 350°F.

Cheese Cake

1	Cream cheese	4	lb
	Hoop cheese	3½	lb
	Egg whites	18	oz
	Egg yolks	30	oz
	Vanilla	to suit	
2	Egg whites	1½	lb
	Salt	80	gr
	Sugar	6	oz
3	Graham cracker meal	5	lb
	Butter	1½	lb
	Sugar, white	12	oz
	Sugar, brown	12	oz

Mix (1) until smooth, and whip it until it is of the proper consistency, then fold (2) into the creamy mass. Scale into spring molds, the bottoms of which are lined with about ¼ inch of the thoroughly mixed (3), and tightly packed. Finally, bake at a temperature of about 350°F.

Cheese Filling for Strudel

Baker's cheese	4	lb
Flour	2½	oz
Egg yolks	11¼	oz
Sugar	25½	oz
Raisins	14½	oz
Lemon rind	to suit	
Egg whites	14½	oz

Mix the cheese with the flour until smooth. Whip up the egg yolks and sugar and fold into the cheese mixture. Add the raisins and lemon rind and mix thoroughly. Finally, whip the egg whites until firm, then fold them into the cheese mixture.

Cheese Pie

Milk	2	lb
Sugar	1	lb
Salt	½	oz
Milk (mix together)	11	oz
Cornstarch (mix together)	5½	oz
Baker's cheese	4	lb
Eggs	21½	oz
Vanilla	to suit	
Egg whites	16	oz
Sugar	10½	oz

Mix the milk, sugar, and salt, and bring to a boil. Add the cornstarch-milk mixture, and continue heating until clear. Blend together the cheese, eggs, and flavor, and continue mixing until smooth. Now add the cooked custard while hot and keep on mixing until smooth. Mix together the egg whites with the sugar and whip until light and firm, then add this to the cheese-custard mixture. Place the batter into pre-baked pie shells. Besprinkle the top with cake crumbs, and bake at 400°F. The batter yields 12 eight-inch pies.

Cherry Oil

No. 1

	oz
Ethyl acetate	6.12
Ethyl acetoacetate	1.50
Ethyl oenanthate	1.50
Ethyl caprate	1.50
Isoamyl butyrate	0.75
Ethyl caproate	0.75
Ethyl caprylate	0.75
Benzaldehyde, F.F.C.	0.75
Essence of bitter almond, F.F.P.A.	0.45
p-Tolyl aldehyde	0.30
Vanillin	0.15
Terpenyl butyrate	0.075
Geraniol, pure	0.075
Geranyl butyrate	0.075
Essence of cloves, Bourbon	0.075
Essence of cinnamon	0.075
Acetyl methylcarbinol	0.075
Essense of wine dregs	0.030

Mix well and allow to stand a week or more.

No. 2

Benzaldehyde, F.F.C.	2.0 oz
Aldehyde C_{17}	2.0 oz
Ethyl acetate	4.0 oz
Isoamyl butyrate	0.5 oz
Tolyl aldehyde	0.5 oz
Allyl benzoate	0.5 oz
Cyclohexyl formate	0.5 oz
m-Methylbenzyl propionate	0.5 oz
Vanillin	40.0 gr

Mix well and allow to stand a week or more.

No. 3

Benzaldehyde, F.F.C.	2.0 oz
Allyl benzoate	0.75 oz
Allyl isovalerate	0.50 oz
m-Methylbenzyl formate	0.50 oz
Cyclohexyl formate	0.75 oz
Benzyl alcohol	0.25 oz
Aldehyde C_{17}	2.00 oz
Ethyl acetate	3.00 oz
Vanillin	40.00 gr

Mix well and allow to stand a week or more.

Chewing Taffy

Granulated sugar	5 lb
Corn syrup	5 lb
Invert syrup	2 lb
Water	1 lb
Vegetable fat, 86 to 96	0.5 lb
Salt	0.5 oz
Color and flavor	to suit

Place the syrups, sugar, and water in a kettle and heat to the boiling point. Wash down the sides of the kettle. Add the fat and cook to medium firm ball (254–262°F.). Pour the batch onto an oiled cooling slab, add the salt, and fold in the edges when partly cool. When sufficiently cool, pull well on the hook. Add the flavor and color while pulling. Spin, cut, and wrap in cellophane or waxed paper.

Chiffon Cake, Plain

1	Cake flour	45.00 oz
1	Baking powder	2.30 oz
1	Sugar, finely granulated	31.66 oz
1	Salt	1.00 oz
	Corn oil	23.33 oz
	Egg yolks	25.83 oz
	Flavor	to suit
	Water	5.00 oz
	Lemon juice	3.33 oz
	Lemon rind, grated	1.67 oz
	Egg whites	46.67 oz
	Granulated sugar	30.00 oz
	Cream of tartar (potassium bitartrate)	91.50 gr

Carefully mix and sift together (1). Stir in the corn oil, egg yolks, and flavor, and continue mixing until a smooth mixture is obtained. Stir in slowly the water, lemon juice, and lemon rind. Now place the egg whites, granulated sugar, and cream of tartar in another mixer and whip slightly—not too firm. Finally, fold the batter, carefully but thoroughly, into the whipped mass. Scale as required, then bake at about 365°F. Invert after the baking is completed. Allow it to cool, then remove from the tins.

Chiffon Pie Fillings

No. 1: Lemon

	Cold water	24 oz
	Gelatin, U.S.P. (50 mesh, high-melting, quick-setting.)	3 oz
1	Sugar, granulated	42 oz
1	Lemon juice	30 oz
1	Lemon peel	1½ oz
1	Water	18 oz
1	Salt	½ oz
1	Eggs	12 oz
1	Egg yolk	24 oz
1	Color	q.s.
1	Egg whites	3¾ lb
1	Sugar, granulated	3 lb

Soak the gelatin in the cold water for 15 minutes or more. Mix (1) and cook over hot water until it begins to thicken, then fold in the softened gelatin and allow the mixture to cool. Whip the egg whites, and, while whipping, add gradually the sugar. Continue whipping until firm. Now fold the whipped mass into the cooled gelatin mixture. Finally, fill into pre-baked pie shells and chill. Use any desired topping.

No. 2: Pumpkin

	Cold water	24 oz
	Gelatin, U.S.P. (50 mesh, high-melting, quick-setting.)	3 oz
1	Sugar, brown	3 lb
1	Evaporated milk	3 lb
1	Salt	¾ oz
1	Pumpkin, cooked	7½ lb
1	Cinnamon	1½ oz
1	Ginger	1½ oz
1	Mace	½ oz
	Egg yolk	27 oz
	Egg whites	3 lb
	Sugar, granulated	3 lb

Soak the gelatin in the cold water for about 15 minutes. Beat the egg yolk until foamy, then add (1) and mix thoroughly. Cook this mixture over hot water for about 10 minutes. Remove from fire, then fold in immediately the softened gelatin. Place in refrigerator for about one hour to chill. Whip the egg whites, and, while whipping, add gradually the sugar. Continue whipping until firm. Now fold carefully the whipped mass into the chilled pumpkin mixture, and fill into pre-baked pie shells. Finally, chill for 3 hours before selling.

No. 3: Squash

Follow the procedure for pumpkin pie filling, except for substituting 7½ lb of cooked squash in place of the pumpkin.

No. 4: Strawberry

	Cold water	24	oz
	Gelatin, U.S.P. (50 mesh, high-melting and quick-setting)	3¾	oz
1	Sugar, granulated	42	oz
1	Strawberry juice, drained of frozen strawberries	30	oz
1	Strawberries, drained	3	lb
1	Egg yolk	2¼	lb
1	Salt	⅜	oz
	Egg whites	3¾	lb
	Sugar, granulated	3	lb

Soak the gelatin in the cold water for 15 minutes or more. Mix (1) and cook over hot water until it begins to thicken, then fold in the softened gelatin and allow the mixture to cool. Whip the egg whites, and, while whipping, add gradually the sugar. Continue whipping until firm. Now fold the whipped mass into the cooked gelatin mixture. Finally, fill into pre-baked pie shells, and chill. Use any desired topping.

Chili Sauce

Ripe tomatoes, finely chopped	8	qt
Sweet red peppers, chopped	4	cups
Onions, chopped	4	cups
Hot pepper, chopped	2	
Celery seed	2	oz
Mustard seed	1	oz
Bay leaf	2	
Whole clove	½	oz
Ginger, ground	½	oz
Nutmeg	½	oz
Cinnamon (3-inch pieces)	4	
Sugar, brown	1	lb
Vinegar (5%–6% acetic acid)	3	pt
Salt	1½	oz

Mix the tomatoes together with the sweet peppers, hot pepper, and onions. Place the bay leaf, celery seed, cinnamon, cloves, ginger, mustard seed, nutmeg in a thin white cloth, and tie top tightly. Add this spice combination to the tomato mixture and boil until the original volume is reduced one-half. Stir frequently in order to prevent sticking. Now stir in the salt, sugar, and vinegar, and boil rapidly with constant stirring for about 5 minutes. Remove the spice bag, and pack into clean, hot, sterile containers. Fill containers to top, and seal tightly.

Chocolate Butter Cream

Butter	30	oz
Icing sugar	3¾	lb
Cinnamon	$\frac{1}{20}$	oz
Heavy cream	12	oz
Chocolate liquor, melted	7–9	oz

Mix the sugar, butter, and cinnamon, and cream thoroughly at slow speed. Add gradually the heavy cream while creaming at slow speed. Finally stir in the chocolate liquor, and make sure that it is thoroughly incorporated. Use this as a filling in layer cakes.

Chocolate Coated Nougat Bar

1	Honey	2¼	lb
	Dried egg albumen	3	oz
	Water	12	oz
2	Sugar	8¼	lb
	Corn syrup	5⅝	lb
	Water	2¼	pt
3	Plastic vegetable butter, 92 degrees	12	oz
	Vanilla flavor	¾	oz
	Nut meats (optional)	½	lb

Dissolve the egg albumen in the 12 oz of water. Heat the honey to 240°F. (the distinctive flavor of honey is lost when honey is heated to temperatures above 280°F.). Pour the honey into the mixing bowl of beater. Mix at slow speed, and when the temperature has dropped to 160°F. or lower, add the dissolved egg albumen. Beat until the batch is light and fluffy. Place (2) in a separate container and heat to 265°F. Put the mixer in second speed, and slowly add (2) to the whipped batch. Continue the beating until the batch begins to stiffen. Add the flavor, melted butter, and nut meats and mix well. Pour the mass onto an oiled cooling slab to a thickness of about ½ inch. As soon as the batch is cold, cut to any desired size and immediately dip in previously prepared chocolate, either by hand or machine. You may replace the dried egg albumen and the 12 oz of water with ¾ oz powdered egg albumen in 15 oz fresh egg whites. Some of the honey may be replaced with invert sugar.

Chocolate Coating for Ice Cream Bars

	oz
Coconut oil	82.00
Sugar, powdered	44.90
Non-fat milk solids	7.50
Non-fat chocolate solids	15.00

Lecithin	0.45
Salt	0.15

Mix the sugar, milk solids, chocolate solids, and salt, very thoroughly. Add the lecithin to the oil, and heat the oil-lecithin mixture to 120°F. Add ⅓ of this oil mixture to the dry mixture and mix thoroughly. Finally, stir in the remaining oil-lecithin mixture, and continue to mix until the resultant product is very smooth. Cool and store the coating until ready to use. Before the dipping is begun, heat the chocolate coating to 150°F., and then cool to 110°F. Dip the ice cream bars at temperatures ranging from 102 to 110°F.

Chocolate Fudge Icing

1	Sugar	18	lb
	Salt	½	oz
	Water	5⅝	pt
2	Bitter chocolate	9	lb
	Invert sugar	4½	lb
3	Powdered XXXX sugar	6¾	lb
4	Shortening	3⅜	lb
	Margarine	1⅛	lb
	Vanilla flavor	1⅛	oz

Boil (1) to 230°F. Remove from fire and add (2), stir until smooth, and then transfer the whole to a mixing bowl. While mixing the batch at low speed, add (3). When the batch stiffens, add (4).

Chocolate Icing

Butter	10	oz
Corn oil	10	oz
Cocoa (partly dutched)	1¼	lb
Fondant	6¼	lb
Emulsifying type shortening	10	oz
Water	10	oz
Vanilla flavor	¼	oz

Mix the butter with the corn oil, and heat to 110°F. Stir in the cocoa and continue to mix until smooth. Add and incorporate thoroughly the fondant, shortening, water, and vanilla flavor.

Use this icing at a temperature of 90–95°F. If the icing is too thin, add simple syrup.

Chocolate Syrup

No. 1

Sugar	3	lb
Corn syrup	1½	lb
Water	3	lb
Cocoa powder	1½	lb
Vanilla extract	¾	oz

Bring the water to a strong boil and dissolve the sugars in it. Add the cocoa powder, rubbing it into a smooth paste. When cool, stir in the vanilla extract and continue stirring until the product is homogeneous.

No. 2

Sugar	2½	lb
Corn syrup	12	oz
Water	5¼	lb
Chocolate liquor, bitter	5	oz
Vanilla extract	½	oz

Place all the ingredients, except the vanilla extract, in a clean kettle and cook to a density of 30° Baumé. Stir in the vanilla extract when cool.

No. 3

Sugar	4	lb
Water	6	lb
Cocoa, good grade	13	oz
Salt	87	gr
Vanilla flavor	½	oz

Mix thoroughly the sugar and cocoa and add the water at 180°F. with constant stirring. Stir in the salt and heat to a rolling boil. Boil for about 3 minutes, cool to room temperature, and stir in the vanilla flavor. Store at 40°F. until used.

Chocolate Topping for Ice Cream, Pies and Bakery Cakes

	oz
Cocoa	3.0
Sugar	11.0
Nonfat dry milk solids	10.0
Vegetable fat	32.0
Water	44.0

Mix thoroughly. Pasteurize at 165°F. for about 30 minutes. Homogenize and cool. Whip it at 40°F. until the desired consistency is attained. Top the ice cream, pies, or baked cakes with this whipped product.

Chop Suey (To Freeze)

1	Onions, sliced	28.12 lb
	Lard	4.50 lb
2	Celery, ¼ inch pieces	18.00 lb
	Water	3.38 gal
3	Meat concentrate (Armour's Vitalox)	3.38 lb
4	Mushrooms, sliced	4.50 lb
	Green pepper, sliced	4.50 lb
	Bean sprouts	13.50 lb

Place (1) in a kettle and lightly brown it. Introduce (2) into (1) and simmer for ½ hour. Now add (3), dissolved in a little water. Next, add (4) and bring to a boil. Finally, thicken the whole batch with the following paste:

Cornstarch	1.50 lb
Cold water	2.25 pt

Mix thoroughly. Fill into suitable containers, and freeze.

Chow Mein Noodles

Flour	23.67 lb
Eggs	4.78 lb
Water	4.84 lb
Salt	8.00 oz

Mix thoroughly to form a smooth dough. Roll out the dough very thin, dry partially and cut into thin strips. Dry the resultant noodles, and then deep-fat fry them at 375°F.

Cinnamon Bun Smear

Sugar, light brown	25 oz
Sugar, granulated	25 oz
Corn syrup	16 oz
Honey	8 oz
Salt	48 gr
Baking soda	80 gr
Shortening	16 oz
Hot water (variable)	6 oz
Flavor	to suit

Mix the first six components thoroughly. Incorporate thoroughly the shortening. Add the hot water, then the flavor, and continue mixing until a smooth product is obtained.

Coconut Filling

1	Granulated sugar	3	lb
	Water	1¼	lb
	Corn syrup	1¾	lb
	Invert sugar	1¾	lb
	Salt	13	gr
2	Macaroon coconut	5	lb
3	Eggs	8	oz

Bring (1) to a rolling boil. Pour the hot mixture over (2) and mix together thoroughly, then set aside to cool. When cool, stir in (3). Use as required.

Coconut Mounds

	lb
Sugar	15.00
Water (variable—the finished mix should be firm)	6.00
Corn syrup	11.25
Invert syrup	15.00
Macaroon coconut, desiccated	30.00

Mix the sugar and water and heat to about 180°F., but do not boil. Add the syrups and mix thoroughly. Finally, incorporate thoroughly the desiccated macaroon coconut. Use a wire cut machine to deposit the cookies, or shape into mounds by hand, on paper-lined pans. Bake at 465°F. only long enough to brown the outside surface.

Do not allow the cookies to be baked through.

Coconut Macaroons

Sugar, granulated	5⅝	lb
Invert syrup	1¼	lb
Corn syrup	10	oz
Coconut, pulverized	6¼	lb
Salt	28	gr
Egg whites (variable)	3¼	lb
Vanilla flavor	to suit	

Mix the sugar, syrups, coconut, and salt, and heat to 170°F. Cool to about 120°F., then gradually work in the egg whites and flavor, and mix the whole mass thoroughly. Roll into balls by hand, and deposit these on paper-covered pans. Bake at about 375°F. Brown the macaroons but do not bake them through. If a softer macaroon is wanted, increase the amount of invert syrup.

Coconut Meringues

1	Egg whites	3.0	lb
	Sugar, granulated	19.2	oz
	Salt	64.0	gr
	Cream of tartar	65.6	gr
2	Cake flour	4.8	oz
	Sugar, powdered	1.5	lb

Whip (1) light. Fold in (2) thoroughly but carefully. Use a pastry bag and a plain tube for depositing mounds on greased and flour-dusted tins. Sprinkle macaroon coconut on the tops, allow them to dry for an hour or more, and then bake them in a cool oven (250–300°F.) until thoroughly dried. Put two units together with a liberal amount of apricot preserves between them.

Coconut Topping

Sugar, granulated	3	lb
Egg whites	6	oz
Macaroon coconut	1½	lb

Mix thoroughly the sugar with the egg whites. Add the macaroon coconut and continue mixing until a good distribution is effected. Spread a layer (about one inch thick) over a greased and flour-dusted pan and bake it until golden brown. Allow it to cool, then crush into small pieces. Use when required.

Coffee Crumb Cake

1	Sugar, granulated	4	lb
1	Honey	10⅔	oz
1	Brown sugar	10⅔	oz
1	Shortening, emulsifying type	2¼	lb
1	Non-fat dry milk	6⅔	oz
1	Eggs	8	oz
1	Salt	1½	oz
1	Flavor	to suit	
	Eggs (part yolks)	30⅔	oz
	Water (variable)	66⅔	oz
	Cake flour	94⅔	oz
	Baking powder	4⅓	oz

Mix the cake flour with the baking powder and sift it. Cream (1) thoroughly. Add while creaming (1) the eggs (part yolks), water, and the sifted flour mixture. Weigh out about 14 oz into tin pans, measuring 5½ x 10⅝ x 1⅝ inches; or into round tins measuring 8 x 1½ inches.

Top each one with about 2½ oz of moistened coconut. Bake at 370°F.

Coffee Crunch

Sugar, granulated	7½	lb
Water	4½	lb
Corn syrup	1⅞	lb
Salt	⅛	oz
Macaroon coconut	1½	lb
Nutmeats, chopped	1½	lb
Instant coffee	18	oz

Mix the sugar, water, corn syrup, and salt, and heat to 280°F. Stir in the coconut and nutmeats, and heat to 300°F. Add the instant coffee and stir thoroughly. Remove from fire, and pour onto pans in thin layers. Allow it to cool, then break into pieces of any desired size.

Coffee Extract

	oz
Ground, roasted coffee	6.0
Glycerin	24.0
Water	12.0

Mix the coffee with the glycerin, and heat to 90°C. Strain, and wash with the water, previously heated to 90°C., then filter.

Cole Slaw

Cabbage, white	14.00	lb
Carrots	2.00	lb
Salad dressing (see Salad Dressing)	3.25	lb
Milk	1.75	lb

Vinegar, white	10.50 oz
Sugar	7.00 oz
Salt	2.50 oz
Pepper, white	193.00 gr
Paprika, Spanish	0.50 oz

Shred the cabbage and carrots slowly in a slicer. Blend the salad dressing, milk, vinegar, salt, sugar, paprika, and pepper, in a small mixer equipped with an agitator. Next, stir in this dressing into the cabbage-carrot mixture, and mix thoroughly. Finally, fill the finished product into trays or into individual containers. Keep this product at a temperature around 36°F. in order to prevent spoilage. If a superior flavor is desired, store the cabbage-carrot mixture overnight in a charred wood barrel.

Concord Grape Oil

	oz
Methyl anthranilate, C.P.	2.00
Ethyl anthranilate	0.25
n-Butyl anthranilate	0.50
Cinnamyl anthranilate	0.50
Isoamyl butyrate	0.25
Ethyl oenanthate	0.80
Geranyl acetate	0.25
Ethyl acetate	8.00

Mix well and allow to stand a week or more.

Corn Muffins

	lb
Sugar	6.75
Invert sugar	1.50
Butter and shortening mixture	4.12
Eggs	3.00
Bread flour	12.00
Corn meal, fine	3.00
Corn meal, coarse	3.00
Baking powder	0.75
Milk	15.00

Cream the sugars and butter-shortening mixture for 5 minutes. Add slowly, while creaming, the eggs. Finally, add successively the bread flour, baking powder, corn meals, and milk, and continue mixing until a smooth batter is obtained. Spoon this batter into greased cups, and bake at 400°F.

Corn Relish

Corn (52–56 ears)	8 qt
Sweet red peppers, diced	4 pt
Green peppers, diced	4 pt
Celery, chopped	4 qt
Onion, sliced	4 cups
Sugar	32 oz
Vinegar (5–6% acetic acid)	1 gal
Salt	3 oz
Celery seed	2 oz
Mustard, dry	3 oz
Flour	4 oz
Water	1 pt

Remove the husks and silks from the corn, and place it in boiling water. Allow to simmer for about 10 minutes, then dip the ears into cold water. Drain and remove corn from the cob, then measure out 8 quarts of it. Mix the peppers with the celery, celery seed, onion, salt, sugar, and vinegar, and boil for about 15 minutes. Mix the mustard with the flour, stir in the water, and add this mustard-flour combination and the corn to the pepper mixture. Stir and boil for about 5 minutes. Pack the mixture into clean, hot, suitable containers, filling to ½ inch from top. Attach the lids and boil containers for about 10 minutes in boiling-water bath. Remove containers, and seal tightly. If more yellow color is desired, mix about 1 oz of curcuma powder with the mustard-flour mixture.

Cream Cheese Filling

1	Cream cheese	3.75 lb
1	Sugar, powdered	21.00 oz
1	Butter	6.00 oz
1	Corn starch	6.00 oz
1	Milk powder	6.00 oz
1	Salt	70.00 gr
1	Vanilla	to suit
	Eggs	9–12 oz

Mix (1) thoroughly. Add the eggs gradually while creaming (1) and continue mixing until the eggs are thoroughly incorporated. Use as required.

Cream Cheese Cookies

Butter	3 lb
Cream cheese	3 lb
Salt	½ oz
Flour, high gluten	1½ lb
Flour, pastry	1½ lb
Vanilla flavor	q.s.
Sugar, powdered	12 oz

Mix all the ingredients very thoroughly at a slow speed until the resultant product is smooth. Give the dough a 4-fold roll as for Danish pastry, then place it in a refrigerator for 20–24 hours. Roll out rather thin, then cut into small triangles, and roll up as for crescents. Place in pans and bake at about 375°F.

Cream Filling for Sugar Wafers

No. 1

Coconut butter	18.75 lb
Icing sugar	36.00 lb
Non-fat dry milk	1.50 lb
Citric acid, powdered	0.75 oz
Flavor	to suit

Stir the coconut butter until it is creamy and smooth. Mix the other ingredients and add them gradually to the cream, incorporating well after each addition.

No. 2

Coconut butter	20.0 lb
Icing sugar	18.0 lb
Non-fat dry milk	2.0 lb
Corn starch	13.0 oz
Salt	175.0 gr
Icing sugar	18.0 lb
Tartaric acid	44.0 gr
Flavor and color	to suit

Cream thoroughly the coconut butter at medium speed. Add very gradually while creaming, the icing sugar, dry milk, corn starch, and salt. Then stir in gradually the rest of the icing sugar until it is thoroughly incorporated, shift the mixer to high speed, and continue creaming until the desired consistency is obtained. Finally, stir in the tartaric acid, flavor, and color.

Cream Topping, Imitation

	oz
Gelatin	0.75
Hot water	7.50
Egg whites	25.50
Powdered sugar	12.00
Whipping cream	48.00
Powdered sugar	6.00

Stir the gelatin in the hot water until solution is complete. Whip the egg whites with the 12 oz of sugar until the batch is firm. Stir the gelatin solution into the egg whites until the mass stands up. Then, in another bowl, whip the cream together with the 6 oz of sugar. Finally, combine the two mixtures, and use as required.

Dehydrated Garlic

Remove the skin from the cloves of garlic, either by hand or by an abrasive machine, and then slice it. Place the sliced garlic into shallow receptacles, allowing 16 to 20 oz per square ft. of drying area, and dry it at a temperature not to exceed 140°F. When the moisture content is about 4%, remove it from the dryer, and finish the drying in a bin. Finally, grind the dried garlic in a hammer-mill, and put it through a sifting machine.

Diabetic Bread

Water	7½ lb
* Gluten flour	9 lb
Butter	5¼ oz
Salt	1½ oz
Yeast	9 oz

* Wheat flour from which a large part of the starch has been removed.

Mix all the ingredients until the dough is fully developed. Allow a rather long mixing period. Remove the dough from the mixer at about 80°F., and allow it to rise and mature (about 1¾ hours before scaling it off). Round out the scaled loaves, and allow them to rest, free from all drafts, for 20 minutes. Mold them into desired shape, and place them in lightly greased pans. Pan-proof them at a uniform temperature of 96–98°F., and a relative humidity of 82%. The pan-proofing period may range from 30 to 60 minutes.

Bake 1-pound loaves for 30 minutes at a temperature of 425°F. Each slice of bread contains about 47 calories.

Dietetic Jam-Like Product

Pitted fresh apricots, crushed	37.50 lb
Glycerin, U.S.P.	4.50 lb
Low-methoxyl pectin (Exchange #466)	9.00 oz
Water	30.00 lb
Citric acid, U.S.P.	4.00 oz
Sucaryl sodium	4.12 oz

Pour the glycerin into a stainless steel kettle and stir in the pectin. Add the water and stir until no lumps remain. Heat and add the fruit. Stir and boil for 5 minutes. Add the sucaryl and citric acid, and boil again for about 5 minutes. Pour into suitable containers while hot and seal immediately.

Doughnut Filling

Icing sugar	6⅖ lb
Butter	24 oz
Shortening, emulsifying type	24 oz
Salt	35 gr
Condensed milk, sweetened	14½ oz
Corn syrup	5 oz
Flavor	to suit

Cream thoroughly the sugar, butter, shortening, and salt. Mix and heat over hot water to 180°F., then stir in slowly the condensed milk, corn syrup, and flavor. Continue creaming at slow speed until the resultant product is of the desired consistency and volume.

Doughnut Glaze

No. 1

Gelatin, U.S.P.	¼ oz
Hot water	2 oz
Corn syrup	2½ oz
Cream of tartar	27½ gr
Water	8 oz
Icing sugar	3 lb
Fondant	8 oz

Dissolve the gelatin in the hot water. Place the corn syrup, cream of tartar, and water in a kettle, and bring the mixture to a boil. Add the gelatin solution and mix thoroughly. Finally, add the icing sugar and fondant, and continue to mix until the glaze is of a smooth consistency.

No. 2

Sugar	1 lb
Agar-Agar, U.S.P.	87½ gr
Pectin	87½ gr
Water (varied to produce the desired consistency of glaze)	8 oz
Powdered sugar	4 lb
Liquid citric acid	⅕ oz

Mix the first four ingredients and bring to a boil. Add the powdered sugar and mix until smooth. Finally, add the citric acid and mix thoroughly.

Dry Spaghetti Sauce Seasoning

Salt, finely ground	5.00 lb
Starch (cold water)	5.50 lb
Sugar, finely ground	2.50 lb
Dehydrated onion powder	1.85 lb
Dehydrated garlic powder	1.85 lb
Sweet basil, finely ground	1.20 lb
Baking soda	0.95 lb
Black pepper, finely ground	2.25 oz
Oregano, finely ground	1.50 oz
Fennel, finely ground	1.50 oz

Mix thoroughly. Add about ½ oz of this powdered seasoning to the following mixture:

Tomato paste	1 6-oz can

Water	2 6-oz cans
Refined corn oil	1 tablespoon

Mix and simmer for 15 minutes. This is sufficient for 8 oz spaghetti (before cooking).

Egg Twist, Jewish

Strong spring wheat flour	25	lb
Water (variable)	13	lb
Yeast	6½	oz
Eggs	26	oz
Corn oil	24	oz
Corn sugar	24	oz
Salt	5	oz
Diastatic malt	2	oz

Mix all the ingredients until a smooth dough is obtained. Remove the dough from the mixer when the temperature reaches about 80°F. Ferment it for about 1¾ hours. Knead the dough and allow to ferment an additional ¾ hour. Scale the dough into 6-oz individual pieces; make them round and allow about 20 minutes for proofing. Shape the individual strips, and braid them together. Brush with egg wash and bake.

English Fruit Cake

Sugar	1½	lb
Butter	1½	lb
Eggs	1½	lb
Flour	1⅞	lb
Currants, thoroughly cleaned	18	oz
Sultanas, thoroughly cleaned	15	oz
Mixed peel, finely cut	6	oz

Cream the sugar and butter and place it in a beating kettle. Add the eggs gradually, stirring and beating well after each addition. Finally, stir in the flour, currants, sultanas, and mixed peel. Blend thoroughly and weigh the mixture into a heavy paper-lined cake mould. Bake at a slow heat for about 3 hours.

Fig Bars

Shortening	3	lb
Sugar, powdered	6⅜	lb
Honey	12	oz
Salt	1	oz
Baking soda	1¼	oz
Vanilla flavor	to suit	
Milk, liquid (variable)	3	lb
Ammonia, U.S.P. (variable)	½	oz
Pastry flour	15	lb
Eggs	30	oz

Mix the shortening, sugar, honey, salt, soda, and vanilla flavor, and cream thoroughly. Add the eggs gradually while creaming. Mix the milk with the ammonia and add this to the cream—just stirring it in. Finally, stir in the pastry flour and continue mixing until the finished product is of smooth consistency.

Fig filling:

Figs (⅗ Smyrna, ⅖ Adriatic Calimyrna)	3½	lb
Invert syrup	28½	oz
Corn syrup	6	oz

Corn sugar	6 oz
Sugar, granulated	22½ oz

Soak the figs in water overnight, drain, and put them through a grinder. Mix the ground figs with the syrups and sugars, and continue mixing until the mass is smooth. Bake the bars in a medium oven. It is best that you have the special dough sheeting and the filling extrusion equipment used by commercial producers of fig bars.

Fig Filling for Cookies

Ground dried Calimyrna figs	6.0 lb
Dextrose	14.4 oz
Corn syrup	14.4 oz
Invert syrup	14.4 oz
Sugar, fine granulated	5.2 oz
Corn flakes, confectioner's (may be varied)	4.8 oz
Lemon and orange oil	to suit

Mix all the ingredients slowly for about 40 minutes. Ground dried apricots or ground dried peaches (or both) may be substituted for the figs, if desired.

Fig Jam for Fig Bars

	lb
Sugar	15.00
Water	4.88
Dextrose, U.S.P.	1.50
Figs, ground	16.13

Place the sugar, dextrose, and water in a clean kettle and boil to 222°F., then stir in the ground figs and continue to boil to 222°F.

Filling for Apfel Strudel

Cake crumbs, partially toasted	¾ lb
Puffed raisins, finely chopped	1⅛ lb
Chopped apples	3¾ lb
Butter	6 oz
Sugar	12 oz

Mix the first three ingredients thoroughly. Roll and stretch the dough gently until it is paper-thin and in an oblong shape. Spread the crumb-apple-raisin mixture and some pieces of butter evenly over the dough, then place on top some sugar and specks of butter. Leave some dough at each end and fold this over to keep the filling in. Brush the top with butter, besprinkle it with sugar, and bake at 400°F.

Filling for Ravioli

Beef, ground	5.250 lb
Parmesan cheese, grated	11.250 oz
Eggs, whipped	1.625 lb
Butter	0.750 lb
Parsley, minced	0.500 oz
Lemon peel, grated	0.250 oz
Salt and pepper	to suit

Blend the ingredients thoroughly into a smooth mixture; package it and freeze.

Flavor Compounds

Use isobutyl furyl propionate and methyl beta-methylthiol propionate as good modifiers in pineapple flavor compositions.

Florentines
(A Continental Favorite)

	oz
Sugar, granulated	21.00
Cream	15.00
Almonds, finely chopped	12.00
Orange peel, candied and finely chopped	9.00
Butter	1.75
Flour	3.00

Mix and cook to 220°F. Bag the mixture out, as pats 1⅛ to 1¼ inch in diameter, onto slightly greased, flour-dusted pans. Place small heaps of the following topping on the distended units:

Topping Mixture

	oz
Sugar, granulated	9.00
Almonds, finely chopped	6.00
Cherries, chopped	6.00
Cream	4.50
Flour	1.50
Egg whites	1.13
Corn syrup	0.75

Mix and cook to 235°F.

Bake the Florentines at about 365°F. Use a spatula to remove the cookies from the pans immediately after baking. Place them on a level surface to cool. When cool, cover with a chocolate coating.

Flour for Frozen Pies

Use a good grade of unbleached pastry flour. Its ash content should run about 0.44%, and its protein should run from 9.0 to 9.5%. The pH of the flour should be about 6.0.

Fluffy Icing

Granulated sugar	4.0 lb
Water	19.2 oz
Dextrose	6.4 oz
Egg whites	1.6 pt
Standardized invert sugar	12.8 oz
Vanilla	3.2 dr

Mix together the sugar, water, and dextrose, and heat to 236–242°F. Brush down the sides of the container to make sure that all sugar grains are thoroughly dissolved. While this combination is being cooked, place the invert sugar, egg whites, and vanilla in a beating kettle. Arrange the time of beating the eggs so that they will be about ¾ beaten up by the time the temperature of 236–242°F. is attained. Pour the boiling syrup into the beaten eggs very slowly, and continue to beat on high speed until the desired consistency is obtained.

For a quick drying surface, stir in from ¾ to 1½ lb of icing sugar before the machine is stopped. Apply this icing while it is warm. It can be used for a wide variety of icings and icing fillings. Any desired type of icing may be produced by adding chopped fruits, jams, preserved fruits, melted chocolate, nuts, or other ingredients.

Fondant

No. 1

Granulated sugar	12.75
Invert syrup	0.75
Corn syrup	1.50
Water	3.38

Place the sugars and water in a kettle, and cook to 240–244°F. As the cooking proceeds, wet a pastry brush with water, and brush this against the sides of the kettle to keep the sugar from graining. When the thermometer registers the proper temperature (240–244°F.), remove from the fire and pour the mass into a fondant beater. Allow the syrup to cool to about 110°F., then agitate. Continue the agitation until the syrup thickens to a firm chalky white mass. Place the finished fondant in sterile containers.

To use fondant for a dipping icing, heat it over a hot water bath to a temperature of approximately 100°F. (If heated much beyond 100°F., the fondant will lose its gloss.) If the fondant is too stiff for easy pouring, thin it to proper consistency with the following simple syrup:

Cane sugar	2 lb
Corn syrup	6 oz
Water	11 oz

Mix the sugar, syrup, and water, and bring it just to boiling. Add color and flavor to fondant icing as required.

No. 2

	lb
Granulated sugar	15.00
Corn syrup	3.00
Invert syrup	1.50
Water	3.75

Place all the ingredients in a kettle, and cook to 242°F. As the cooking proceeds, wash the sugar from the sides of the kettle in order to prevent graining. When the proper temperature is reached, remove from the fire and pour the mass into a fondant beater. Let the syrup cool to about 125°F., then agitate. Continue the agitation until the syrup thickens to a firm chalky white mass. Place the finished fondant into sterile containers.

No. 3

	lb
Sugar, granulated	15
Water	4½
Corn syrup	2⅝

Mix and cook to a temperature of 240°F. Wash down the sides of kettle as cooking proceeds. Remove from the fire and pour the mass into a mixing bowl. Besprinkle the top of the syrup in mixing bowl lightly with cold water, and then allow it to stand until it has cooled to about 110°F. Start to agitate at slow-to-medium speed until the batch becomes chalky white and firm. As soon as fondant turns white and begins to harden, remove it from the mixing bowl and place it in sterile containers. Allow the fondant to mellow for several day before using it.

Food Antioxidants

Butylated hydroxyanisole and propyl gallate are excellent preservatives for natural peanut oil.

Hydroquinone is best for hydrogenated oil.

Butyl-*p*-hydroxybenzoate is excellent for coconut oil.

Di-*tert*-butyl-*p*-cresol may be used as an antioxidant and preservative to prevent rancidity in lard and shortenings—all animal fats. This compound meets all requirements of the Food and Drug Administration as a food additive. It can be obtained from the Koppers Co., Pittsburgh, Penn.

The following anti-oxidants should retard or inhibit the development of rancidity in batches of cream:

Butylated hydroxyanisole (BHA): 0.02% in propylene glycol without propyl gallate.

Brewers' yeast: 1–1.5%.

Add about 1% of glycerin as a protection against the development of free fatty acids (hydrolytic rancidity).

Frappé

Corn syrup	15	lb
Invert sugar	15	lb
Egg albumen	4¾	oz
Water	9½	oz

Cook the corn syrup to 245°F. Add the invert sugar and mix thoroughly. Dissolve the egg albumen in the water, and beat it into the hot mixture. The resultant product yields about 6 pounds to the gallon, and its moisture content is about 16 per cent. This frappé will not separate, nor grain prematurely, nor ferment.

French Creme Icing

1	Icing Sugar	7½	lb
1	Butter	3½	lb
1	Salt	¼	oz
1	Vanilla extract	1	oz
	Condensed milk (variable)	1¼	pt

Mix (1) thoroughly at medium speed, and heat to 140°F.; then stir in the condensed milk very slowly and at slow speed. Continue creaming at slow speed until the resultant product has the proper consistency for icing.

French Fried Popcorn

Place some coconut oil (m.p. 76°F.) in a steam-jacketed kettle, and heat it to 380°F. Place the corn in a sieve and submerge it in the hot oil. When the corn stops popping, remove the sieve from the oil, and empty the popped corn on a metal-topped table. Add some salt, and separate the unpopped corn. Finally package into moisture-proof, heat-sealable bags.

Frozen Dessert of the Mellorine Type

Cocoanut oil	13½ lb
Powdered skim milk	41⅗ lb
Sugar	41 lb
Irish moss stabilizer	4⅓ oz
Glyceryl monostearate (Aldo 33)	4⅓ oz
Water	171 lb

Mix all the components, pasteurize and homogenize them, then cool to below 40°F., and store at that temperature. All kinds of fruits may be added to this product.

Fruit Cookies

1	Sugar	2¼ lb
	Shortening	2¼ lb
	Eggs	12 oz
	Mace	3/16 oz
	Vanilla	⅜ oz
	Baking soda	¾ oz
	Salt	1 oz
	Water	6 oz
	Cake flour	4½ lb
	Raisins	2¼ lb
	Candied cherries, finely chopped	12 oz
	Ground orange	6 oz

Cream (1), then stir in the flour and water. Finally stir in the cherries, ground orange, and raisins. Cut the dough into pieces the size of a walnut, flatten them with the hand, brush them with egg wash, and bake at about 380°F.

Fudge

No. 1: Vanilla

Sugar	6 lb
Corn syrup	2 lb
Sweet cream, 18%	4 pt
Butter	4 oz
Evaporated milk	2 pt
Vanilla flavor	to suit

Mix all the ingredients and cook to 242°F. Remove from the fire and keep stirring while adding the vanilla flavor. When the mass is thick, pour it onto oiled wax paper spread over a wooden tabletop. When cold, mark with cutter and cut into squares.

This recipe may be used for making chocolate fudge by adding 16 oz of sweet chocolate and 8 oz of chocolate liquor at the end of the cooking.

No. 2: Chocolate

1	Granulated sugar	45.00 lb
	Water	12.00 lb
2	Corn syrup	22.50 lb
	Invert sugar	7.50 lb
	Skim milk solids (in solution)	0.75 lb
	Salt	1.50 oz
3	Extra-high-strength gelatin in 2¼ lb of hot water	0.60 lb
4	Chocolate liquor and flavor	9.00 lb

Bring (1) to a boil and add (2). Continue to boil to 236°F. Cool the batch to 165°F. and add (3). Stir the mass thoroughly and add

(4). Whip the whole at 130°F. until the weight per gallon is 9 lb, and deposit it in trays.

No. 3: Maple

Sugar	18.0	lb
Sugar, dark brown	7.5	lb
Corn syrup	4.5	lb
Sorbitol solution	3.0	lb
Vegetable butter, m.p. 92° (refined coconut oil)	18.0	oz
Cream (20%)	9.0	pt
Evaporated milk	3.0	pt
Maple flavor		q.s.
Butter	1.5	lb
* Mazetta	18.0	oz
Salt	0.75	oz
Walnuts or pecans	6.00	lb
Egg whites, fresh	3.00	oz

Mix the sugars, syrup, sorbitol, vegetable butter, and cream, and heat to boiling point. Add the evaporated milk and flavor and cook until the temperature reaches 244°F. Remove from fire and pour into a clean cream beater (preferably ball-type). Allow it to cool to 150°F., then add the butter, mazetta, and salt and start the beater. As soon as signs of graining appear, add the walnuts. When it appears that the batch would hold its shape if the beating were stopped, add the egg whites, and allow about four more turns. Ladle the mass out immediately in "globs" on paper-lined trays, and slice these "globs" for packaging.

* Mazetta

Caramel starch	3.50	oz
Water	1.50	pt
Glucose	4.50	lb
Sugar	2.25	lb
Albumen	2.00	oz
Water	4.00	oz

Mix the starch with the water and bring to a slow boil for about 30 minutes. Cook the glucose and sugar to 236°F. Add the albumen to the water in a separate container and whip it. Finally, add the glucose-sugar solution, then the starch solution, and stir thoroughly.

Fudge Bar

Cane sugar	36	oz
Milk solids, non-fat	28	oz
Cocoa powder	6	oz
Gelatin, U.S.P.	1	oz
Water	1	gal

Place all the ingredients in a clean kettle, stir constantly and heat to 238°F. Remove the heat and stir the mass until it begins to thicken. Pour it into molds and freeze.

Fudge Base

Microfine cocoa (10–12% fat)	9	lb
Shortening	8	lb
Corn syrup, 43° Baumé	4	lb
Seaken Type 104 Stabilizer	1	oz
Icing sugar	10	oz
Lecithin	¾	oz
Vanillin	54	gr
Ethyl vanillin	55	gr

Melt the shortening at 120°F., add the corn syrup, and cream thoroughly. Mix the stabilizer with the icing sugar and add these with one-half of the lecithin and the cocoa. When the mass is stiff, add the remaining lecithin and then the vanillins. Use this fudge base for making icings.

Such an icing may be prepared as follows:

Fudge base	8 oz
Hot water	8 oz
Icing sugar	30 oz

Blend this mixture until the resultant product is smooth.

Fudge Icing

No. 1

1	Fresh milk	17.0 oz
	Granulated sugar	3.0 lb
	Corn syrup	8.0 oz
2	Water	3.0 oz
	Gelatin, U.S.P.	0.5 oz
3	Bittersweet chocolate, melted	1.0 lb
	Shortening	7.0 oz
	Cocoa butter	2.0 oz
	Corn oil	0.5 oz
4	Fondant	3.0 lb
	Vanilla	q.s.

Cook (1) to 226°F. Add (2) and stir thoroughly. Cool this mixture to about 110°F., then add (3), and mix thoroughly. Finally add (4), and mix until a smooth product is obtained. Use this icing at 95° to 100°F.

No. 2

Sugar	6.0 lb
Sugar, brown	1.0 lb
Corn syrup	4.0 lb
Milk and cream	4.8 pt
Chocolate base	1.8 lb
Salt	0.5 oz
Butter	6.4 oz
Vanilla	0.5 oz
Agar-Agar solution	2.4 oz

Mix thoroughly all the components and boil to 228°F. Reheat as required.

Agar-Agar Solution

Agar-Agar, U.S.P.	88 gr
Water	1 pt

Mix thoroughly, and bring solution just to boiling.

Fudge Type Icing

Fondant	7.50 lb
Chocolate liquor, melted	19.50 oz
Condensed milk, sweetened	6.00 oz
Butter, melted	6.00 oz
Corn oil, refined	0.75 oz
Salt	40.00 gr
Vanilla flavor	to suit

Mix ingredients thoroughly. Place in a double boiler and heat to 100°F. before using it. If thinning is necessary, add simple syrup to get the desired consistency. Do not use water under any circumstances.

Ginger Ale Oil

Oleo-Resin ginger	6.0 oz
Ginger oil	2.0 oz

Citral, C.P.		2.0 oz
Aldehyde C_8	10% in alcohol	1.0 dr
Aldehyde C_9	10% in alcohol	2.0 dr
Aldehyde C_{10}	10% in alcohol	1.0 dr

Mix well and allow to stand a week or more.

Gingerbread

1	Sugar	45 oz
1	Shortening	15 oz
1	Eggs, mixed	5 oz
1	Baking soda	1¾ oz
1	Salt	½ oz
1	Ginger, ground	1¼ oz
1	Cinnamon, ground	¾ oz
	Eggs, mixed	22½ oz
	Light molasses	88 oz
	Cake flour	5 lb
	Bread flour	22½ oz
	Cream of tartar	⅝ oz
	Water (variable)	60 oz

Mix and cream (1) thoroughly. While creaming, add gradually, first the eggs and then the light molasses, and incorporate them thoroughly. Sift together the cake flour and bread flour, and add it to the mixture, alternating with the cream of tartar dissolved in the water. Continue the mixing until the batter is smooth. Scale as required, and bake at about 375°F.

Glaze for Baked Goods

1	Granulated sugar	1⅓ lb
1	Corn syrup	⅔ lb
1	Water	1 lb
1	Potassium bitartrate, U.S.P. (cream of tartar)	⅙ oz
	Gelatin, U.S.P.	⅔ oz
	Icing sugar	5⅓ lb

Bring (1) to a boil. Cool slightly, then stir in the gelatin which has been soaked in 5½ oz of water. Finally, stir in the icing sugar and any desirable flavor. Thin down with the following hot simple syrup if necessary.

Simple Syrup

Sugar	2 lb
Corn syrup	8 oz
Water	1 pt

Mix and stir, and heat just to boiling.

Glaze for Banana Cream Pies

Water	3⅛ lb
Sugar, granulated	23 oz
Agar-Agar, U.S.P.	1 oz
Glycerin	5 oz
Vegetable oil	2 oz
Apricot pulp	3¼ lb
Sugar, granulated	3¼ lb
Corn syrup	8 oz
Lemon juice	½ oz

Soak the agar-agar and sugar in the water for about 11 hours, then place them in a copper kettle and cook until the agar-agar is in solution. Add the glycerin and oil, mix thoroughly for five seconds, and then remove from the fire. Place the pulp, sugar, corn syrup, and lemon juice, in a separate kettle and bring them to a boil. Stir frequently while cooking, and continue to cook until the mass thickens. Now add the agar-agar mixture, and cook quickly for a few minutes. Remove from the fire, and pass the mass through a fine sieve. Use as required.

Never use a metal knife for slicing bananas; use a string or a wooden blade.

Glaze for Fruit Cakes

Sugar, granulated	2 lb
Acacia, U.S.P.	8 oz
Apricot jam	1⅓ lb
Corn syrup	1⅓ lb
Water	34⅔ oz

Mix the sugar and acacia thoroughly. Stir in the jam, corn syrup, and water, and bring slowly to a boil. Finally, remove from the fire, and force the mass, while hot, through a fine screen.

Glaze the cakes as they are removed from the oven.

Glaze for Hams

Karo corn syrup (2 5-lb cans)	10 lb
Gelatin, U.S.P.	4 lb
Paprika	12 oz
Cloves	8 oz
Water	2 gal
Caramel, N.F.	4 lb

Place the first five ingredients in a jacketed kettle and heat to about 125°F. Add the caramel, for its caramelizing effect, and mix well. You may increase or decrease the amount of caramel, depending on the color desired. Dip the hams into this glaze or apply it with a brush. This glaze sets immediately.

Grape Oil

	oz
Methyl anthranilate, C.P.	2.000
Ethyl oenanthate	0.800
Cinnamyl anthranilate	0.500
Iso-butyl caproate	0.250
Geranyl acetate	0.125
Ethyl acetate	8.000

Mix well and allow to stand a week or more.

Halvah Candy

Sugar	30.0 lb
Water	38.4 oz
Glucose	6.0 lb
Cobee 92 coconut fat	3.6 lb
Sesame seed	36.0 lb
Salt	2.4 oz

Place the water, sugar, and glucose in a double-action, agitator-type, steam-jacketed kettle, and cook to 268–270°F. Stir in the coconut fat. Finally, shut off the steam, and add the sesame seed and salt. Pour the finished batch onto a cooling slab. Flatten it to desired thickness and cut to any desired size.

Hard Candy (Coffee)

Granulated sugar	7.00 lb
Water	1.68 lb
Invert sugar	11.20 oz
Dry, soluble coffee (this can be varied to suit one's taste)	6.00 oz

Place the sugars and water in a gas-fired copper vessel and gradually bring to a boil. Wash down the sugar crystals adhering to the sides while bringing it to a boil. Cover the boiling syrup for 3 minutes. Remove the cover, and quickly heat to 320°F. Pour the batch onto a greased cooling slab. Wait 3 minutes, then turn in the cool edges. When partly cooled, fold the batch, add the dry coffee, and then work it into the hot portion of the batch. Finally, form into suitable shapes and cut. Allow it to cool, and then wrap.

Honey Cake

Honey	7½ lb
Eggs	2⅝ lb
Water	3 lb
Rye flour, medium	3¾ lb
Cake flour, good grade	3¾ lb
Baking soda	1⅛ oz

Mix and sift the flour and baking soda. Mix thoroughly the honey with the eggs. Add the water and the flour mixture alternately and mix thoroughly to effect a smooth mass. Weigh as required and then bake at approximately 370°F.

Honey Chiffon Cake

Cake flour	40½ oz
Baking powder	2$\frac{1}{16}$ oz
Honey	1½ lb
Salt	¾ oz
Egg yolks	21 oz
Corn oil	21 oz
Water	19½ oz
Vanilla	to suit
Water (variable)	6 oz
Egg whites	42 oz
Cream of tartar	⅜ oz
Sugar	30 oz

Mix thoroughly by sifting the flour, baking powder, honey and salt. Add the egg yolk, corn oil, and water and stir until thoroughly blended. Add the vanilla and water and stir thoroughly, but do not over-aerate. Beat the egg whites, cream of tartar, and sugar at medium speed until stiff. Finally, fold the batter into the beaten egg whites, thoroughly but carefully. Scale as needed and bake at 350°F.

Honey Cookies

1	Diamalt	24 oz
	Honey	24 oz
	Egg yolks	6 oz
	Allspice	41 gr
	Salt	½ oz
	Baking soda	1⅛ oz
	Ammonium bicarbonate	¾ oz
	Water	10½ oz
	Cake flour	39 oz
	Bread flour	39 oz
	Sugar	1½ oz

Blend (1) together. Dissolve the baking soda and bicarbonate in the water, and stir this into (1). Finally, stir in the flour and sugar and mix thoroughly. Roll out the finished dough and cut with a cookie cutter. After baking, brush slightly with the following icing:

Egg whites	3 oz
Water	9 oz
Sugar, 6X	q.s.
Vanilla	to suit

Whip the egg whites lightly. Dissolve enough sugar in the water to

make a thick syrup, then add the hot syrup to the beaten egg whites, and whip up light. Stir the vanilla into the hot syrup.

Honey Cake (German)

1	Shortening	24 oz
1	Safflower oil	1½ oz
1	Sugar, granulated	2¼ lb
1	Sugar, brown	24 oz
1	Honey	12 oz
1	Baking soda	1⅛ oz
1	Molasses	9 oz
1	Cinnamon	⅜ oz
1	Ginger	⅜ oz
1	Salt	½ oz
	Eggs	24 oz
	Pastry flour, unbleached	4½ lb

Mix (1) and cream thoroughly. While creaming add the eggs gradually. Finally, add the flour and continue mixing until the batch is smooth. Place it in a cool room to age for an hour, then roll it out and cut it as desired. Bake at about 375°F.

Honey Flavor (Synthetic)

	oz
Ethyl phenylacetate	5.250
Propyl phenylacetate	4.500
Phenyl ethyl salicylate	1.500
Phenyl ethyl phenyl acetate	1.050
Allyl phenylacetate	0.750
Ethyl pelargonate	0.750
Vanillin	0.300
Protovanol "C"	0.150
Dimethylbenzylcarbinyl acetate	0.150
Rose oil, Bulgarian	0.150
p-Methyl tetrahydroquinoline	0.225
Methylnonyl acetaldehyde, 5%	0.075
Cyclotene, 10%	0.075
Exaltolide, 2%	0.075

Mix and shake well. Allow it to stand a week or more with frequent shaking.

Honey Paste

		oz
1	Sugar, granulated	12½
1	Sugar, brown	12½
1	Baking soda	⅛
1	Salt	⅛
1	Corn syrup	5
1	Honey	5
1	Water, hot (variable)	3
	Butter	4
	Margarine	4½

Mix (1) together, then stir in the butter and margarine, and continue to mix until a smooth paste is obtained.

Hydroxymethylcyclopentenone

Hydroxymethylcyclopentenone is a crystalline solid having a maple-licorice taste with a walnut note. It is sold under the trade name of Cyclotene. Use 10–15 parts of Cyclotene per million parts to give a maple flavor; and only 5 parts of cyclotene per million parts for a walnut flavor.

Ice Cream Mix

No. 1: 4% Fat

Cream, 40%	7½ lb
Concentrated skim milk, 30%	31½ lb
Cane sugar	9 lb
Corn syrup solids	4½ lb
Stabilizer	6 oz
Water	22⅛ lb

No.2: 4% Fat

	lb
Butter	3.53
Dry skim milk	8.51
Sugar	12.00
Gelatin, U.S.P.	0.38
Egg yolks (fresh yolks)	0.75
Water	49.85

No. 3: 6% Fat

	lb
Butter	5.25
Dry skim milk	9.19
Sugar	12.00
Gelatin, U.S.P.	0.34
Glyceryl monostearate (Aldo 28)	0.11
Water	48.07

No. 4: 10% Fat

	lb
Butter	8.81
Dry skim milk	8.50
Sugar	12.00
Gelatin, U.S.P.	0.34
Glyceryl monostearate (emulsifier)	0.11
Water	45.24

No. 5: 10% Fat

Cream, 40%	57½ lb
Skim milk	125½ lb
Nonfat dry milk solids	11¼ lb
Sugar	34½ lb
Stabilizer	10 oz
Emulsifier	5 oz

Mix together all the ingredients in a pasteurizing tank and heat to 155°F. for 30 minutes. Homogenize at 2500 lb pressure, then cool to below 40°F., and store at that temperature.

No. 6: 10½% Fat
(Soft)

Cream, 40%	21.0 lb
Concentrated skim milk, 30%	29.0 lb
Liquid sugar	17.0 lb
Water	20.0 lb
Egg yolk, powdered	8.0 oz
Stabilizer	4.4 oz

Mix the skim milk with the water and stir in the liquid sugar, powdered egg yolk, and stabilizer. Now stir in the 40% cream, and mix well. Pasteurize this mixture and then homogenize it. Allow it to cool, then place the mixture in a freezing tank where it is beaten until smooth. Finally, stir in any desired flavor.

Pasteurize at 165°F. for about 30 minutes. Homogenize at 3500 pounds pressure.

No. 7: 12% Fat

	lb
Butter	10.50
Dry skim milk	8.10

Sugar	12.00
Gelatin, U.S.P.	0.30
Emulsifier	0.11
Water	44.17

Disperse the emulsifier and gelatin in hot water. Dissolve the sugar and skim milk in the water. Finally, add the butter and proceed as outlined under Ice Cream Mix, 14% Fat.

No. 8: 12% Fat

Cream, 40%	24 lb
Concentrated skim milk, 30%	24⅘ lb
Cane sugar	10⅖ lb
Corn syrup solids	3⅕ lb
Stabilizer	4½ oz
Water	16⅘ lb

No. 9: 12% Fat

Cream, 40%	73.6 lb
Nonfat dry milk	15.6 lb
Stabilizer	9.6 oz
Sugar	33.2 lb
Water	61.0 lb

Dissolve the dry milk, stabilizer, and sugar in the water, then stir in the cream and mix well.

No. 10: 14% Fat

Cream, 40%	28 lb
Concentrated skim milk, 30%	21⅗ lb
Cane sugar	10⅖ lb
Corn syrup solids	3⅕ lb
Stabilizer	4⅒ oz
Water	16⅗ lb
Flavor	to suit

Mix the skim milk with the water, and dissolve in it the sugar, corn syrup solids, and stabilizer. Stir in the 40% cream, and mix well. Pour this mixture into a tank in which it is mixed and pasteurized, then homogenized. Allow it to cool, then place the mixture in a freezing tank where it is beaten until smooth. Stir in the flavor, and nuts or fruits if so desired. Remove the ice cream from the freezing tank when partially frozen, and pack it into containers which are then stored in a refrigerating room until the cream is hard.

Ice Cream

	lb
Butter, unsalted	25.0
Nonfat dry milk solids	22.0
Sugar	32.0
Stabilizer and emulsifier	1.0
Water	120.0

Ice Cream, Chocolate

Cream, 36%	125.0 lb
Nonfat dry milk solids	7.0 lb
Sugar	37.0 lb
Corn syrup solids, dried	5.0 lb
Cocoa	10.0 lb
Whole milk	5.0 lb
Stabilizer	4.0 oz
Water	60.0 lb

Pasteurize all the components at 160°F. for about 30 minutes, homogenize at 2500 lb pressure, and cool quickly to 40°F. or lower. Use water that is free of excessive amounts of iron and sulfur. See procedure as outlined under Ice Cream, 14% fat.

Ice Cream with Vegetable Oil

	lb
Sugar	6.00
Corn syrup solids	2.50
Milk solids, nonfat	6.25
Stabilizer	0.20
Vegetable oil (Safflower oil)	4.50
Water, enough to make	50.00

Mix the milk solids with the water, and dissolve in it the sugar, corn syrup solids, and stabilizer. Stir in the vegetable oil, and mix thoroughly. Pasteurize and homogenize in the same manner as for regular ice cream.

Ice Cream Stabilizers

Commercial stabilizers contain one or more of the following colloids:

Carboxymethylcellulose, Irish moss derivatives, gelatin, locust bean gum, guar seed gum, algin derivatives.

Icing for Cookies

Fondant	3¾ lb
Invert syrup	1½ oz
Corn syrup	1½ oz
Butter, melted	3 oz
Corn oil, refined	2¼ oz

Blend together all the ingredients. Heat to 105°F. before applying this icing. If necessary, thin down with simple syrup.

Icing for Dipping

Fondant	9⅜ lb
Butter, melted	1½ lb
Non-fat dry milk	3 oz
Corn oil, refined	¾ oz
Salt	18 gr
Simple syrup	3¾ oz

Mix all the ingredients thoroughly at a slow speed until smooth. Heat this icing to 100°F. before using it. If too thick, thin it down with simple syrup.

Icing for Doughnuts, etc.

Granulated sugar	4 lb
Water	2 lb
Corn syrup	9⅓ oz
Gelatine, U.S.P.	2–3 oz
Cold water	10⅔ oz
Icing sugar	4 lb
Fondant	4 lb
Salt	36 gr
Flavor	to suit

Bring the granulated sugar, water, and corn syrup to a rolling boil, and cook for about 3 minutes.

Soak the gelatine in the cold water for about 20 minutes. Add the gelatine to the solution of sugar-water-corn syrup, and stir until all is in solution. Now add the icing sugar, and mix thoroughly for about 5 minutes. Finally add the fondant, salt, and flavor, and mix for about 5 minutes until a very smooth product is obtained. Use the icing while warm. If too thick, thin it down with simple syrup.

Icing for Layer Cakes

Sugar, powdered	10 lb
Shortening	2 lb
Butter	1 lb
Nonfat milk solids	12 oz
Salt	1 oz
Vanilla	1 oz
Water	2 lb

Place all the ingredients except the water in a beater-type mixer, and cream thoroughly for about 5 minutes. Finally add slowly the water, and continue to cream until the batch is light.

Icing for Wedding Cake

	oz
Sugar	37
Water	16
Cream of tartar	1/8
Agar-Agar, powdered	1/16
Egg whites	17
Sugar	4
Flavor	to suit
Icing sugar	24

Bring the water to a boil and dissolve the cream of tartar in it, then add the sugar-agar mixture slowly and cook to 240°F. Mix the egg whites, sugar, and flavor, and whip lightly. Add the cooked syrup to this, and continue the beating until meringue is of proper consistency. The beating of the egg white mixture should be timed so that its consistency is reached at the same time the syrup reaches the desired temperature. Allow the meringue to cool to about 100°F., then stir in vigorously the icing sugar. Use a trace of certified liquid Marine Blue color in order to enhance the whiteness of the icing.

Vanilla (Synthetic) (Army and Navy Specifications)

Vanillin	3/4 oz
Ethyl vanillin	1/4 oz
Protovanol "C"	5 1/2 cc
Propylene glycol, U.S.P.	1 1/2 pt
Caramel	1 1/4 dr
Water, to make	1 gal

Heat the propylene glycol, and dissolve in it the vanillin, ethyl vanillin, and Protovanol "C". Dissolve the caramel in the water, and add this to the vanillin solution with vigorous stirring.

Icing for Cakes and Pies

1	Sugar	3 1/3 lb
	Fresh milk	1 1/6 lb
	Corn syrup	9 1/3 oz
2	Butter	10 1/2 oz
	Bitter sweet chocolate, melted	17 1/3 oz
	Fondant	3 1/3 lb
	Flavor	to suit

Place (1) in a clean kettle and cook to 228°F., then remove from the fire and allow it to cool to about 115°F. Stir in (2) and mix thoroughly. Use icing while warm. If necessary, thin it down with simple syrup.

Invert Syrup

Sugar	15	lb
Water	5	lb
Tartaric acid, U.S.P.	3/8	oz
or		
Cream of tartar, U.S.P.	3/4	oz
dissolved in water	12	oz

Place the sugar and water in a steam-jacketed kettle and bring the contents to a boil. As soon as the boiling point is reached, add the tartaric acid or the cream of tartar previously dissolved in the 12 oz of water. Allow the mass to boil slowly for 30 minutes more. Remove the heat and cool as quickly as possible.

Jams

To prevent crystallization in jams, add about 1/2 oz of glycerin to each pint of jam. The resultant product will be more transparent and less sugar will be required.

Jelly Rolls

Eggs	4	lb
Sugar	4	lb
Salt	1/2	oz
Cake flour, high moisture content	4 3/4	lb
Sugar	10 1/2	oz
Baking powder	2	oz
Butter	1 1/3	lb
Milk	29 1/3	oz
Flavor	to suit	

Mix the eggs, sugar, and salt, and heat over hot water to 140°F., stirring constantly to prevent coagulation of the eggs. Then whip until the beaten mass will hold a crease for a few seconds when drawing a spatula through the top of the batter. The crease should not close completely for 25 seconds. Mix and sift the cake flour, baking powder, and sugar, and fold this carefully into the whipped mass. Finally, mix the butter, milk, and flavor, heating slowly until the butter is melted, and then fold this in, carefully but thoroughly. Scale into standard sheet pans, 18 by 26 inches and bake at 380°F. Roll as usual. This makes a jelly roll of excellent keeping qualities.

Jumble Cookies

1	Sugar, granulated	4 1/2	lb
1	Butter	3	lb
1	Shortening, vegetable	1 1/2	lb
1	Salt	1/4	oz
1	Flavor	to suit	
	Eggs	18	oz
	Milk, liquid	12	oz
	Cake flour	7 1/8	lb
	Baking powder	3/8	oz

Cream (1) thoroughly. Add the eggs during creaming, and continue creaming until light. Stir in the milk. Sift together the flour and baking powder, and incorporate the mixture into the creamed mass. Continue to mix until smooth. Deposit on paper-covered pans through a star-shaped tube into any desired shape and size. Bake at about 390°F.

Kaiser Rolls

Hard bread flour	20	lb
Water (variable)	10	lb
Yeast	8⅘	oz
Sugar	8⅖	oz
Malt	8	oz
Salt	3	oz
Corn oil, refined	11⅗	oz
Egg yolk	12	oz

Mix all the ingredients until a smooth dough is obtained. Remove the dough from the mixer at about 78°F., and allow it to ferment for about 2½ hours. Puncture, then take the dough to the work-bench after about 45 minutes, and shape it as required. Bake, in the presence of low-pressure steam, at about 425°F.

Kisses

Sorghum syrup	4½	lb
Sugar	3	lb
Vinegar	4½	oz
Butter	6	oz
Vanilla flavor	¾	oz

Place the first four components into a kettle, and cook to 245°F. Remove kettle from fire, stir in the flavor, and pour onto a greased slab. As soon as the candy can be handled, pull it on a candy hook, and cut into any desired size.

Lemon Chiffon Pie

Boiling water	7½	lb
Gelatin, lemon flavored	2¼	lb
Eggs	1⅞	lb
Egg yolks	6	oz
Salt	55	gr
Lemon juice (variable)	21	oz
Lemon rind	1⅛	oz

Dissolve the gelatin in the boiling water. Add slowly the eggs, egg yolks, and salt to the hot gelatin solution while beating it lightly. Stir in the lemon juice and lemon rind, then chill while stirring occasionally until the mass thickens. When thickened, fold this mass into the meringue which is made as follows:

Meringue

Egg whites	3	lb
Granulated sugar	1½	lb

Whip the egg whites to a foam. Add the sugar gradually and continue whipping until wet peaks form. Fill about 1½ lb of the finished product into prebaked pie shells. Chill thoroughly. If desired, top with whipped cream.

Lemon Cream Filling

1	Water	4	pt
	Corn syrup	14	oz
	Sugar	26	oz
	Salt	96	gr
	Lemon rind, grated	½	oz
2	Water	8	oz
	Cornstarch	5⅓	oz
	Tapioca starch	1⅓	oz
	Eggs	9	oz
	Butter	2¼	oz
	Lemon juice	3½	oz
	Egg whites	9	oz
	Sugar	9	oz

Mix (1) and bring to a boil. Mix (2) and stir it into (1). Continue to stir until the mass thickens. Now remove it from the fire and stir in the butter and lemon juice. Whip the egg whites and sugar to a wet peak, fold it into the cooked filling, then pour this into pre-baked shells while warm.

Lemon Cookies

1	Sugar	45	oz
	Butter	10	oz
	Shortening	10	oz
	Salt	110	gr
	Eggs, mixed	10	oz
	Milk	10	oz
	Baking soda	7/8	oz
	Lemons (peeling and juices)	2½	
	Cake flour, good grade	55	oz
	Cream of tartar	7/8	oz

Mix and cream (1) until it is of light consistency. Add the egg mixture in small portions, whipping well after each addition. Now stir in the milk, lemons, and baking soda. Finally, sift together the cake flour and cream of tartar, and add this to the batter. Continue mixing until smooth. Spread out with a rolling pin and cut with a 3-inch cutter. Brush with egg wash, and bake at about 380°F.

Lemonade Powder

Powdered sugar	5	lb
Powdered citric acid	1½	lb
Terpeneless lemon oil	2	dr

Rub the sugar up with the lemon oil. Allow it to dry a little and then mix thoroughly with the citric acid.

Lemon Oil Stabilizers

The following compounds will preserve lemon oils from citral oxidation for 30 to 120 days:

Ethyl gallate 0.01 to 0.04%

or

Propyl gallate 0.01 to 0.04%

The removal of closures from citrus oil containers permits the air to enter, thus oxidizing the unsaturated constituents of the oil. The oftener the closure is removed, the greater the deterioration. This oxidation can be prevented by dropping a small piece of dry ice into the container before closing. The carbon dioxide gas will form a protective blanket.

Lemon Crunch

1	Sugar, granulated	7½	lb
	Water	4½	lb
	Salt	55	gr
	Lemon gratings	4½	oz
	Corn syrup	30	oz
	Macaroon coconut	3	lb
	Lemon juice	12	oz

Mix (1) and heat to 280°F. Stir in coconut and lemon juice and heat to 300°F. Remove from the fire, and pour into pans in thin layers. Allow the candy to cool, then break it into pieces of any desired size.

Linzer Torte

Powdered sugar	2⅔ lb
Butter	3 lb
Eggs	1½ lb
Almonds, finely ground	2 lb
Cake flour	5⅓ lb
Baking powder	1⅓ oz

Mix the sugar with the butter, and cream thoroughly. While creaming, stir in the eggs. Finally add the ground almonds, cake flour, and baking powder. Continue to mix until a smooth product is obtained. Chill, then scale as required. Shape into balls, then roll these fairly thin as for cookies. Line the bottom and sides of round pans with this rolled paste. Fill with preserves or any desired fruit fillings. Cover with lattice strips made from this paste. Now brush with egg wash, and bake at 375°F. Cool, and besprinkle with powdered sugar.

Low-Calorie Soft Drinks

Use calcium cyclamate instead of sugar in compounding low-calorie soft drinks, and use algin, pectin, methoxycellulose, or carboxymethylcellulose as a bodying agent. These hydrophilic colloids improve the carbonating ability of the beverages.

L-Lysine

The protein content of many cereal products can be boosted by direct addition of the essential amino acid L-Lysine monohydrochloride. The addition of this amino acid has no effect on the flavor texture, or processing of the product. This essential amino acid balances the protein of wheat bread and cookies. It also improves breakfast cereals, rice, rye flour, etc.

Add about 0.25% of this water-soluble amino acid to cereal foods. The cost of this addition ranges from ½ to 2 cents per pound of product.

Macaroon Coconut Cookies

	lb
Sugar	7½
Water	3
Invert syrup	7½
Corn syrup	5⅝
Flavor	to suit
Macaroon coconut, desiccated	15

Heat the sugar and water to about 180°F.—do not boil. Remove from the fire and stir in the syrups and flavor. Finally, add the macaroon coconut and mix thoroughly—the product should be fairly stiff. Cut with wire-cut cookie machine or shape into balls by hand. Bake at a somewhat high temperature for a short time. This cookie should be toasted, not baked.

Macaroon Crunch Topping

Almond paste	7½ lb
Sugar, granulated	6⅜ lb
Macaroon coconut	6 lb
Egg whites (variable)	1½ lb
Non-fat dry milk solids	18 oz

Salt	1/8 oz
Cocoa butter, melted	6 oz
Flavor	to suit

Mix all the ingredients very thoroughly, then place in a revolving heated compartment until the batch has been toasted to a golden brown color. Cool, then break up the product into pieces of any desired size, or shape into balls by hand. Bake at a somewhat high temperature for a short time. This cookie should be toasted—not baked.

Maple Cream or Butter

Maple syrup can be made into maple cream by boiling it. The cream made from the maple syrup is a candy-like spread that is good on bread, pancakes, toast, and waffles. Maple syrup consists principally of sucrose with a little invert sugar. It is the sucrose that crystallizes to make the cream. Sucrose and invert sugar are made up of the same simple sugars, namely, dextrose and fructose. In sucrose these sugars are united, whereas in invert sugar they occur separately. Because of this difference, sucrose crystallizes easily and invert sugar does not. Invert sugar tends to prevent the crystallization of sucrose. The degree of prevention depends on the amount of invert sugar present. If too much invert sugar is present, the sucrose in the maple syrup will not crystallize to make the cream. Maple syrup needs but a small amount of invert sugar in order to be made into cream. This small amount aids in the formation of extremely small sucrose crystals. Syrup containing 0.5–2% invert sugar is suitable for making a fine-textured cream; 2–4% invert sugar can be made into cream if the syrup is heated until it is 2–4°F. hotter than temperature specified in instructions for making the cream. Syrup containing 4% or more of invert sugar is not suitable for making maple cream.

Place the maple syrup in a clean kettle and heat it to 232°F. Cool rapidly to about 70°F., and stir continuously until the sucrose in the syrup crystallizes or "creams."

Avoid using maple syrup of a high invert sugar content, because cream made from it will be too fluid and more likely will separate a few days after it is made.

Marshmallow

No. 1

Water	7½ lb
Gelatin, medium strength	12 oz
Sugar	18 lb
Plastic invert sugar	7½ lb
Corn syrup	7½ lb

Place the water in a kettle and, while mixing, sift the gelatin into it. Apply a little heat and continue to stir until the gelatin is in solution. Add at once the sugar, and continue the heating and stirring until the sugar is dissolved. Remove the heat, stir in the invert sugar and corn syrup, and mix thoroughly. Transfer the batch to a beater and whip until light. Add color and flavor if so desired. Use this marshmallow for bagging on top of biscuits, cakes, crackers, sugar wafers, etc.

No. 2

Water	28½ oz
Gelatin	6 oz
Granulated sugar	9⅜ lb
Water	43½ oz
Invert syrup	2¼ lb
Corn syrup	12 oz
Vanilla	q.s.

Place the gelatin in the 28½ oz water, and allow it to soak for about 20 minutes. Dissolve the sugar in the 43½ oz water, and cook to 225°F. Stir in the syrups and bring the temperature back to 225°F. Remove from the fire, stir in the gelatin mixture, and continue stirring until the gelatin is in complete solution. Pour into a sterile container and allow it to cool. Use any amount required at a time for beating and continue beating until the desired consistency is reached. Add the vanilla flavor just before the beating is completed.

Marshmallow Creme

	lb
Corn syrup	6¾
Invert syrup	3⅛
Cane sugar	5
Corn starch	½
Egg albumin	½
Gelatin, U.S.P.	¼
Water	8⅞

Mix the gelatin, albumin, and corn starch, and stir in the cane sugar. Then very carefully, with a minimum of agitation, stir this dry mixture into the water. Allow it to soak for 15 minutes and work out any lumps that may have formed. Mix the syrups and heat to 110°F. Then slowly blend the sugar-gelatin mixture with the heated syrups. Pasteurize the mass with very little agitation, then cool. Partially freeze this cream while whipping it.

Marshmallow Powder

	oz
Sugar 4X	43.85
Corn syrup, powdered (Frodex)	26.00
Dextrose, powdered	26.00
Gelatin, 200 bloom, 100 mesh, or finer	0.50
Kelcoloid	0.15
Soy albumin	2.50
Salt	0.16
Vanilla sugar	0.50

Have all ingredients in a finely powdered form and mix thoroughly, then store in moisture-proof containers. To use, dissolve 9 oz of this mixture in 3 oz of hot water and whip it for about 4 minutes at high speed.

Marshmallows

Gelatin (225 bloom)	14.00 oz
Granulated sugar	20.75 lb

Corn syrup	10.75 lb
Sorbo	7.00 lb
Water	10.75 lb

Mix the gelatin with 3.5 lb of the water and set it aside. Place the remaining 7.25 lb of the water in a kettle with a beater, add the corn syrup and sugar, and keep on mixing and heating, but do not boil. Remove the heat and stir in the sorbo and the soaked gelatin. Continue mixing until the gelatin is completely dissolved, then beat the batch until it is white. Flavor with vanilla if so desired.

Marshmallows

Cold water	18	oz
Gelatin, U.S.P.	6	oz
Sugar	8¼	lb
Water	75	oz
Invert syrup	39	oz
Corn syrup	36	oz

Mix the gelatin with the cold water, allow it to soak for about 15 minutes, then heat it to 145°F. on a hot water bath to effect solution. Mix the sugar with the water and heat to about 160°F. Stir in the invert and corn syrups and mix thoroughly. Finally, add the gelatin mixture and whip the batch to the desired consistency. Pour on a slab previously powdered with XXXX sugar. Allow it to stand about 4 hours, then cut into the usual size for marshmallows.

During the winter season reduce the amount of sugar by about 25%, and increase the amount of invert syrup by about 100%. It may also be necessary to decrease slightly the amount of water employed.

Marshmallow Powder

	lb
Powdered sugar	7.62
Powdered, edible gelatin	0.24
Powdered egg albumin	0.24
Powdered gum arabic, U.S.P.	0.24

Mix thoroughly and flavor to suit with vanillin. Use 2.25 lb of this powder to a quart of warm water, and beat up stiff.

Marshmallow Topping

Sugar, granulated	2½	lb
Water	1	lb
Cream of tartar, U.S.P.	⅛	oz
Corn syrup	1	lb
Invert sugar	1	lb
Water, warm	18	oz
Gelatin, U.S.P.	2	oz
Egg whites	8	oz

Mix the sugar, water, cream of tartar, and cook to 240°F. Add the corn syrup and invert sugar, and mix thoroughly. Dissolve the gelatin in the warm water, add to it the egg whites, place this mixture in a beater and whip it. As soon as the gelatin-egg white mixture begins to thicken, add, while whipping, the syrup-sugar mixture to it. Continue to beat until the mass becomes of the desired consistency. Use this topping immediately.

Matzoth Sponge Cake

1	Eggs	6.00 lb
	Egg yolks	6.00 lb
	Sugar, granulated	6.00 lb
	Honey or invert syrup (variable)	1.00 lb
	Salt	1.00 oz
	Almonds, ground	2.86 lb
	Matzoth flour	2.30 lb

Mix (1) and whip light. Fold in, thoroughly but carefully, the mixture of ground almonds and matzoth flour. Scale as required, then bake in a fairly hot oven.

Meringue

No. 1

		oz
1	Egg whites	12.75
	Cream of tartar (potassium bitartrate)	0.19
2	Granulated sugar	15.00

Whip (1) to the point where the egg whites are no longer a foam but begin to stiffen. Add (2) and continue the whipping until the batch is stiff. Add sufficient vanilla (or other) flavor. Color may be added with the flavor if desired.

No. 2

		oz
1	Granulated sugar	25½
	Tapioca flour	1⅞
	Salt	1/10
2	Egg whites	25½
	Flavor	to suit

Blend together (1) by sifting several times. Place (2) in a mixing bowl and whip with a wire whip until light and firm. When (2) is firm, fold in (1) and add the flavor. Use this meringue as a topping for pies, and brown it at 425°F.

No. 3

		oz
1	Gelatin, 200 bloom	¾
	Cold water	3
2	Egg whites	25½
	Sugar, granulated	18
3	Flavor	to suit
	Sugar, granulated	12

Allow the gelatin to soak in the water for 20 minutes, then heat it to 140°F. over a hot water bath. Mix (1) and (2) and whip until light. Now add (3) slowly while whipping, and continue to whip until the meringue is firm.

Meringue Powder

	oz
Powdered albumen	10.000
Cornstarch	4.500
Powdered sugar	6.000
Gelatin, U.S.P. (powdered)	0.125
Aluminum sodium sulfate, U.S.P. (powdered)	1.500
Salt, powdered	0.500

Blend together all the powders by sifting several times. Add 3 oz of this mixture and 1½ lb of sugar to a pint of water, and whip until stiff. Flavor to suit.

Meringue Shells

Sugar, granulated	4½ lb
Water	38¼ oz
Egg whites	37⅛ oz

Mix the sugar and water, and boil until the temperature reaches 242°F. Beat the egg whites until firm, then add the cooked syrup to the egg whites while beating slowly all the time. Continue the beating until the batch is cool. Do not add the hot syrup faster than the egg white can take it up. Decorate through a star tube as desired. Allow the meringue to cool for a few hours, then brown it in an oven at about 225°F.

Milk Sponge Cake

Sugar, granulated	5 lb
Eggs, mixed	4 lb
Salt	¾ oz
Flavor	to suit
Milk, hot (140°F.)	1 lb
Cake flour	5¼ lb
Starch	8 oz
Baking powder (variable)	2 oz
Milk, hot (140°F.)	1¾ lb
Butter, melted	1 lb
Invert syrup	1 lb

Mix the sugar, mixed eggs, salt, and flavor, and whip at medium speed until light. While whipping, add slowly the hot milk. Continue the beating until the batter holds a crease for about 20 seconds (made by drawing a spatula through it). Mix the cake flour, starch and baking powder by sifting, then fold this carefully into the batter. Now mix thoroughly the hot milk, melted butter and invert syrup, and fold this carefully into the batter. Finally, scale into pans, and bake at 390°F.

Mincemeat

1	Raisins	18.00 lb
	Currants	2.50 lb
	Orange peel	2.40 lb
	Evaporated apples	10.00 lb
	Citron peel	1.00 lb
2	Water	3.60 gal
	Sugar	20.00 lb
	Corn syrup	10.00 lb
	Molasses	3.20 pt
	Vinegar	1.60 pt
	Salt	8.80 oz
	Benzoate of soda	1.40 oz
3	Cinnamon	5.60 oz
	Dry mustard	1.80 oz
	Allspice	0.70 oz
	Nutmeg	0.35 oz
	Cloves	0.20 oz
	Ginger	0.15 oz

Grind (1) and soak overnight. Place (2) in a steam-jacketed kettle and mix thoroughly. Add (1) to the kettle and bring it to a boil. Turn off the steam and blend (3) into the batch. While the batch is cooling, stir in 6.40 oz of rum and 6.40 oz of artificial rum flavor.

Allow this mincemeat to age in a wooden barrel.

Molasses Spice Cookies

1	Sugar	21	oz
1	Dark honey	12	oz
1	Shortening	15	oz
1	Baking soda	$2\frac{1}{4}$	oz
1	Salt	$\frac{3}{4}$	oz
1	Cinnamon	$\frac{3}{4}$	oz
1	Ginger	$\frac{9}{16}$	oz
1	Cloves	$\frac{3}{16}$	oz
1	Eggs	9	oz
	Molasses, light	$2\frac{1}{4}$	lb
	Water (variable)	21	oz
	Pastry flour	6	lb

Mix (1) thoroughly. Add the light molasses and stir in the water. Finally, stir in the flour and continue to mix until it is thoroughly incorporated. Cut out the cookies with wire-cut machine, and top them with sugar. Bake at 375°F., using steam freely while baking them. If there is no steam, brush the cookies with water before baking.

Mushroom Chop Suey

Brown rice, cooked	35	lb
Pork (1-in. cubes)	$11\frac{5}{8}$	lb
Veal (1-in. cubes)	$11\frac{5}{8}$	lb
Chicken gravy	$11\frac{1}{2}$	lb
Bean sprouts (not drained)	$5\frac{7}{8}$	lb
Celery, chopped	$4\frac{5}{8}$	lb
Mushrooms, sliced	6	lb
Onions, chopped	19	oz
Soy Sauce (Chinese, made from fermented soybeans)	$1\frac{3}{4}$	lb
Salt	to suit	

Mix thoroughly. Pack into suitable containers and freeze it.

Niacin in Coffee

(J. Sci. Food Agr.)

Niacin (Nicotinic acid amide) is one of the important vitamins of the B complex.

Coffee prepared by infusion, using $\frac{1}{3}$ oz of ground coffee bean for each $3\frac{1}{3}$ oz of water, gave 3.4 mg of niacin per $3\frac{1}{3}$ oz of liquid coffee.

Noodles

Yolks	25 oz
Salt	1 oz
Water (variable)	15 oz
Hard wheat flour, unbleached	5 lb
Soya flour	20 oz

Mix the yolks, salt, and water, and beat to a light froth. Add the mixed flours, and continue mixing until the dough is smooth and pliable and can be rolled very thin without breaking.

Nut Brittle

	lb
Butter	45.00
Granulated sugar	50.00
Invert sugar	5.00
Water	1.25
Nuts	15.00

Melt the butter in a steam-jacketed kettle. Add the sugars and the water, and cook, with continuous stirring, until the temperature reaches 300°F., then add the nuts and pour the mixture to 1/4-inch thickness on an oiled slab. When the batch is somewhat cooled, turn it upside down. Allow it to become cold, then coat both sides with milk chocolate and sprinkle it with sliced nuts. Finally, break it into suitable pieces and package them.

Oatmeal Cookies

1	Sugar	49	oz
1	Shortening	18 2/3	oz
1	Raisins, ground	20	oz
1	Eggs	1	lb
1	Milk	4	oz
1	Baking soda	1 2/3	oz
1	Salt	1/3	oz
	Honey	18 2/3	oz
	Pastry flour	5	lb
	Oats, rolled	1 5/8	lb
	Cinnamon	1/2	oz

Blend (1) and mix thoroughly. Stir in the honey; then add the flour, rolled oats, and cinnamon, and continue mixing until the mass is of smooth consistency. Cut the cookies with a 2 1/2-inch cutter, and place them on baking sheets about 1 inch apart. Bake at 350°F.

Orange Syrup

	oz
Tween 20	7.68
Orange oil, U.S.P.	1.28
Glycerin, C.P.	12.80
Citric acid solution	1.00
Syrup, enough to make	128.00

Mix the orange oil with the Tween 20 and the glycerin, and incorporate this mixture with the acidulated syrup. This syrup will substitute for the U.S.P. product.

Orange Glaze

Icing sugar	7.50 lb
Whole oranges, ground	1.50 lb
Gelatin	2.25 oz
Water	12.00 oz

Mix the sugar with the ground oranges until smooth and free of lumps. Soak the gelatin in the water for about 18 minutes, then heat it to 140°F. Stir the gelatin solution into the sugar mixture, and continue to mix at a slow speed until the finished product is smooth.

Use this glaze hot (115°F.). If necessary, thin it down with simple syrup.

Pastry Shells

Water	3 3/8	lb
Shortening	18	oz
Salt	1/8	oz
Bread flour	27	oz
Cake flour	9	oz
Eggs	2 3/8	lb
Egg whites	18	oz
Milk, liquid (variable)	9	oz
Ammonia	2 1/4	dr

Mix the water, shortening, and salt, and bring to a rolling boil. Add the flours and stir vigorously until the whole mass forms a ball following the stirring paddle. Place it in a cake mixer, mix at medium speed until slightly cool, then add the eggs and egg whites in four (4) portions, mixing thoroughly after each addition. Finally, dissolve the ammonia in the milk, add it to the mixing bowl, and continue to mix until smooth. Bake at 425°F., using a small amount of steam at the beginning of the baking period.

Peach and Apricot Oil

Aldehyde C_{14}	4.00 oz
Aldehyde No. 15	2.00 oz
Allyl cyclohexane valerate	1.00 oz
Allyl butyrate	1.00 oz
Ethyl acetate	1.00 oz
Allyl cyclohexane acetate	0.50 oz
Isobutyl ketone	0.25 oz
Ethyl sebacate	0.25 oz
Rhodinol	15.00 min
Allyl cinnamate	0.50 oz
n-Propyl cinnamate	0.50 oz
Benzaldehyde, F.F.C.	0.20 oz

Mix well and allow to stand a week or more.

Peanut Butter Biscuits

	oz
Sifted flour	16
Baking powder	1
Salt	¼
Shortening	1¾
Peanut butter	4⅖
Milk	12

Mix and stir the dry ingredients, then work in the shortening and peanut butter. Add the milk slowly and keep on stirring until a soft dough is formed. Knead the dough on a lightly floured board, then roll it to the desired thickness, and cut it into 2-inch biscuits. Place them on an ungreased baking sheet and bake at 450°F. for about 15 minutes.

Peanut Bread

Sifted flour	1½ lb
Sugar	8 oz
Baking powder	1 oz
Salt	⅜ oz
Shortening	2½ oz
Milk	30 oz
Eggs	3
Peanuts, finely chopped	3 cups

Mix and sift the dry ingredients. Work in the shortening. Beat the eggs with the milk and stir this into the dry mixture. Finally, stir in the chopped peanuts. Put into lightly-greased loaf pans (8½x4½x2½ inches) and bake at 350°F. for about one hour.

Peanut Brittle
No. 1

Liquid sugar	9.94 lb
Corn syrup	3.75 lb
Spanish peanuts	5.25 lb
Butter	3.75 oz
Baking soda	2.25 oz
Salt	0.50 oz

Mix the sugar with the corn syrup, and bring to a boil. Stir in the Spanish peanuts, and cook to about 290°F. Now stir in the butter and cook to 295°F. Remove from the fire and stir in the baking soda and salt. Continue the stirring until the baking soda is thoroughly mixed and the whole batch becomes soft and fluffy. Pour this onto a greased slab and spread it out as thin as possible. When the batch is somewhat cool and stiff enough to handle, cut it into pieces of desired size, and stretch out to the desired thickness. Finally, when the batch becomes brittle and cool, break it into pieces of the desired size suitable for packing.

No. 2

1	Granulated sugar	8	lb
1	Water	35	oz
1	Corn syrup	57½	oz
1	Molasses, New Orleans	13	oz
1	Spanish peanuts, raw	6⅖	lb
	Butter	6⅖	oz
	Salt	350	gr
	Baking soda	350	gr

Bring (1) to a boil, and allow it to boil for two minutes with occasional stirring. Continue the cooking, stirring occasionally, until the peanuts become light brown in color. (The temperature at this stage should be 315°F.) Now stir in the butter and mix thoroughly. Remove from the fire and stir in the salt and baking soda. Mix thoroughly and pour onto an oiled surface, spreading the mass as thin as possible with a heavy knife. When cooler, turn the batch upside down and stretch the sheet as thin as possible. When cooled to about 95°F., mark and break the candy into pieces of the desired sizes and pack them into air-tight containers.

Peanut Butter Cookies, Filled

Shortening	5⅓	oz
Peanut butter	8¼	oz
Sugar, brown	10½	oz
Eggs	2	
Milk	5⅓	oz
Vanilla	⅙	oz
Baking powder	⅔	oz
Salt	⅙	oz
Sifted flour	1⅛	lb
Peach filling or raisin filling		

Mix and cream together the peanut butter, shortening, and sugar. Stir in the eggs, milk, and vanilla, and mix thoroughly. Now mix and sift the dry ingredients and stir this into the first mixture. Chill. Roll the dough thin and cut it into rounds with a 2-inch cooky cutter. Drop a spoonful of the chosen filling in the center of one round and cover with another round. Then press the edges together. Finally, place them on an ungreased baking sheet and bake at 425°F. for about 10 minutes.

Peach Filling

Peaches, dried and ground	1½	cups
Sugar	5⅓	oz
Water	1	pt

Lemon juice	1/6 oz
Lemon rind, grated	1/2 oz
Peanuts, finely chopped	1/2 cup

Raisin Filling

Raisins, ground	13 1/2 oz
Sugar	6 oz
Water	8 oz
Lemon juice	1 1/2 oz
Lemon rind, grated	1/2 oz
Peanuts, finely chopped	3/4 cups

For both: Mix all the ingredients except the peanuts and cook on a slow fire until thickened, with frequent stirring. Finally, remove from the fire and stir in the finely chopped peanuts.

Peanut-Oatmeal Cookies

Shortening	12 oz
Sugar, brown	1 1/2 lb
Eggs	3
Milk	3 oz
Vanilla	1/4 oz
Sifted flour	1 1/4 lb
Salt	1/8 oz
Baking soda	5/8 oz
Rolled oats, quick-cooking	3 cups
Peanuts, finely chopped	1 1/2 cups

Mix and cream the shortening and brown sugar. Stir in the eggs, milk, and vanilla, and mix thoroughly. Mix and sift the flour, salt, and baking soda, and stir this combination into the first mixture. Finally, add the rolled oats and chopped peanuts, and mix well. Cut cookies with a 2 1/2-inch cutter, place them on baking sheets about 1 inch apart, and flatten them with a fork. Bake at 375°F. for about 8 minutes.

Peanut Butter Muffins

Sifted flour	1 1/2 lb
Sugar	6 oz
Baking powder	1 1/2 oz
Salt	1/4 oz
Peanut butter	8 3/4 oz
Eggs	6
Milk	1 1/2 pt
Vegetable oil	3 1/4 oz

Mix and sift the dry ingredients and work in the peanut butter. Beat the eggs, mix them with the milk, then pour this into the dry mixture. Add the vegetable oil and stir just enough to moisten the ingredients. Finally, put the batter into greased muffin pans 2/3 full, and bake at 400°F. for about 25 minutes.

Pecan Cookies

Sugar, brown	24 oz
Sugar, powdered	24 oz
Butter	19 oz
Shortening	24 oz
Salt	1/2 oz
Vanilla flavor	to suit
Eggs	18
Cake flour	3 1/2 lb
Nutmeats	12 oz

Mix and cream the first six. Add the eggs gradually while creaming. Finally, stir in the cake flour and nutmeats, and continue to mix until a smooth batter is obtained. Deposit pats about the size of a large hazelnut on lightly greased and flour-dusted pans. Decorate the tops with finely chopped nuts, and bake at about 370°F.

Pecan Pies

1	Sugar	3⅓ lb
	Corn syrup	2⅔ lb
	Honey	2 lb
	Eggs	3⅓ lb
	Butter	1½ lb
	Salt	1½ oz
	Vanilla	to suit
2	Pecans, chopped	4 lb
	Macaroon coconut	1⅓ lb

Mix (1) thoroughly, then heat it to 110°F. over a hot water bath. Add (2) and stir well together. Finally, fill into pie shells and bake at about 350°F. If desired, sprinkle the pie shells with graham cracker crumbs.

Pecan Wafers

		lb
1	Granulated sugar	3.00
	Margarine	1.50
2	Whole eggs	1.12
	Melted chocolate	0.58
	Cake flour	0.75
3	Chopped pecans	0.38

Cream (1); mix (2) and add to (1); then add (3) and mix all until smooth. Weigh 2½ lb dough into each 18x24 inch bun pan. Bake light. Mark into 1-inch squares, while warm. This batch produces 2 sheets.

Pectin Glaze

1	Water	1 pt
2	Fruit pectin (100 grade)	1 oz
	Granulated sugar	3 oz
3	Corn syrup	2¼ lb
	Granulated sugar	2¼ lb
	Water	3⅜ lb

Boil (1); mix (2) and stir it into the boiling water. Mix (3), stir it into the hot mixture, and boil for 3 minutes. Finally, stir in enough lemon juice (or ¼ to ⅜ oz of citric acid solution) to thicken the mass to the desired consistency. Use it on fruit tarts.

Pepper-Onion Relish

Onions, finely chopped	4 qt
Sweet red peppers, finely chopped	8 cups
Green peppers, finely chopped	8 cups
Salt	2½ oz
Sugar	32 oz
Vinegar (5–6% acetic acid)	1 gal

Mix all the ingredients, bring slowly to a boil, and cook until slightly thickened. Finally, pour into clean, hot, sterile containers; fill containers to top, and seal tightly.

Piccalilli

Green tomatoes, chopped	4 qt
Sweet red peppers, chopped (medium size)	8

Green peppers, chopped (medium size)	8	
Onions, mild, chopped (large)	8	
Cabbage, chopped (small head)	4	
Salt	12	oz
Vinegar (5–6% acetic acid)	6	pt
Sugar, brown	4	lb
Mixed pickle spices	½	cup

Mix the tomatoes with the peppers, onions, cabbage, salt, and allow them to stand overnight. Put the vegetable mixture in a clean, thin, white cloth and squeeze out all the liquid. Dissolve the sugar in the vinegar. Put the pickle spices in a thin, clean, white cloth and tie top tightly. Place this spice bag in the vinegar mixture and bring to a boil. Stir in the vegetable mixture and simmer for about 30 min. Finally, remove the spice bag, and pack the piccalilli into clean, hot, sterile containers. Fill containers to top, and seal tightly.

Pie Crust

Pastry flour, unbleached, low protein	30	lb
Shortening	20	lb
Salt	12	oz
Dextrose	7⅕	oz
Non-fat dry milk	7⅕	oz
Ice water (variable)	9	lb

Mix the flour, shortening, dextrose, and non-fat dry milk and rub them together sufficiently to reduce the particles of shortening to almond-like size. Dissolve the salt in the water, add it to the shortening-flour mixture, and mix only enough for thorough incorporation. Chill, and use as required.

Pie Meringue

Granulated sugar	1½ lb
Cold water starch	1½ oz
Egg whites	25½ oz

Blend together the sugar and the cold water starch. Mix the egg whites with half of the sugar-starch mixture, and whip at medium speed until the mass begins to thicken, then change to high speed, and keep on whipping until the mass is firm. When the consistency of the meringue is satisfactory, add slowly the remaining sugar-starch mixture. Mix only a minute or two after the last portion has been incorporated. Top pies with the meringue, and brown the meringue in the oven at 400 to 425°F.

Pineapple Glaze

		lb
1	Unsweetened pineapple juice	7.50
	Sugar	5.25
2	Cornstarch	9.75
	Unsweetened pineapple juice	1.50

Bring (1) to a boil. Mix (2) and add it to the boiling juice and sugar. Stir and cook until clear.

Pineapple Oil

No. 1

Allyl caproate	1.0 oz
Allyl cyclohexane propionate	2.0 oz
Methallyl caproate	1.0 oz
Cyclohexyl caproate	0.5 oz
Ethyl acetate	1.0 oz
Allyl heptoate	0.5 oz
Aldehyde No. 19	1.5 oz
Vanillin	25.0 gr

Mix well and allow to stand a week or more.

No. 2

Allyl caproate	2.00 oz
Allyl cyclohexane propionate	1.00 oz
Allyl cyclohexane acetate	0.50 oz
Aldehyle No. 19	2.00 oz
Ethyl acetate	1.00 oz
Methyl beta-methyl thiolpropionate	0.06 oz
Ethyl heptanoate	0.50 oz
Amyl valerianate	0.25 oz
Isobutyl butyrate	0.25 oz
Butyl propionate	0.25 oz
Allyl caprylate	0.33 oz
Propyl propionate	0.33 oz
Allyl heptoate	0.50 oz
Vanillin	20.00 gr

Mix well and allow to stand a week or more.

Pineapple Pie Filling

	lb
Crushed pineapple	24.75
Sugar	10.50
Salt	0.25
Water	9.50
Cornstarch	1.50
Water	4.25

Place the pineapple, sugar, salt, and water in a suitable vessel, and bring to a boil. Dissolve the cornstarch in the 4¼ lb of water, and add it to the boiling fruit. Cook until clear.

Pizza Pie Crust

Bread flour	20 lb
Sugar	1 lb
Corn oil	13 oz
Eggs	3 oz
Non-fat dry milk solids	10 oz
Salt	6 oz
Water (variable)	9½ pt
Yeast (variable)	7 oz

Mix all the ingredients until a smooth product is obtained. Remove the dough from the mixing bowl at 82°F. Allow it to ferment for about 52 minutes, then scale as required, and make up in the usual manner.

Pizza Pie Dough

No. 1

Spring wheat flour	8.0 lb
Water	4.6 lb
Yeast	3.2 oz
Salt	1.0 oz
Corn oil	5.2 oz
Corn syrup	3.2 oz
Eggs	3.2 oz

Dissolve the yeast, corn syrup, and salt in some of the water. Place the flour in a mixing bowl and add the rest of the water. Finally, stir in the yeast mixture, then the eggs and corn oil, and continue mixing until a smooth dough is obtained. Remove the dough from the mixer at about 82°F., and allow about 50 minutes for fermentation before making it up.

No. 2

Flour	6 lb
Water	6 lb
Yeast	2 oz
Salt	1 oz
Shortening (8 tablespoons)	4 oz
Olive oil	enough for kneading

Dissolve the yeast and salt in some of the water. Place the flour in a mixing bowl, make a depression, and add the rest of the water. Stir in the yeast-salt solution, and mix thoroughly. Now stir in the melted shortening, and knead the dough until it is elastic. Pour a little olive oil over the dough and knead for several minutes more. Finally roll the dough into thin sheets the size of the baking pans.

Pizza Filling

Chopped garlic sausage	4 lb
Tomatoes, peeled and cut	4 lb
Olive oil	8 oz

Cook the chopped sausage for 5 minutes in the olive oil. Pour the oil-cooked sausage over the dough, add the cut tomatoes, and press this mixture into the dough. Bake about ¾ hour at 350°F. Sliced, fresh mushrooms may be substituted for half of the garlic sausage.

Popcorn Balls

Sorghum syrup	6 lb
Sugar	2 lb
Butter	4 oz
Salt	1½ teaspoon
Popped corn	q.s.

Place the first 4 components in a kettle and cook to 230°F. Stir in the freshly popped corn, and form the popcorn into balls by molding them with the hands, previously dipped in cold water.

Potassium Metabisulfite

Add 2 oz of potassium metabisulfite per 1000 lb of wine-making grapes to control the activity of undesirable micro-organisms.

Pound Cake

		oz
1	Shortening	28½
	Sugar, granulated	40½
	Non-fat dry milk	2¼
	Cake flour	6
	Salt	1
2	Eggs	33
	Flavor	q.s.
3	Sugar	18
	Water (variable)	30
4	Cake flour	54
	Baking powder	3/16

Mix and cream (1) thoroughly. Add (2) gradually while creaming. Make a solution of (3), add it alternately with the mixture (4), and continue to mix until the finished product is smooth. Scale as required, and bake at 340°F.

Pound Cake Flavor

Lemon oil	1 oz
Orange oil	1 oz
Mace oil	1 dr
Nutmeg oil	1 dr
Vanillin	1 oz
Alcohol, U.S.P.	8 oz

Mix and shake well. Allow to stand overnight. Use an amber bottle, and keep it well corked.

Powdered French Salad Seasoning

Salt, finely ground	9.00 lb
Sugar, finely ground	4.50 lb
Black pepper, finely ground	1.50 lb
Dehydrated onion powder	1.20 lb
Monosodium glutamate, finely ground	1.20 lb
Soluble celery (sugar base)	9.50 oz
Dehydrated celery stalk, finely ground	9.50 oz
Mustard flour	8.00 oz
Red pepper, finely ground	3.25 oz
Curcuma, finely ground	2.25 oz

Mix all thoroughly. Add 3/5 oz of this powdered seasoning to the following liquid mixture:

	oz
Vinegar, 10% acetic acid (100 gr)	2 1/6
Water	1
Corn oil, refined	5

Mix and shake well. The resultant product is a good French dressing.

Puff Pastry

1	Bread flour	7 1/2 lb
	Butter	1 7/8 lb
	Salt	1 oz
	Water, cold (variable)	5 1/4 lb
	Color	q.s.
	Pastry butter	5 5/8 lb

Mix (1) at low speed for about 2 minutes. Add the cold water and color and mix until the dough is mature. Remove dough from the agitator with a scraper, then add the pastry butter, and stir only enough to incorporate it. Roll and fold the dough a few times. Now roll out the finished dough to a thickness of about 1/7 inch, then cut from it disks five inches or more in diameter. Brush the outside edge with egg wash, then fill center with the following mixture:

Currants or raisins	3.75 lb
Cake crumbs	15.00 oz
Juice and rind of	5 lemons
Cinnamon	0.75 oz
Raspberry or other jam, enough to make a paste.	

When the disks of puff paste are filled, fold the edges into the center, with minimal overlapping. Flatten them by pressing down, then turn them over and place on wet pans. Allow them to rest for one hour, then bake at 375°F. When baked and cool, cover the tops with powdered sugar.

Pumpkin Pie Filling

No. 1

1	Non-fat dry milk	16	oz
	Dark brown sugar	24	oz
	Flour	6	oz
	Salt	½	oz
	Cinnamon	¾	oz
	Cloves	54	gr
	Allspice	55	gr
	Ginger	55	gr
	Butter, melted	4	oz
2	Pumpkin, No. 10 can	1	can
	Water	2	lb
	Corn syrup	24	oz
3	Eggs	2	lb
	Water (variable)	60	oz

Blend (1) together. Add (2) and mix thoroughly. Mix (3), stir it into the other mixtures, and continue to stir until the mass is rather firm. Allow it to stand for about 60 minutes, then stir well, and continue to stir while the pie shells are being filled. Bake in deep tins in a moderately hot oven for about 30 minutes. Remove the pies from the oven when they quiver like a gelatin dessert when tested. Do not overbake because it will impair the pies.

No. 2

Sugar	3	lb
Corn starch	6	oz
Cinnamon, ground	⅔	oz
Cloves, ground	⅙	oz
Ginger, ground	⅓	oz
Nutmeg, ground	⅓	oz
Salt	½	oz
Corn oil, refined	6	oz
Eggs	3	lb
No. 10 can pumpkin	1	can
Non-fat dry milk	18	oz
Water (variable)	10	pt

Blend together the sugar, corn starch, spices, and salt. Add the corn oil, eggs, and pumpkin, and mix well. Finally, stir in the dry milk and water. Pour this filling into the pastry shells, and bake at 425°F. for 45 minutes.

Pure Vanilla Flavor

No. 1

	oz
Oleoresin vanilla	6.0
Propylene glycol, U.S.P.	48.0
Simple syrup	26.0
Water	48.0

Mix the oleoresin vanilla with the propylene glycol, and stir well. Stir in the simple syrup, then add the water slowly with vigorous stirring. Allow the mixture to stand 2 to 4 days and filter clear.

No. 2

Chopped vanilla beans	2.50	lb
Glycerin	1.25	gal
Water	1.25	gal

Mix the glycerin with the water and heat to about 75°F. Add the vanilla beans, and allow to stand for 2 to 3 weeks. Stir occasionally. Then press and strain the batch through muslin and add enough glycerin to make 3¾ gals.

No. 3

Oleoresin vanilla	6	oz
Glycerin	½	gal
Hot water	½	gal

Heat the glycerin to 230°F. Stir in the oleoresin vanilla, and gradually add the hot water, with constant agitation. Allow to stand for several hours, and strain through cheese cloth.

Raspberry Oil

	oz
Ethyl methyl phenyl glycidate	2.00
Aldehyde No. 20	2.00
Isobutyl acetate	0.40
Amyl acetate	0.20
Beta-ionone	0.25
Ketone No. 18	0.50
p-Methylbenzyl propionate	0.25
Ethyl acetate	0.65
Vanillin	0.25
Propyl acetate	0.50

Mix well, and allow to stand a week or more. As beta-ionone is found in fresh raspberries, it must be incorporated in all synthetic raspberry oils.

Roast Beef Loaf

Chuck meat, boneless	50	lb
* Plate beef	16½	lb
Bay leaf, crushed	1	
Onions, grated	1½	lb
Tomato catsup	6½	lb
Salt	1¼	lb
White pepper, ground	5	oz
Worcestershire sauce	2	oz
Non-fat milk solids	8	lb
Broth	26½	lb

* A thin cut from the lower end of the ribs.

Grind the meat, transfer it to a steam-jacketed kettle with enough water to cover it, and bring it to a boil. Now stir in the bay leaf, onions, salt, tomato catsup, white pepper, and Worcestershire sauce, and cook at a slow heat until the meat becomes tender. Transfer the ingredients to a mixing machine and, while mixing, sprinkle with the non-fat milk solids, and add the broth from the kettle. While mixing thoroughly, fill into 6-lb shallow pans to chill. When the product becomes somewhat hard, stuff it into artificial casings.

Rum Chiffon Cake

		oz
1	Cake flour	40½
	Sugar	15
	Sugar, light brown	12
	Baking powder	2¹⁄₁₆
	Salt	¾
2	Corn oil	21
	Egg yolk	21
	Water (variable)	1½
3	Rum	7½
4	Egg whites	42
	Sugar	28½
	Cream of tartar	⅜

Mix (1) thoroughly by sifting. Add (2) and stir until the mix is smooth. Add the rum (3) and stir thoroughly, but do not over-aerate. Now mix (3), beat this to a firm peak, and fold the batter portion into this whipped mass, thoroughly but carefully. Scale as required, and bake at 365°F. Remove the cake from oven, allow it to cool, then dip it in the following rum glaze:

Rum Glaze

Sugar	4½	lb
Corn syrup	12	oz
Cream of tartar	64	gr
Water	19½	oz
White rum	3¾	oz

Mix all the ingredients except the white rum and bring just to boiling. Remove the heat and allow it to cool to 110°F., then stir in the white rum.

Rum Cake Finish

1	Sugar, granulated	6.0	lb
	Water	1.5	lb
	Corn syrup	1.5	lb
	Invert syrup	3.0	oz
	Salt	20.0	gr
	Rum or rum flavor	q.s.	
	Butter flavor	q.s.	

Mix (1) and bring it to just boiling. Remove from fire, allow it to cool, and then stir in the flavors. Dip the cakes in this rum syrup, then allow them to drain on screens long enough for excess syrup to run off.

Rye Flour Bread (Without Shortening)

(Soft Sponge)

1	* Sour dough	3	lb
	Rye flour, medium	1⅔	lb
	Water	6	lb
	Yeast	5⅓	oz

(Dough)

2	Rye flour	15	lb
	Water (variable)	6	lb
	Salt	5	oz

Mix (1) thoroughly until smooth. Allow it to ferment until sponge drops. Mix (2) thoroughly until smooth. Add (2) to (1) and mix until dough is of smooth consistency. Remove the dough from the mixer at about 80°F., and allow it to attain a full rise. Scale into 18 oz units, round them, and allow them to rest, free from all drafts, for 18 minutes before molding them into loaves.

Mold the dough into any desired shape, and place it in greased 24x24x4 inch tins. Brush the sides and ends with molten butter. Place them in a pan proofing cabinet and allow one-half proof before baking. While in the proofer, wash the loaves with water in order to prevent tearing. Bake at 400°F. for about 55 minutes. As soon as the loaves are set, break them apart and return them to the oven for 18 minutes more at 375°F. This procedure will prevent gumminess.

* Sour Dough

1	Rye flour, medium	16	oz
	Water	16	oz
	Yeast	1	oz
2	Rye flour	2	lb
	Water	3	lb

Mix (1) thoroughly, and allow it to ferment for 24 hours. Mix (2) thoroughly and add it to (1). Allow the batch to ferment for 4 hours more. Rye flour is rich in Vitamin B and has considerable of Vitamins A and E. It is lower than wheat in protein, carbohydrates, fat and minerals.

Salad Dressing

	oz
Cornstarch	1.25
Water	22.50
Corn oil, refined	13.00
French mustard	6.00
Salt	1.00
Sugar	2.50
Vinegar, white	10.50

Mix the cornstarch with a little cold water. Heat the remaining water and stir in the cold cornstarch mixture. Boil this mixture until it stiffens, then allow it to cool. Place the mustard into a bowl and gradually add the corn oil with constant stirring. Finally, stir in the salt, sugar, vinegar, and the cooled-down starch.

Salt Substitute

	parts by weight
Calcium formate	10.0
Calcium citrate	9.0
Lithium formate	1.0
Magnesium formate	10.0
Starch	1.5

Mix thoroughly.

Magnesium citrate may be substituted for the Magnesium formate. Add this salt substitute to dough before baking and to other foods before cooking, except when prolonged boiling is necessary.

Shelf-Life of Butter Cream Candies

One or two per cent of glycerin added to butter cream candies will lengthen their shelf-life by suppressing the formation of free fatty acids.

All the ordinary butter cream candies show the presence of about 1 per cent of free fatty acids after 5 to 10 weeks in storage. This small amount imparts a disagreeable taste and odor to the butter creams.

Butter cream candies with 1 per cent glycerin, stored at 86°F., had their shelf-life prolonged from 9 weeks to 14 weeks; 2 per cent glycerin indicated a much longer time.

Shelf Life of Baked Goods

The shelf life of biscuits and other baked goods may be lengthened by adding the following antioxidants:

	fat weight
Butylated hydroxyanisole (BHA)	0.005%
Dodecyl gallate	0.01%

Wrappers impregnated with antioxidants were also effective, but less so than incorporating the antioxidant directly in the fat used for baking. Brushing with very dilute (0.025%) aqueous solutions of propyl gallate has also given good results.

Sherbet Powder

Cane sugar	15 lb
Dextrose	4½ lb
Citric acid	4⅕ oz
Non-fat dry milk solids (soluble in cold water)	3¾ lb
Stabilizer (soluble in cold water)	6 oz
Color and flavor	to suit

Mix the color and flavor with the dextrose. Stir in the other ingredients, and mix thoroughly. Use 8 oz of this powder to 17½ oz of water.

Sherbet Mix with Yogurt

Cane sugar	5.25 lb
Corn syrup solids	5.25 lb
Pectin	3.00 oz
Yogurt (a thick, fermented liquor made from milk)	13.50 lb
Fruit juice	2.00 qt
Water, enough to make	3.75 gal

Mix together the sugar, corn syrup solids, and pectin in a small amount of water and heat sufficiently for complete solution. Cool to about 50°F., stir in the yogurt, then the fruit juice, and water enough to make 3.75 gal. Use a mixing machine for this operation. If additional tartness is desired, stir in a small amount of a 50% solution of citric acid. Run the mixture into molds, and put these in a refrigerator or pack them in ice and salt until frozen. If desired, coat the finished product with chocolate.

Simple Syrup

	lb
Sugar	12
Corn syrup	3
Water	3

Bring the water to a boil. Remove from the fire and stir in the sugar and corn syrup. Continue to stir until solution is complete.

Sorghum Syrup

Sorghum syrup is obtained from a certain variety of sorghum—a tall, earless, corn-like grass with a head of small seeds forming the tip. Sorghum is cultivated in Africa, Southern Europe, China, and the United States as a livestock food, and for the syrup made from its sweet juice. Sorghum syrup has the following composition:

	average %
Sucrose	39.72
Invert sugar	29.27
Mineral matter	2.03
Organic non-sugars	4.97

Sorgo and the Manufacture of Sorgo Syrup

Sorgo is a member of the grass family, which is grown most extensively for syrup in the Southeastern states. The stalks put out side branches 12 to 15 inches long, but these side branches should not be used for syrup production. Sorgo syrup is a product of good quality; it is light colored and mild, and it has a good, sweet flavor. It is a healthful food, and it is used as a table syrup.

The percentage of juice extracted depends chiefly upon the juiciness of the stalks and the milling equipment. The yield of syrup is determined by the total content of soluble solids in the juice.

All commercial varieties of sorgo are subject to some diseases. A good variety should be resistant to disease; a satisfactory one should grow rapidly enough to mature before the first killing frost.

The following table gives brief descriptions of some varieties of sorgo known to yield a syrup of good quality; and the approximate number of days required for sorgo to mature:

Variety	*Gal. Yield per Acre %*	*Days to Maturity*	*Quality of Syrup*
Hodo	100	129	Excellent
Atlas	62	100	Good
Honey	85	115	Excellent
Iceberg	63	106	Excellent
Sart	107	126	Excellent, mild
Sugar drip	76	100	Good
Tracy	88	106	Good
White African	78	106	Fairly good
Wiley	124	—	Good
Williams	86	106	Excellent

In a fairly fertile soil a small quantity of fertilizer to assist this early growth may be all that is necessary for the entire season. Most of the fertilizer used for sorgo is a 4–8–4 or 5–10–5 mixture of nitrogen, phosphorus, and potassium, respectively.

The best planting time is from early April to the middle of May. The late-maturing varieties usually produce the highest yields of syrup per acre. Under the most favorable conditions of moisture and temperature sorgo seeds germinate within 3 to 5 days.

The plants should be spaced from 8 to 12 inches apart. It is very important that the farmer be skilled in judging the right time for harvesting. The plants are generally considered mature when the seeds are firm, sometimes hard, and not easily crushed with the fingers.

Use the following procedure in the making of sorgo syrup:

Cut the stalks close to the surface of the soil. If cut higher there is a loss in the production of syrup. Remove all the leaves before milling, or else the yield and quality of syrup will suffer. Use a small, upright, 3-roller mill propelled by animal power to crush the stalks, or a larger mill, consisting of 3 horizontal rollers, and propelled by motor power. 100 pounds of stripped and topped stalks should furnish 50 to 60 pounds of juice.

Use a continuous-type, shallow, open evaporator, made of copper or galvanized-iron. Use a direct fire to heat the bottom of the evaporator, or place steam coils in the evaporator to heat the juice. Clarify the juice in the evaporator by removing all skimmings (coagulated proteins and nonsugar substances), which rise to the surface. After clarification, evaporate the juice to the density of syrup as quickly as possible. Determine the desired density by means of a syrup hydrometer, 35 to 36° Baumé, or a good thermometer, 226°F. Use the thermometer test instead of the hydrometer, because it provides an accurate and continuous observation of the syrup density. Filter the finished syrup as efficiently as possible, cool to the right temperature, and store in suitable containers. Fill half-gallon and smaller containers with syrup at a temperature of 190°F., gallon containers, at 180°F., and barrels at 120°F.

Soft Freeze Mix 6%

	lb
Sugar	6.50
Non-fat dry milk	6.00
Vegetable fat	3.00
Stabilizer and emulsifier	0.25
Water	34.25

Use the same procedure as outlined under "Ice Cream Mix, Soft." This mixture will yield 5½ gal.

Soy Flour

Wheat flour is especially deficient in the amino acid, lysine, whereas soy flour, being rich in lysine, will satisfy this deficiency and supplement the other amino acids as well. The following table shows the percentages of the important amino acids in the protein of soy flour:

Amino Acid Content

	%
Arginine	6.99
Cystine	1.48
Glycine	5.49
Histidine	2.40
Isoleucine	5.46
Leucine	7.42
Lysine	6.36
Methionine	1.31
Phenylalanine	4.80
Threonine	3.71
Tryptophane	1.31
Tyrosine	3.06
Valine	5.24

Soy flour will enrich the protein composition of cakes, as it contains about 50% protein. Soy flour, being rich in vitamins and minerals, will improve the properties of any cake in numerous ways.

As it is naturally hydrophilic, soy flour will absorb and retain moisture, thus prolonging the shelf life of the baked product. It not only produces a more uniform, richer, appearance, but it also imparts a rich golden sheen to the crust because of the carmelizing of its proteins.

Soy flour imparts a finer texture and a better firmness to cakes. It minimizes shrinkage and adds more stability. It increases the bulk of the batter and produces larger volumes, since its absorption values are high. Soy flours are classified according to their fat or oil content.

The following tables give the amounts of vitamins and minerals, respectively, found in soy flour used in cakes.

Vitamins in One Pound of Soy Flour, mg.

	High Fat	*Low Fat*	*Extracted*
Vitamin A (I.U.)	204.00	110.00	71.00
Niacin	10.10	11.30	11.50
Pantothenic acid	10.50	11.80	12.00
Pyridoxine	3.40	3.70	3.80
Riboflavin	1.53	1.36	1.58
Thiamine	5.37	6.04	6.13
Biotin	0.29	0.26	0.30
Choline	1171.00	1308.00	1330.00
Inositol	1518.00	1706.00	1730.00

Minerals in Soy Flour, %

Calcium	0.33	0.38	0.38
Copper	0.001	0.001	0.001
Iron	0.009	0.010	0.010
Magnesium	0.250	0.280	0.280
Manganese	0.004	0.004	0.004
Phosphorus	0.680	0.760	0.780
Potassium	1.640	1.840	1.870

The high-fat flour is generally preferred for all-around bakery production, because its high oil content supplies additional fat for lubrication. The low-fat or extracted flours are mostly used for the production of white cakes.

The extracted soy flour, being lowest in fat content, has the highest protein value. Soy flour, being a natural vegetable protein product, is an excellent ingredient for enriching baked products. It is best that the baker start with low percentages of soy flour and increase the amount as he familiarizes himself with the use of it.

Use from 5 to 10% of soy flour in the various cakes. As soy flour has a high absorptive power, add from 1 to 1½ lb of water for each pound of soy flour; the high-fat flour uses the lower proportion of water, and the low-fat or extracted flour uses the larger proportion of water. Increase the leavening and salt by 1 oz and ¼ oz, respectively, for each pound of soy flour. Incorporate the soy flour by creaming it with the sugar, shortening, and egg, stirring in some water if necessary.

Soy flour improves the taste and texture, and adds much to the nutritional value of cakes at very little cost.

Spice Cake

1	Sugar	3	lb
	Shortening	1⅛	lb
	Baking soda (variable)	1¾	oz
	Salt	¼	oz
	* Mixed spice	9/16	oz
	Eggs	1 5/16	lb
	Ground raisins (soaked before grinding)	2¼	lb
	Buttermilk	1½	lb
	Milk, liquid	15	oz
	Cake flour	3¾	lb

Cream (1) thoroughly. Add the eggs while creaming, then add the ground raisins. Finally stir in the buttermilk, milk and cake flour, rotating successively. Apportion in pans as required and bake at about 375°F.

* Mixed Spice

Cinnamon, ground	4	oz
Cloves, ground	1	oz
Ginger, ground	28	gr
Mace, ground	¼	oz

Mix thoroughly, and pack in suitable containers.

Spice Combination for Apple Butter

	lb
Cassia (Chinese cinnamon), ground	84.0
Allspice, ground	18.0
Cloves, ground	18.0

Mix thoroughly and run it through a No. 14 sieve.

Spice Mixture for Stuffings

No. 1

	oz
Sage	5.0
Black pepper	12.0
Nutmeg	4.0
Marjoram	3.0
Salt	8.0

No. 2

	oz
Sage	2.0
Black pepper	8.0

Celery salt	8.0
Onion salt	8.0
Marjoram	2.0
Nutmeg	4.0
Mono-sodium glutamate	6.0

Mix thoroughly the ground ingredients, and use as required to suit the taste.

Sponge Cake

1	Eggs	33	oz
	Egg yolk	16½	oz
	Sugar	3	lb
	Corn syrup	4	oz
	Water	1	pt
	Cake flour	3¼	lb
	Baking powder	⅝	oz
	Anise oil, U.S.P.	1½	oz

Mix (1) and heat over a hot water bath to 115°F., then whip at medium speed until the batch holds a crease (made by drawing a spatula over it) for 20 seconds. Now add the mixture of cake flour, baking powder, and anise oil, and mix thoroughly. Exercise great care not to destroy the air cells created during the beating operation. Scale into pans and bake in a moderate oven (350°F.).

The thickness of the crust may be reduced by baking at a slightly higher temperature, thus reducing the tendency to form a skin.

Sponge Drops

Sugar, granulated	39	oz
Eggs	28½	oz
Salt	⅛	oz
Vanilla	to suit	
Milk, hot (140°F.)	21	oz
Cake flour } sift	3¾	lb
Baking powder } together	½–¾	oz

Mix the sugar, eggs, salt, and vanilla, and heat to about 110°F., then whip the mass light as for sponge cake. Finally, stir in alternately the hot milk and the mixture of cake flour and baking powder, and continue mixing until smooth. Drop onto papered pans and bake at about 385°F. Cool and then ice with fondant.

Stabilized Caramel

Corn syrup	15.00	lb
Sugar	7.25	lb
Sweetened condensed whole milk	12.50	lb
Standard vegetable shortening	2.50	lb
Butter	1.25	oz
Salt	1.00	oz
Lecithin	0.63	oz
* Ammonium carbonate solution	1.25	oz

* 3 oz to 1 pt water.

Place all the ingredients in a kettle equipped with scrapers, and cook to 190°F. Now prepare a dry blend of 5 oz of sugar and 224 gr of Sea Kem Irish moss extractive, and dissolve this blend in 1½ lb of water previously heated to 180°F. Finally, stir the solution of Irish moss and sugar into the main batch, and cook to about 240°F. Allow it to cool, and stir in 7 dr of vanilla flavor. Pour the mass onto a greased slab and cool. While cooling, cut into small blocks of any desired size.

Stock Icings

No. 1: Water Icing

Gelatin, U.S.P.	0.50	oz
Hot water	10.00	oz
Glucose	10.00	oz
Confectioners' sugar	5.00	lb
Vanilla	0.25	oz

Use a small part of the water cold to dissolve the gelatin. Add the rest of the water hot and stir until solution is complete. Finally, mix all of the ingredients together until the whole mass is smooth. Use this icing as is for transparent glacé effects, or beat the whole mass to desired consistency. Other flavors, and colors, may be used if desired.

No. 2: Simple Icing

Gelatin, U.S.P.	3/4	oz
Water	12	oz
Invert sugar	18	oz
Confectioners' sugar	5 5/8	lb
Flavor and color	to suit	

Soak the gelatin in the water and then heat it to 170°F. Stir the invert sugar into the dissolved gelatin. Finally, stir in the confectioners' sugar, flavor, and color, and beat this whole mixture until it is of the proper consistency for use.

Sour Cream Doughnuts

1	Sugar	2 1/2	lb
1	Baking powder	2 1/2	oz
1	Baking soda	1 1/4	oz
1	Salt	1 1/4	oz
1	Non-fat dry milk	5	oz
1	Pastry flour, unbleached	10	lb
	Sour cream	35	oz
	Eggs	1 1/4	lb
	Buttermilk (variable)	4	pt

Mix (1) thoroughly by sifting. Add the sour cream, eggs, and buttermilk, and continue mixing until a smooth dough is obtained. Roll out and cut to the desired size or run through a machine. (Increase the amount of buttermilk if a machine is used.) Cook in hot oil at 370°F.

Strawberry Chiffon Pie

Boiling water	3 3/8	lb
Strawberry juice	1 1/8	lb
Gelatin, strawberry flavored	2 1/4	lb
Eggs	1 7/8	lb
Egg yolks	6	oz
Salt	55	gr
Crushed, drained strawberries	3	lb
Lemon juice	6	oz

Mix the strawberry juice with the hot water and dissolve the gelatin in it. Add slowly the eggs, egg yolks, and salt to the hot gelatin mixture while beating it light. Stir in the crushed strawberries and lemon juice, and then chill, stirring occasionally until the mass thickens. When thickened, add this mass slowly to the following meringue and mix until smooth:

Meringue

	lb
Egg whites	3
Granulated sugar	1½

Follow the same procedure as for meringue under Lemon Chiffon Pie. Fill about 1½ lb of the finished product into pre-baked pie shells. Chill thoroughly. If desired, top with whipping cream.

Strawberry Oil

	oz
Ethyl methyl phenyl glycidate	4.00
Ethyl butyrate	0.50
Isoamyl acetate	0.10
Isoamyl butyrate	0.25
Ethyl benzoate	0.10
Propyl acetate	0.25
Isobutyl anthranilate	0.25
Octyl acetate	0.50
Ketone No. 22	0.25
Nerol	0.10
Vanillin	0.20
Ethyl acetate	1.00
Ethyl valerate	0.33

Strawberry Pie Glaze

1	Water	2 lb
2	Sugar	1 lb
	Pectin (100 grade)	1½ or 2 oz
3	Apricot pulp, finely ground	7 or 8 oz
	Sugar	7 lb

Bring (1) to a strong boil. Mix thoroughly (2) and then add this mixture to (1). Place (3) in a double boiler, add the (1) and (2), and bring the entire mixture to a boil. Use this glaze while hot; it will set fairly firm.

Strudel Dough

Water (variable)	30	oz
Bread flour	4	lb
Eggs	1	lb
Corn oil (warm)	1	lb
Salt	½	oz

Mix all the ingredients until the mass is smooth and pliable. Allow the finished dough to rest for about 30 minutes before sheeting, stretching, and filling.

Strudel Filling

Apples, finely chopped	3.25 lb
Cake crumbs, partially toasted	0.50 lb
Raisins, soaked and drained	0.50 lb
Currants	0.25 lb
Sugar	0.25 lb
Maraschino cherries, chopped	0.25 lb
Fruit peel, candied	0.25 lb
Almonds, finely chopped	0.13 lb
Cinnamon	28.00 gr

Mix all together thoroughly. Stretch a piece of dough, very thin, brush it with butter, and place on it a generous portion of this filling.

Stuffing For Turkey (To Freeze)

1	Oleomargarine	7.50 lb
	Celery (including leaves and stalks), finely chopped	7.50 lb
	Onions, finely chopped	7.50 lb
2	Stale bread, diced	39.00 lb
	Salt	3.75 oz
	Pepper, ground	0.50 oz
3	Turkey broth	30.00 lb

Place (1) in a kettle and brown it. Blend (2) into (1). Then moisten the whole batch with (3) until thoroughly mixed. Stuff into dressed, disemboweled turkey, and freeze.

Sugar Substitute

Sodium cyclohexylsulfamate is a new sweetening agent which is thirty to fifty times sweeter than cane sugar. This compound has no caloric value, and it can be cooked or heated without losing its sweetening properties.

Tabasco Sauce

Tabasco pulp	15.0 gal
Salt	2.5 lb
Vinegar, 10% (100 grain) acetic acid	3.0 gal

Cook the tabasco pulp together with the salt until volume is reduced to 12¾ gal. Add the vinegar and cook for 5–6 minutes more. Finally, fill the sauce into suitable bottles, and pasteurize it (*i.e.*, expose it to temperature of 160°F., for 30 minutes, to prevent fermentation). To make tabasco pulp, cook Tabasco peppers until thoroughly disintegrated, and then run the mass through a sieve to remove seeds and skins.

Taffy

Sorghum syrup	6¾ lb
Sugar	4½ lb
Butter	3 oz
Vinegar	1½ oz
Sodium bicarbonate, U.S.P.	a pinch

Place the first 3 components in a kettle, and cook to 250°F. Remove kettle from fire, add the vinegar and the soda, and stir in any desired flavor. Pour the mass onto a greased slab, and as soon as it can be handled, pull it on a large candy hook. Cut it into 2-inch lengths.

Tapioca Flour Glaze

Water	4 lb
Sugar	2 lb
Corn syrup	2 lb
Corn starch	5 oz
Tapioca flour	3 oz
Icing sugar (dissolved in a little water)	2½ oz
Citric acid	¼ oz
Color	as desired

Stir together the corn syrup, sugar, and water and bring to a boil. When solution is complete, add the corn starch, tapioca flour, and dissolved icing sugar, and boil for about 2 minutes to thicken. Finally, add the citric acid and the color, and mix thoroughly. Increase the amount of starch and tapioca flour if a thicker glaze is desired.

Tartare Sauce

Mayonnaise	1.0 gal
Capers	5.6 oz
Olives	5.6 oz
Onions	4.8 oz
Parsley	5.6 oz
Pickles	5.6 oz

Have the vegetables finely chopped and mix them thoroughly with the mayonnaise. Fill into jars, cap, and label.

Vanilla Chiffon Pie (Light, fine quality)

1	Gelatin, U.S.P.	1½ oz
	Milk, liquid	6 oz
2	Milk, liquid	4½ lb
	Sugar	21 oz
	Butter	15 oz
	Salt	83 gr
3	Eggs	30 oz
	Milk, liquid	12 oz
	Starch, U.S.P.	6 oz
4	Whipping cream	4½ lb
	Vanilla flavor	to suit

Soak (1) for some time. Bring (2) to a boil and stir it until it is thick and smooth. Remove from the fire and stir in the gelatin mixture. Now add (3) and mix thoroughly. Cool this mixture to about 145°F., then fold in (4). Fill pre-baked shells with this finished product, and chill for a few hours.

Vanilla Flavor, 16-Fold (Synthetic)

Vanillin	8 oz
Ethyl vanillin	1 oz
Protovanol C	1 oz
Heliotropine	⅓ oz
St. John's Bread extract	2½ oz
Pure vanilla 10-fold	1 oz
Propylene glycol, U.S.P.	3½ pt
Caramel	2¾ oz
Water, to make	1 gal

Heat the propylene glycol, and stir into it the vanillin, ethyl vanillin, heliotropine and Protovanol C. Keep on stirring until solution is complete. Stir vigorously while adding about 2½ pts of water, then add the St. John's Bread extract and the pure vanilla 10-fold. Dissolve the caramel in some water and add it to the vanillin solution with constant stirring. Stir in more water to make 1 gallon. If desired, add 40 minums of caprylate solution to the finished gallon. This gallon, when mixed with 15 gallons of water, will yield 16 gallons of standard imitation vanilla flavor.

Vanilla Oil (Synthetic)

		oz
1	Vanillin	4.50
	Heliotropine	0.30
	Vanillidine acetone (F. Ritter & Co.)	0.75

2	Protovanol C (Florasynth)	0.30
	Anisic alcohol	0.75
	Anisyl acetate	0.33
	Absolute resin vanilla	0.75
	Absolute resin Peru	0.75
3	Benzyl alcohol	6.00

Mix (2) and (3). Add (1) and shake well. If necessary, apply a slow heat to aid solution. Allow this to stand a week or more before using it. Use 1–1½ oz of this oil to make 1 gallon of standard, imitation vanilla.

Vanillin Solvent

	oz
Glucose (43° Bé)	77.56
Water	16.77
Glycerin, U.S.P.	33.67

Mix thoroughly and heat to 25°C. This vehicle will dissolve 1.53 oz of vanillin.

Vichysoisse Soup (To Freeze)

Potatoes, sliced	50.00 lb
Onions, sliced	7.50 lb
Leeks, sliced	5.00 lb
Water	6.25 gal
Chicken bouillon cubes, granulated	1.25 lb
Pepper, white	2.50 oz
Celery salt	0.88 oz
Light cream	2.50 gal

Place the first 7 components into a jacketed kettle, and boil slowly until all the vegetables are cooked. Next, run the batch through a pulper, and finally stir in the light cream into the pulp. Fill into cans or liquid-holding paper containers, and then freeze.

Vitamins

Avidin, a substance in raw egg white, destroys one of the B vitamins, namely, Biotin or Vitamin H, thus greatly increasing the daily requirements of Vitamin B if much egg white is ingested.

All the Vitamin C in food products is destroyed or rendered ineffective when prepared in a copper cooking utensil.

Iron salt contained in medicinal preparations destroys Vitamin E.

Vitamin C (Ascorbic Acid)

The following table shows minimum and maximum levels of Vitamin C in commercially canned juices. All figures are in milligrams per 100 grams of juice.

	Min	*Max*
Apple juice	0.2	3.6
Grape juice	0.0	4.7
Grapefruit juice	10.00	49.0
Orange juice	9.7	70.0
Pineapple juice	5.4	18.0
Tomato juice	2.5	32.0

The National Research Council recommends 75 milligrams as the daily allowance for adult males and 70 milligrams daily for adult females. These levels are supported by many controlled nutrition studies.

Whip Meringue Powder

Egg albumen, powdered	26.0 lb
Tapioca flour	8.4 lb
Icing sugar (10X)	4.0 lb
Aluminum ammonium sulfate, U.S.P., powdered	12.8 oz
Gelatin, U.S.P., powdered	6.4 oz
Salt	6.4 oz
Vanilla, powdered	0.8 oz

Mix the powders thoroughly, and use 6 oz of this powder to each quart of cold water. Whip fairly light, then gradually add:

Granulated sugar	3.0 lb

Continue whipping until a stiff meringue is obtained.

Wheat Flour

A good wheat flour for baking should have high absorption, a medium dough-development time, and good endurance in mixing. The dough should be elastic and stable during the entire baking process. The resultant bread should have good crumb color, grain and texture, and loaf volume.

Tests for quality can be divided roughly into the following categories: Physical grain tests, chemical tests, and physical dough tests performed on flour.

PHYSICAL GRAIN TESTS:

The test weight is one of the oldest. Wheats of high test weight are superior to wheats of low test weight. They have better keeping qualities.

CHEMICAL TESTS:

The quality of flour is determined mainly by the quantity and quality of protein. The quantity of protein is determined by the Kjeldahl procedure.

Another chemical test is the ash test: A weighed sample is burned to ash in a muffle furnace at1100°F. overnight, and the amount of ash is expressed as a percentage of the original sample. The ash test shows the thoroughness of the separation of bran and germ from the rest of the wheat kernel. Certain millers do not use wheat that is high in ash even though it may be of superior quality. Usually high-protein flour has a high ash content, yet it claims a premium on the market. The simplest and best single indicator of quality in flour is the amount of protein it contains.

PHYSICAL DOUGH TESTS:

Many factors other than the variety of wheat affect the characteristics of flour. As the protein content increases, the absorption, the time for dough-development, and the stability also increase, but the mixing tolerance index (MTI) decreases. Flour with a short time of dough-development and good stability to mixing is in great demand by bakers, as less power is required for mixing. Two instruments, the Brabender Farinograph, and the National Swanson Working Mixo-

graph, are now widely used to measure the characteristics of dough. A wheat with a high protein content and a good mixing tolerance is very much in demand.

Whole Wheat Cake

1	Sugar, granulated	3¾ lb
	Butter	22½ oz
	Shortening	22½ oz
	Salt	1 oz
	Flavor	to suit
2	Eggs	3⅛ lb
	Corn syrup	10 oz
3	Milk, liquid (variable)	1½ lb
4	Whole wheat flour, extra fine-ground	4⅜ lb
	Baking powder	137 gr

Cream (1) thoroughly. Mix (2), and add this gradually while creaming. Finally, add alternately (3) and (4), and continue to mix until smooth. Scale as required, and bake at about 335°F.

Whipped Cream Filling or Topping

Gelatin, 200 bloom	1½ oz
Water, hot, 180°F.	33 oz
Heavy cream, 40% butter fat	1½ gal
Sugar, powdered	15 oz
Salt	40 gr
Flavor	to suit

Allow the cream to age for about 30 hours. Dissolve the gelatin in the hot water. Add the heavy cream (after aging it) and mix well with a wire whip. Allow this mixture to stand for about 15 hours, then place it in a clean, cold, bowl and whip at medium speed until the mass is of a medium firm consistency—do not overbeat. Finally, incorporate the powdered sugar, salt, and flavor, and the cream is ready to use. Add any fruit to the filling, if desired, provided the fruits are thickened as for pie filling.

Whole Wheat Doughnuts

		oz
1	Fine granulated sugar	24.75
	Honey	2.25
	Shortening	3.37
	Salt	0.40
	Non-fat, dry milk	4.88
	Baking soda (sodium bicarbonate, U.S.P.)	0.75
	Lemon oil	0.33
	Mace oil	0.33
	Egg yolk	9.00
	Water, cold (variable)	45.00
	Whole wheat flour, fine	33.75
	Cake flour	45.00
	Cream of Tartar	1.69

Cream (1) thoroughly. Add, while creaming, the powdered egg yolk and stir in the cold water. Sift the flour with the cream of tartar, and add this to the creamed mass. Continue to mix until the batch is of a smooth consistency. Cut out the doughnuts and cook them in hot fat at 375°F.

Wiener Coatings

A 0.0025-inch coating of acetostearin on wieners will inhibit loss of moisture and rancidity. The coated wieners lost only 2% of moisture by weight when stored for nine days at 39°F., whereas uncoated wieners lost 39%. The coating itself is highly resistant to rancidity and will, if unbroken, prevent the growth of mold spores.

Wine Clarifier

Bentonite	1½ lb
Gelatin	2 oz

Mix thoroughly and use this mixture to treat 500 gallons of wine. Have the treated wines refrigerated before filtering, as this procedure is more effective than the usual practice of filtering before refrigerating.

Yeast-Raised Doughnuts

Water (variable for desired consistency of dough)	6	pt
Yeast	12	oz
Soft wheat flour	3	lb
Bread flour	9	lb
Potato flour	6	oz
Non-fat dry milk	3	oz
Salt	2	oz
Baking powder	⅜	oz
Sugar, fine granulated	15	oz
Shortening	33	oz
Eggs	18	oz
Lemon oil	30	min
Mace oil	30	min

Mix all the ingredients thoroughly to produce a smooth dough. When the dough in the mixer is at 80°F. take it out of the mixer and allow it to reach a full rise. Then take it to the worktable for rolling and cutting. Work some scraps back into each piece of dough before each rolling and cutting. Fry at 375°–380°F.

Yellow Cake Mix

	oz
Cake flour	46.08
Sugar	55.68
Emulsifying type shortening	16.00
Non-fat milk solids	3.84
Egg yolk	4.00
Baking powder	2.56
Salt	1.00
Vanilla flavor	to suit

Gingerbread Mix

	oz
Cake flour	41.73
Sugar	48.00
Emulsifying type shortening	16.00
Molasses solids	8.96
Non-fat milk solids	3.84
Whole egg solids	4.60
Baking powder	2.56
Salt	0.90
Cinnamon, ground	0.41
Mace, ground	0.25
Ginger, ground	0.51
Cloves, ground	0.25

For both:

Have all dry ingredients finely powdered, and mix them thoroughly. Blend well with the shortening in a mixer for 15 minutes at low speed.

Paraffin wax	10⅔ oz
Morpholine	9$\frac{1}{9}$ oz
* White spirits	25 lb
Water	25 lb

* A turpentine substitute: a petroleum product, having a flash point and degree of evaporation similar to turpentine; the fraction of distillate boiling at 150–250°C. is called white spirit.

Mix the first six ingredients together and heat slowly until solution is complete. Heat the water to the same temperature and add it slowly to the solvent-oil-wax mixture with extremely vigorous agitation. If a paste polish is desired, stir 8⅓ lb of an abrasive, such as bentonite, into the liquid polish.

No. 2: Semi-Liquid

Carnauba wax	4 lb
Stearic acid	2⅓ lb
Paraffin wax	2 lb
Beeswax	1⅓ lb
Triethanolamine	14½ oz
* White spirits	16⅔ lb
Water	16⅔ lb

* See note under No. 1.

Mix the waxes and stearic acid with the white spirit, and heat slowly until solution is complete. Dissolve the triethanolamine in the water and heat this to the same temperature. Stir the aqueous solution into the wax-solvent mixture, and continue stirring until the resultant product is cold. If a more pasty consistency is desired, use less of water or solvent, or both.

No. 3: Paste

	oz
Mineral oil (60–80 viscosity)	7.68
Naphtha	7.68
Oleic acid	2.56
Carnauba wax	1.28
Infusorial earth	14.10
Aminomethylpropanol	1.28
Water	93.42

Melt the first four ingredients together and stir in the infusorial earth to make a thick paste. Mix the aminomethylpropanol with the water and heat to about 75°C. Stir this aqueous solution into the solvent-oil-wax mixture, and continue stirring until cold. For perfect results, use a colloid mill for this operation. You may vary the proportions of the infusorial earth, mineral oil, and naphtha within a reasonable range.

No. 4: Paste

	oz
Rosin	9
Carnauba wax	12
Paraffin wax, 140°F.	21
* White spirits	108
Bentonite	18
Soda ash	9
Glycerin	9
Water	114

* See note under No. 1.

Melt the waxes and rosin and thin with the white spirit. Make the bentonite into a paste with a small amount of water, adding more water gradually. Dissolve the glycerin and soda ash in the remaining water and add this to the bentonite mixture. Finally, slowly add the bentonite mixture to the wax-solvent combination with continuous stirring and stir until it is cold. The resultant product is a smooth, soft paste with mild abrasive action. The glycerin controls the rate of evaporation, and its proportion may be increased if the paste dries too rapidly. This product is a rapid polisher which gives good results on old, worn paint, as well as on metal parts.

No. 5

	oz
Carnauba wax	8.0
Ouricury wax	2.0
Beeswax	4.0
Ceresin	3.0
Petrolatum	0.5
Stearic acid	8.0
Benzin (naphtha)	70.0
Triethanolamine	3.0
Water	80.0
Tripoli	54.0

Melt the waxes, petrolatum, stearic acid, and triethanolamine, and slowly stir in the benzin. Keep the temperature at 90–95°C. When the solution becomes clear, add the tripoli and mix thoroughly. Heat the water in a separate container to the same temperature, and pour it into the hot naphtha solution with vigorous stirring until an emulsion of proper consistency is obtained. Continue to stir slowly until the product is cold.

No. 6: Silicone

	oz
Microcrystalline wax, high melting	6.40
Silicone oil	1.92
White mineral spirits	119.68

Dissolve the wax and silicone oil in the mineral spirit at about 140°F., and then cool fairly rapidly with good agitation. This polish produces a film of good appearance and durability. Wipe the polish over the surface with a cloth and let the solvent evaporate. Remove excess wax; a good shine is obtained by comparatively moderate rubbing.

Brass and Copper Polish

Carbowax polyethylene glycol 1500	7.0 lb
Tergitol nonionic NPX	9.6 oz
Water	5.0 lb
Citric acid	1.0 lb
Sodium chloride	1.0 lb
Kieselguhr	3.8 lb
Bentonite	25.6 oz
Perfume oil	to suit

Mix the Glycol 1500 and Tergitol in the water, and stir until a clear solution results. Add the citric acid and sodium chloride and stir until dissolved. Finally, stir in the bentonite, kieselguhr, and perfume oil, and continue the mixing until a smooth paste forms.

Chromium Polish

	oz
Kieselguhr	11½
Amorphous silica	4
Oleic acid	10¼
Ammonia (0.88)	2⅗
Glycerin	12¾
Powdered soap	2⅗
Water	84½

Mix the soap, glycerin, and ammonia in the water, and stir in the oleic acid. Continue stirring, and, while stirring, incorporate the silica and kieselguhr.

Dust-Attracting Cloths

No. 1

	oz
Crude oleic acid	96.00
Petrolatum	3.00
Stearic acid	3.00
Methyl salicylate	2.75

No. 2

	oz
Crude oleic acid	36.00
Petrolatum	12.00
Stearic acid	18.00
Methyl salicylate	1.25

For both: Melt the first three components, remove from fire and stir in the perfume oil. Cut good-weight canton flannel (a strong cotton cloth with one side soft and fleecy) into any desired size, and dip each piece into the warm mixture until it is thoroughly saturated; then pass it through tight wringer rolls. Finally, fold and wrap each one in oiled paper or acetate film. This cloth is excellent for removing dust and restoring the luster to car finishes.

Floor Polishes

No. 1

Wax O M	10.88 oz
Wax O P	0.64 oz
Wax F	0.64 oz
Cresin (mp 70°C)	0.64 oz
Paraffin (mp 54°C)	25.60 oz
* Mineral spirits	89.22 oz
Perfume oil	3.00 dr

No. 2

Wax O	7.76 oz
Wax F	2.56 oz
Ceresin	0.64 oz
Paraffin	24.32 oz
* Mineral spirits	94.34 oz
Perfume oil	3.00 dr

* A petroleum product intermediate between gasoline and kerosene.

For both: Mix the waxes, ceresin and paraffin in the mineral spirits, and heat slowly until solution is complete. Remove the heat and incorporate the perfume oil at 40°C. Continue the mixing until cold.

Furniture (Cream) Polish

No. 1

	oz
Mineral oil	18.0
* Stoddard Solvent	12.8
Sodium lauryl sulfate	1.3
Gum karaya	1.3
Glycerin	2.5
Triethanolamine	5.1
Water	87.0

* A high flash point petroleum naphtha.

Mix the lauryl sulfate, gum, glycerin, and triethanolamine with the water, and agitate until the mass is homogeneous.

Mix the oil with the Stoddard Solvent, and pour this slowly into the aqueous solution with constant stirring. This preparation polishes bone dry.

No. 2

Wax S	7.68 oz
Wax BJ (unbleached)	5.12 oz
Paraffin	6.40 oz
Balsam turpentine oil	43.52 oz
Silicone oil, 350 CS (centistokes)	5.12 dr
Triethanolamine	5.12 dr
Water	63.62 oz
Perfume oil	3.00 dr

Mix the first five components and heat slowly until solution is complete. Dissolve the triethanolamine in the water and heat to the same temperature. Add the aqueous solution, with vigorous stirring, to the solvent-wax-oil mixture. Remove the heat, and incorporate the perfume oil at 40°C. Continue the mixing until cold.

Furniture Polish

A simple but quite up-to-date furniture polish may be made as follows:

	oz
Mineral oil	51
* Ethofat 60/20	6⅖
Water	70⅕

* From Armour Chemical Division, Chicago, Ill.

Mix the Ethofat with the mineral oil, then add the water with moderate agitation.

General Purpose Polish

Carbowax (polyethylene glycol 1500)	20.0 lb
Tergitol nonionic NPX	1.2 lb
Water	11.6 lb
Borax	4.0 oz
Trisodium orthophosphate	2.0 oz
Bentonite	3.6 lb
Kieselguhr	8.4 lb
Perfume oil	to suit

Use the same procedure as outlined under Brass and Copper polish.

Liquid Metal Polish

	oz
Infusorial earth	6.40
Silica dust	5.12
Powdered red iron oxide	5.12
Benzin	24.32
Kerosene	12.80
Oleic acid	2.56
Triethanolamine	0.64
Ammonia, 26° Bé	1.92
Water	69.12

Mix the ammonia and water. Mix the oleic acid with the benzin and kerosene, and stir in the abrasives. Continue stirring and add the aqueous solution of ammonia and the triethanolamine. You may increase the proportion of water by about 10% if so desired.

Liquid Solvent Polish

Low molecular weight polyethylene (ACP-6)	10 oz
Silicone (500 centistokes)	6 oz
Naphtha	3 gal

Mix and heat slowly until a clear solution is obtained. Continue to stir until cold.

Polishing Paste

Low molecular weight polyethylene (ACP-6)	15 oz
Paraffin wax	42 oz
Ceresin	1 oz
Mineral spirits (a petroleum product)	8¾ pt

Melt together, stir occasionally, pour into cans.

Shoe Polish

Low molecular weight polyethylene (ACP-6)	12 oz
Beeswax	14 oz
Carnauba wax	24 oz
Mineral spirits (a petroleum product)	10½ pt

Mix and heat by water bath until melted. Remove the heat and continue to stir until uniform.

Silicone Automobile Polish

	oz
* Silicone oil	0.7
Petroleum ether (Benzin)	2.7
Water	12.3
Octadecylamine acetate	0.3

* From Dow Corning Corp., Midland, Michigan.

Mix the oil with the benzin, add the amine acetate, then the water, and shake well.

Silicone Furniture Polish (Paste)

	oz
SF-96-300 Silicone fluid (General Electric Co.)	6.40
Carnauba wax	32.00
Mineral oil	3.33
* Mineral spirits	75.39
Turpentine	10.88

* See note under Floor Polish.

Mix the silicone fluid with the mineral spirits and turpentine. Melt the carnauba wax with the mineral oil, and slowly pour the silicone mixture into the molten wax, stirring all the time until cold.

Silicone-Wax Polish

	oz
Carnauba wax	2.56
Dimethyl silicone MS200/500 CS	2.56
Oil of turpentine	122.88

Mix the wax with the oil of turpentine and heat on a water bath until solution is complete. Stir in the silicone and mix thoroughly. The resultant polish produces a high gloss and it has very little tendency to smear. The polish is very durable, and is water-repellent and stain-resistant. The polished surface is resistant to heat and sunlight, and it can be easily cleaned.

Inks

Inks for Ruling

The acid and basic dyes are the only dyes having the necessary characteristics for ruling work. The acid dyes are much more suitable for ruling than the basic dyes, because they are more soluble in water, they keep well in solution without preservatives, and they are much more stable to light than the basic dyes are. Stronger solutions of the acid dyes must be used, however, because they have less tinctorial power than the basic dyes.

Acid dyes are suitable for such ruling work as records and ledgers; basic dyes are suitable for cheaper grades of paper, such as writing tablets, pads, etc.

Use the following acid and basic dyes for ruling inks:

Color	*Acid Dye*	* *C. I. No.*
Blue	Cyanol Extra F F	715
Brown	Resorcin Brown	235
Green	Naphthalene Green V	735
Red	Croceine Scarlet 3B	252
Red	Fast Crimson	31
Violet	Wool Violet 4 BN	698
Yellow	Tartrazine Wool Yellow extra, concentrated	640

Color	*Basic Dye*	*C. I. No.*
Blue	Methylene Blue 2B (zinc free)	922
Brown	Bismarck Brown R or Y	332
Green	Malachite Green	657
Green	Acid Green B	666
Red	Croceine Scarlet 3B	252
Violet	Methyl Violet 2B	680
Yellow	Chrysoidin Y	20

* Color Index.

Dissolve about ¼ oz of the desired dye in one gallon of hot (not boiling) distilled water. Allow the solution to stand for a few hours before using it.

Paper that is poorly sized, especially with greasy sizing, will not take the ink. This can be overcome by substituting alcohol or acetic acid for part of the water. This substitution increases the brightness of the color, and decreases the spreading of the ink over the paper. Excessive acidity of inks should be avoided, because it corrodes the pens and tends to destroy the paper on which the rulings are made.

The following tests will help to distinguish between basic and acid dyes:

(1) Dissolve some of the dye in water and add a small amount of tannic acid solution. If the dye is basic, it will show a precipitate; if the dye is acid, it will not be affected. Eosin, which is both basic and acidic, can be easily identified by its fluorescence when dissolved in water.

(2) Dye a fresh piece of woolen yarn. If the dye is basic, most of it can be rinsed out with water; if the dye is acid, it remains fixed on the wool.

Most of the manufacturers reduce their dyes to a standard strength. For basic dyes, the reducing material is dextrin; for acid dyes, the reducing material is sodium sulfate, U.S.P. Dextrin has a tendency to retard the flow of ink, and moreover, if too much dextrin is used, the ink solution tends to mold, particularly in warm weather. This can be remedied by the use of preservatives, yet these, too, may cause trouble, as some preservatives cause the precipitation of the dyes. Most acid dyes are not precipitated by preservatives.

Black Ink for Ruling

The following formula will produce a satisfactory black ink for ruling. It produces blue-black rules, but dries deep-black, which is fast to light, and resistant to water when completely dried:

Tannic acid, U.S.P.	6⅝ oz
Gallic acid, N.F.	2⅛ oz
Ferrous sulfate, U.S.P.	8½ oz
Hydrochloric acid, C.P. 10% solution	7 oz
Phenol, U.S.P.	¼ oz
Soluble Blue A (C. I. No. 707)	⅝ oz
Water, enough to make	2 gal

When purchasing the blue dye, specify that it must not react with the phenol.

Dissolve the gallic and tannic acids in warm water, at about 65°C. Dissolve the ferrous sulfate in ½ gallon of water, add to it the hydrochloric acid solution, and then the gallic-tannic acid solution. Dissolve the blue dye in ½ gallon of water, and add it to the ink solution. Finally, stir in the phenol, dilute the mixture to 2 gallons, and shake well.

Water-Resistant Inks for Ruling

Make these inks according to the following formulas:

Victoria Blue base (Blue), C. I. No. 729: 69 gr to ½ gal solvent.

Rhodamine base B (Red), C. I. No. 749: ¼ oz to ½ gal solvent.

Methyl Violet base D, C. I. No. 680: 123 gr to ½ gal solvent.

Auramine base (Yellow), C. I. No. 655: ⅛ oz to ½ gal solvent.

Make the solvent as follows:

	oz
Acetic acid, 28%	12
Distilled water	108

Mix thoroughly. Dissolve the desired dye in this solvent. The ruling ink made from Rhodamine base B is not completely water-resistant.

Black Ink for Ruling (Water-Resistant)

	oz
Fast Black A, extra dye	9/16
Ammonium hydroxide, 28%	3
Distilled water	94

Mix thoroughly. Do not use this ink with brass pens or disks, because copper is soluble in ammoniacal solutions.

The inks used in ruling machines usually flow by capillary attraction from the ink fountain, through wicks and felts, to the ruling pens which draw the lines on the pages of account books, ledgers, forms, and pads.

Marking Ink for Porcelain (Permanent)

	gm
Potassium carbonate	4.0
Borax	4.0
Lead monoxide	8.0
Cobalt nitrate	8.0
Glycerin	sufficient

Dry the cobalt nitrate at 100°C. for about one hour, mix it with the other chemicals, and grind and pulverize all to form a very fine powder. Add to this powder 20 to 24 drops of glycerin until the product is of proper consistency to flow from a pen.

Write lightly on the ceramic ware and heat the piece to redness for a minute or two over an oxidizing flame. On cooling, a clear, permanent blue mark appears on the porcelain surface.

Insecticides and Rodenticides

Anti-Midge Cream

Stearic acid	5.4 oz
Sodium hydroxide	1.5 gm
Glyceryl monostearate	1.0 oz
Water	2.5 oz
Dimethyl phthalate	8.5 oz
Citronella oil	5.0 cc

Melt the stearic acid and glyceryl monostearate, and add to this hot mass the hot solution of caustic soda, with constant stirring. While still warm, add the dimethyl phthalate, and finally the citronella oil. Continue stirring until cold. Regulate the consistency of this cream by increasing or decreasing the water content.

Anti-Midge Oil

	oz
Dimethyl phthalate	126.72
Citronella oil	1.28

Mix thoroughly. Apply to arms, legs, neck, and chest with a piece of cotton.

Ant Poison

1	Sugar	2 lb
	Honey	6 oz
	Glycerin	3 oz
	Water	2 pt

Mix and dissolve the ingredients, and boil for about 5 minutes.

2	Thallium sulfate	61.73 gr
	Water, lukewarm	2 pt

Dissolve the thallium sulfate in the water. Add (2) to (1) and shake well. Place this mixture in small containers, such as pillboxes, and punch quarter-inch holes in them. This poison is particularly effective in reducing ant colonies when the actual colonies cannot be located.

Carpet Beetle

The larvae of the carpet beetle destroy carpets and other woolen materials. Use

Chlordane	2.0%
or	
Dieldrin	0.5%

Dissolve in any common organic solvent. Paint or spray either of these solutions on baseboards, in cracks, and on shelves where woolen materials are stored.

Control of Chiggers

The red bugs called Chiggers are a species of mites. They are so small that one cannot see them without a magnifying glass. Two types of chiggers commonly attack man. Their bites cause intense itching and small reddish welts on the skin. Chiggers are especially troublesome in the south.

If an area is infested with chiggers, use repellents to prevent their attack, or get rid of the infestation by spraying or dusting the area with an insecticide. The following compounds are highly effective repellents:

Dimethyl phthalate
Dimethyl carbate
Ethyl hexanediol
Benzyl benzoate

These compounds do more than repel; they kill chiggers that attempt to crawl over clothing or skin areas treated with them. Use these repellents individually or in combination. Apply any repellent to clothing by rubbing it on, pouring it directly from the bottle, or spraying it over the fabric. (Do not use repellents on rayon fabrics.)

Apply repellent lightly to bare arms or legs. Use an ordinary hand sprayer for spraying.

Long-lasting protection is effected by impregnating clothing with an emulsified repellent or by spraying an undiluted repellent on the clothing. For best results use dimethyl phthalate or benzyl benzoate.

To Impregnate Clothing

Soap powder (don't use synthetic detergents)	292 gr
Benzyl benzoate	2 oz
Water	1 qt

Put the soap in the water and shake until the soap is in complete solution. Take 8 oz of the soapy water and mix with the benzyl benzoate, stirring vigorously. Pour the benzyl benzoate mixture into the rest of the soapy water and stir vigorously. This emulsion will treat one set of clothes consisting of shirt, trousers, and socks. Place the clothes in a container and slowly pour on the emulsion. Wet them uniformly but don't let them soak. Wring them and hang out to dry.

Benzyl benzoate lasts longer than dimethyl phthalate, and it washes out less readily. Clothing should be retreated after it has been laundered twice.

To Spray the Clothing

Dimethyl phthalate or Benzyl benzoate	2 oz

Use a hand sprayer and apply a fine mist of the repellent to the inside and outside of the clothing until it is slightly moist, but not wet. Do not use more than 2 oz of the undiluted repellent to a set of clothes. Allow the clothes to dry for several hours before wearing them. Sprayed-on repellent loses its effectiveness sooner than when applied by the impregnation method.

To Reduce Itching

Take a soapy bath immediately, then rinse it off. Repeat this several times. Next, dab any kind of antiseptic on each welt. Then apply the following anesthetic to allay the itching.

Anesthetic Lotion

	oz
Ethyl aminobenzoate, U.S.P.	1.0
Methyl salicylate, U.S.P.	0.4
Salicylic acid, U.S.P.	0.1
Specially denatured alcohol	14.6
Water	3.9

Dissolve the first three components in the alcohol, stir in the water, and shake well. Filter if necessary. Apply this anesthetic to each welt with a piece of cotton. Repeat the treatment as often as necessary.

Insecticide Dust

Infestation by chiggers can be wiped out by spraying an insecticide dust in the infested area. Chlordane and lindane are recommended.

No. 1: Chlordane Dust

	oz
Chlordane	5.0
Talcum powder	95.0

No. 2: Lindane Dust

	oz
Lindane	1.0
Talcum powder	99.0

For both: Mix ingredients thoroughly, and apply at the rate of 1¼ lb to every 1000 sq feet. Use a rotary hand duster for small areas, and a power duster for large areas. Apply the insecticide dust to grass, logs, and ground litter. Put it around high weeds and bushes. One dust treatment lasts from 1 to 4 weeks.

Chlordane and lindane are poisonous; hence you must exercise great care in handling them. Treat skin or clothing with repellents only. Do not allow livestock to graze on a treated area within two weeks after the treatment.

Insecticides

No. 1

Dusts containing the following mixture:

Pyrethrins	0.1%
Piperonyl butoxide	1.6%

when applied as a daily light dusting, were found to be the most effective treatment against house flies that resist chlorinated hydrocarbons.

Use this mixture of pyrethrins and piperonyl butoxide to impregnate bags containing cereals. The impregnated bags will protect the cereal against the flour beetle for about nine months if stored in the dark, or six months if exposed to daylight.

No. 2

A mixture of paradichlorobenzene and naphthalene showed very good results in small scale tests on control of clothes moths.

No. 3

	parts by weight
Pyrethrum	1.0
Sesamolin	1.0

Mix well.

Sesamolin, a derivative of sesame oil, is the most potent synergist (cooperator), or booster, known for pyrethrum insecticides. Sesamolin greatly increases the killing power of pyrethrum insecticides against houseflies (31 times) and certain other insects, although it does not increase their extremely low toxicity to humans and warm-blooded animals. Sesamolin may be extracted from the oil of sesame seeds (no commercial process yet developed).

No. 4

Basil, a sweet herb, characterized by a pleasant aromatic odor and taste, can be used as a repellent for flies and mosquitoes. Sweet basil is an annual plant native to the East Indies. It grows to a height of about one foot, and it has egg-shaped or oblong leaves. Put the plants in pots, and place them at strategic points.

Insect Repellents

The following effective chemicals may be used for repelling mosquitoes, flies, gnats, and other insects:

Dimethyl carbate, dimethyl phthalate, ethyl hexanediol, and indalone.

These compounds have little odor and provide protection for several hours. They do not kill the insects, but merely repel them. Rub these repellents on the skin in order to make them most effective. Do not use them on skin abrasions or other sensitive spots. These chemicals may stain clothing and may damage rayon, nylon, plastics, and paints. Ethyl hexanediol and dimethyl phthalate are by far the best mosquito repellents. Mosquitos prefer landing on dark-colored clothing rather than on light-colored clothing.

Diethyl-meta-toluamide, an organic chemical, is about the best all-purpose insect repellent. It provides long-lasting protection against mosquitoes, chiggers, ticks, fleas, and biting flies. It can be safely applied to the skin or clothing, and it is remarkably long-lasting. Clothing and other fabrics can be treated with diethyl-meta-toluamide, by saturating them with a solution containing this insect-repellent chemical. Diethyl meta-toluamide, has a higher repellency and more lasting effectiveness than either the ortho- or the para- form.

Insect-Repellent Liquids

No. 1

	oz
Isopropyl alcohol, 99%	104.0
Diethyl toluamide, meta	24.0

Mix and shake well.

No. 2

	oz
Methyl phthalate	9.0
Indalone	3.0
Dimethyl carbate	3.0

Mix thoroughly. This mixture is very effective in repelling insects when applied to the human body.

Insect-Repellent Cream

Stearic acid	4⅛	lb
Lanolin, anhydrous	3	oz
White mineral oil (65/75 viscosity)	6	oz
Potassium hydroxide	2$\frac{7}{16}$	oz
Glycerin	6	oz
Water	13½	pt
Diethyl-meta-toluamide	37	oz

Heat the acid, lanolin, and mineral oil at 170°F. Heat the hydroxide, glycerin, and water at 175°F., and add it to the melted fats slowly while stirring rapidly for several minutes until emulsification is complete. Allow the mixture to cool while stirring slowly. When the temperature has dropped to 140–130°F., add the diethyl toluamide, and stir intermittently at low speed until cold.

Pack in air-tight jars.

Mexican Bean Beetle Control

The Mexican bean beetle is the most serious insect enemy of beans in this country. The adult beetle is copper-colored, with 16 black spots on its rounded back. It is nearly ¼ inch long and ⅕ inch wide. The adult beetle and the larvae feed on the under surface of the leaf. If the leaves have been destroyed or have become unpalatable, the beetles will feed on the young pods; they may even eat the stems. The Mexican bean beetle propagates by eggs deposited in clusters of about 60 on the lower surface of a leaf. This beetle prefers the common (green or string) bean, kidney, pinto, navy, and lima beans, to other varieties.

The adult beetle lives through the winter, hibernating in woodlands near bean fields, where they collect in small colonies. In certain areas of this country the adult beetle may fly several miles to hibernate.

The following two insecticides will protect the plants from injury by the Mexican bean beetle:

No. 1

Rotenone Dust

	oz
Rotenone	1.5
Talcum powder	148.5

Mix thoroughly, and apply at the rate of 30 lb per acre, or 2 ounces per 50 feet of row. This insecticide dust is the most effective material that is not hazardous to the person applying it, and it does not leave any harmful residues on the plants.

No. 2
Methoxychlor Dust

	oz
Methoxychlor	7.5
Talcum powder	142.5

Mix thoroughly, and apply at the rate of 30 lb per acre, or 2 ounces per 50 feet of row. Methoxychlor is related to DDT, but is less toxic to man and animals. Do not apply this dust within 7 days before a harvest. It is of extreme importance that the insecticide dust be directed to the under sides of the leaves, as both the adult and the larvae feed on this under surface.

Apply the insecticide dust immediately upon noticing any damage to the foliage. Look for eggs on the under sides of the leaves. As the plants grow, cover the new foliage with the dust. If the beetles are plentiful, make another application within a week or 10 days. Protect lima beans over a longer period.

After the beans have been picked, destroy the remains of the crop. A large percentage of all stages of the beetle will be destroyed by plowing the fields about 6 inches deep and covering all the foliage with soil. Thus the destruction of crop remnants after harvest will greatly reduce the need for insecticides.

Pea Aphid Control

The pea aphid (pea louse) is one of the most destructive insect enemies of peas in this country. It sucks the sap from the leaves, stems, blossoms, and pods of the plants on which it feeds. Infested pea plants become stunted and produce fewer and smaller pods than uninfested plants. The pea aphid is nearly $\frac{3}{16}$-inch long and one-third as wide. This insect also feeds on alfalfa.

Use insecticides in order to control the pea aphid. Apply them before the peas develop buds, and before the aphids have become sufficiently abundant to damage the peas.

Rotenone (the principal active constituent of derris root or cube root) or DDT (dichloro-diphenyl trichloroethane) may be used as dusts or sprays.

Rotenone Dust

	parts by wt
Rotenone, powdered	1.0
Talcum powder	99.0

Mix thoroughly, and apply at the rate of 35 lb per acre.

Rotenone dust continues to kill pea aphids for several days after application. It is highly poisonous to insects, but practically non-toxic to man and animals.

DDT Dust

	parts by wt
DDT, powdered	5.0
Talcum powder	95.0

Mix thoroughly, and apply at the rate of 35 lb per acre.

DDT Spray

DDT	1.6 oz
Stoddard Solvent (petroleum distillate)	1.0 gal

Dissolve and mix well. Apply at the rate of 10 gallons per acre.

DDT continues to kill pea aphids for several days after application. This prolonged activity is known as residual effectiveness. As DDT is highly poisonous, great care should be exercised in handling it. Use hand equipment or power equipment for dusting or spraying. Do not apply DDT to varieties of peas with edible pods after the pods have taken shape. Do not feed plants treated with DDT to livestock.

Pea Weevil Control

The pea weevil is a small grayish or brownish-gray beetle, about $\frac{1}{5}$ of an inch long and marked with black and white spots. It is one of the most injurious insect pests of cultivated peas in the world as it attacks all varieties of edible and field peas. It does serious damage wherever peas are grown on an extensive scale.

These weevils damage peas by the larvae feeding within the seeds. The rapidly growing larvae consume a large part of the substance of the pea, thus destroying the life of the seed, and making the peas unfit for human consumption.

Infestation by pea weevils may be controlled by means of dusts containing rotenone or methoxychlor during the early blooming period, before the eggs are laid. Prepare the dusts by thoroughly mixing the following ingredients:

No. 1

Rotenone	6.0 oz
Talcum powder or infusorial earth	49.5 lb

No. 2

Methoxychlor	2.50 lb
Talc or infusorial earth	47.50 lb

Rotenone is highly toxic to insects both by contact and through the stomach, but at the recommended dosage, it is practically non-toxic to man, warm-blooded animals, and all plants. It is also highly toxic to fish. The effectiveness of rotenone is reduced by sunlight to about 24 hours.

Rotenone, however, does irritate the mucous membrane of the nose and throat; it is therefore advisable to wear a respirator when using it. Rotenone should be stored in tightly closed containers, as it deteriorates slowly upon exposure to light and moisture.

Methoxychlor is fully effective against the pea weevil and it is relatively harmless to warm-blooded animals. It should not be applied to peas with edible pods within 7 days before a harvest.

Use one to three applications at 15 to 30 pounds per acre. Dust the peas between the appearance of the first blossoms and the first pods in order to kill the adult weevils before they begin to lay their eggs. In general, start dusting a little early. Do the dusting at a temperature above 65°F., since weevils are inactive at lower temperatures, and they do not lay eggs at temperatures below 65°F. Use a hand duster for pea weevils in farm and home gardens. Cover the entire plant completely with a thin layer of the dust. Use ¼ pound to each 150 linear feet of row.

When handling insecticides, be careful to keep the materials out of the mouth and eyes. Cover the body well and wear goggles to protect the eyes, and a respirator to protect the mouth.

Termite Repellents

Termites (soft-bodied insects, often called white ants) cause extensive damage to a wide variety of materials, such as fabrics, paper, wooden structures, buildings, etc. The best mode of attack is by treating these materials chemically. It can be accomplished by dipping, painting, spraying, or impregnating the material by pressure with a suitable vehicle in which the toxic agent or repellent is incorporated. The vehicle in most cases is a ketone, such as acetone, or an alcohol. Of the many chemical compounds tested, the following were found to be most effective in repelling attacks of termites:

	%
Pentachlorophenol	1–2
Copper pentachlorophenate naphthenate	2
Zinc pentachlorophenate naphthenate	2
Hexachlorophenol	2
Zinc dithiocarbamate	2

Mildew Prevention and Removal

Molds that cause mildew are always present in the air. They grow on anything from which they can obtain food—on cellulose materials like cotton, linen, paper, and wood, and on protein products such as leather, silk, and wool. These molds require moisture and certain temperatures in order to flourish. They grow wherever it is damp, warm, poorly ventilated, or poorly lighted. As they thrive they discolor fabrics and leather; they cause decay in wood and leave a musty odor. Sometimes the molds eat into cloth causing it to rot and fall to pieces.

Prevention of Mildew

Keep all places and things clean, well aired and dry. Use adequate ventilation only when the outside air is cooler and drier than that inside. Burn a small electric light continuously in poorly ventilated closets. Leave closet doors and dresser drawers open occasionally. Ventilate linen closets in bathrooms. Use chemicals, such as silica gel, activated alumina, or calcium chloride to absorb the moisture from the air.

SILICA GEL: These porous granules hold half their weight of water, and feel dry even when saturated. They are not harmful to fabrics, and they can be used over and over. Silica gel is blue when dry, but turns pink when full of moisture. Put the silica gel in cloth bags and hang them in clothes closets, or place an open container of silica gel on the floor or on a shelf of the closet. Keep closet doors closed. Dry the moist silica gel by simply placing the granules in a vented oven at 300°F. for several hours. When dry, put the material in an air-tight box and cool it before reusing it.

ACTIVATED ALUMINA: This chemical is used in the same way as silica gel. Activated alumina holds moisture without dripping, and it is not harmful to fabrics.

CALCIUM CHLORIDE: This compound is the cheapest of the three described here. It holds twice its weight of water and liquefies as it absorbs moisture. Do not allow calcium chloride to come in contact with clothing or textiles. Put the granular substance on a non-rusting screen supported in a special container, place it in the closet, and keep the doors closed. As it liquefies, replace it with fresh calcium chloride.

Do not allow damp or wet clothing or other articles to lie around. Wash or dry-clean clothing or textiles before storing. Do not store textiles in damp basements. Sun and air articles stored in closets.

If musty odors persist in basements and cellars, sprinkle chloride of lime over the floor, and allow it to remain until all mustiness disappears. Then sweep it up, scrub the floor, and dry it.

Mildew-Resistant Chemicals

FOR COTTON: Articles such as awnings, sails, shower curtains, tents, etc., may be treated with chemicals to make them resistant to mildew.

Dip the article in hot soapsuds prepared by dissolving a good neutral soap in soft water. Soak for several minutes to make sure the article is thoroughly wet. Then remove the article, without rinsing, and put at once into a hot solution of the following mixture:

Cadmium chloride	1½ oz
Water	1 gal

Stir and turn the article in this solution for about 15 minutes; then wring it and hang it to dry using a twine clothesline. Articles so treated will withstand about three launderings. Cadmium chloride is poisonous; hence wash all utensils thoroughly.

FOR LEATHER: Protect leather against mildew by sponging it with either of the following solutions:

Paranitrophenol	1/3 oz
Specially denatured alcohol	1 qt

or

Thymol	1/3 oz
Specially denatured alcohol	1 qt

Test a small area of the leather to make sure that the solution does not change its color.

Protect leather shoes with a good wax dressing.

FOR PAINTED SURFACES: Protect indoor wood surfaces from mildewing by using a paint containing 20 per cent or more of zinc oxide.

FOR BOOKS: Protect books in closed bookcases by dusting them with paraformaldehyde powder. Use this powder sparingly, as it may be irritating to some persons.

Removal of Mildew

FROM WASHABLE CLOTHING or Household Articles: Fresh mildew stains may be removed by washing the articles in a solution of soap and water, then rinse them well and dry them in sunlight. If the mildew stain persists, prepare the following solution:

Sodium perborate	½ oz
Water, lukewarm	1 pt

Sponge the stain with this solution and allow it to stand a minute or two; then rinse well. Use extreme care on colored goods.

FROM UNDYED FABRICS: Old mildew stains may be removed from undyed cotton, linen, or rayon by dipping them into a chlorine bleach for about one minute. Then dip the stains into the following vinegar solution to counteract the effect of the chlorine:

	oz
Vinegar	1.0
Water, soft	8.0

Finally, rinse well with water. Do not use chlorine bleach on silk or wool.

Remove mildew stains from upholstered articles, mattresses, rugs by brushing them outdoors with a whisk broom and running a vacuum cleaner over the surface. Then wipe the articles with a cloth wrung out of dilute alcohol:

	oz
Specially denatured alcohol	16.0
Water, soft	16.0

Dry the articles thoroughly in the sunlight.

FROM LEATHER: Remove mildew stains from leather goods by wiping with a cloth wrung out of dilute alcohol, then dry them in a current of air. If necessary, wash with thick soapsuds, wipe with a damp cloth, and dry in an airy place.

If the mildew has grown into the articles, fumigate with formaldehyde gas. Place the articles in a sealed closet or room and burn formaldehyde candles. Use extreme care not to inhale the formaldehyde fumes.

Remove mildew stains from wood by wiping with a cloth dipped in water to which some kerosene has been added or wash it with warm soapsuds, and wipe dry thoroughly. If the mildew stain has grown into the wood under the paint, remove the paint and bleach the stain with the following oxalic acid solution:

	oz
Oxalic acid	1½
Water, soft	16

Apply the solution, and rinse well with water. Have it thoroughly dried before repainting it.

FROM PAPER: Loose mold may be removed from paper by brushing and then drying with a clean, soft cloth. If the paper is washable, wipe it with a cloth wrung out of thick soapsuds, then with clear water. Air the pages of books and, if they are very damp, sprinkle pure talcum powder between the leaves to absorb the moisture. Leave the powder there for several hours, then brush it out.

If wallpaper has mildewed, be sure to dry both the paper and the plaster beneath it. This is best accomplished by heating the room for several hours, or even days.

Mushroom Spray

Chlorine	1 oz
Water	78⅛ gal

Mix thoroughly and use the solution as a spray. This chlorinated water will control effectively some common diseases of mushrooms, and will improve their yield and appearance. Chlorine is effective against some disease-producing fungi, yet it is nontoxic to the mushroom, which also is a fungus.

Polyvinylpyrrolidone-Iodine (PVP)

PVP combines with iodine to form a compound in which the iodine is detoxified without losing its therapeutic property. It is effective as a fungicide, insecticide, nematocide (killer of thread-like worms) and soil pesticide.

As a pesticide PVP-Iodine compound has the following advantages:

It is water-soluble and the solution is very stable. It has a low vapor pressure, thus allowing fumigation of the soil to continue over a longer period. Concentrations even as high as 20% by weight, are not toxic to man, to warm-blooded animals, and to plants in general. The use of PVP-Iodine does not necessitate any costly equipment, as the aqueous solution is merely sprayed or dusted on the soil.

For control of nematodes (thread-like worms), root knot nematodes, leaf spots, etc., make a solution or a dust composition of 0.1–5.6% by weight of the PVP-Iodine compound.

Rodents and their Control

Man's carelessness in handling foodstuffs has attracted populations of rats and mice into such close proximity to his home that they are called "domestic" rodents. Because of this relationship man suffers from rat bites and rodent-borne diseases.

Three varieties of rodents which infest the homes of man are the Norway rat, the most common and largest of the domestic rats; Roof rat, middle-sized and an agile climber found abundantly in the temperate or tropical areas; House mouse, smallest of the rodents, widespread and abundant throughout the United States.

Rats and mice are habitually nocturnal and secretive, and are rarely seen.

Poison Baits

No. 1

Red squill	12	oz
Bait	6¾	lb

Use bacon, canned fish, ground meat, cereals, grains, or a combination of these as the bait. Use fish oil or molasses as a binder to hold the poison and dry bait together. Mix the bait and poison thoroughly. If large quantities of bait are to be mixed, use a mechanical mixer.

Red squill is a natural emetic with a bitter taste, which contributes to its safe use for control of Norway rats. It kills them by a digitalis-like action, causing heart paralysis, because rats cannot vomit the poison.

This poison is ineffective against roof rats and mice.

No. 2

Warfarin, pival, or protopine	12	oz
Yellow corn meal	14¼	lb
or		
Warfarin, pival, protopine	12	oz
Corn meal	7	lb
Rolled oats	3¾	lb
Corn oil	12	oz
Granulated sugar	12	oz

This latter mixture is more acceptable to the rodents. Stir in a discoloring agent, such as charcoal, Mix thoroughly, using a mechanical mixer.

These poisons kill in a different manner from the older single-dose poisons; they must be ingested for several days before they become effective. To be fatal, repeated doses must be consumed by the rodent for a period of five or more days. These poisons cause internal hemorrhages, so the rodents literally bleed to death.

These poisons are effective against both rats and mice.

No. 3

Arsenic trioxide, powdered	9 oz
Bait	18 lb
Tartar emetic	1⅛ oz
Corn oil or molasses	optional
Charcoal	optional

The bait consists of bacon, fish, ground meat, cereals, grains, or a combination of these, and water. This poison is effective against Norway rats and Roof rats.

No. 4

Zinc phosphide	3 oz
Bait	18¾ lb
Tartar emetic	1⅛ oz

Use the same bait as with red squill, and mix thoroughly.

Zinc phosphide is often used to coat ½-inch cubes of sweet potato or apple as bait. Gently whirl the freshly cut, moist cubes in a bucket with the zinc phosphide until all of the poison has been absorbed by the cubes. Zinc phosphide is effective against both rats and mice. Most animals will not touch baits prepared with zinc phosphide, but rats and mice seem to like the taste and pungent odor of phosphorus.

No. 5

Thallium sulfate	1⅞ oz
Bait	22½ lb
Tartar emetic	1⅛ oz

Use the same bait as with red squill, and mix thoroughly. This poison is effective against both rats and mice.

No. 6

Sodium monofluoroacetate	⅜ oz
Water	98 oz

Dissolve the fluoroacetate in the water, and mix well. Sodium fluoroacetate is a fast-acting rodenticide; it is very effective against both rats and mice.

Both sodium fluoroacetate and thallium sulphate are extremely toxic and dangerous to use. They are best left for professional operators.

Add a small amount of molasses, syrup, or raisins to dry or watery baits, because rats and mice are attracted to sweets.

CAUTIONS: Have all poisons and all mixing equipment clearly labeled. Do not use this mixing equipment for other purposes. Keep all poisons and equipment under lock. Avoid inhaling powders, or getting poisons on hands, clothes, or utensils. Always do your mixing in a well ventilated room, especially when mixing dry components.

If rodents die in inaccessible places and cannot be removed, use the following preparation as a deodorizer:

	oz
Isobornyl acetate (Fritzsche Bros.)	1
Isopropyl alcohol	64

Mix thoroughly, and apply with an atomizer or with a fine-mist sprayer.

If dead rodents are located between partitions or walls, bore a hole in the wall and pour in the following mixture:

Zinc chloride	7 oz
Sodium chloride	5 oz
Water	4 pt

Dissolve the chlorides in the water and mix thoroughly. Apply the preparation as close as possible to the source of the odor of dead rodent.

Wood Preservative

Decay (rot) in wood is caused by low forms of plant life called fungi. This decay can be stopped by poisoning the food supply in this case, the wood itself. The wood can be preserved by putting into it poisonous chemicals that will either kill the decay fungi outright, or keep them from growing. The same preservative is effective in controlling attack by termites. These insects are most abundant in moist, warm soil where there is a plentiful supply of food in the form of wood.

Zinc chloride, commercial	54	oz
Sodium dichromate, commercial	11½	oz
Water	10	gal

Dissolve the chemicals in the water and shake well. Soak either green or seasoned wood in this chromated zinc chloride solution for 1 or 2 weeks. If time is very limited, shorten the soaking period to 4 or 5 days. This steeping treatment has been found to be definitely beneficial to posts made of ash, jack pine, lodgepole pine, ponderosa pine, red pine, and Scotch pine.

Chromated zinc chloride is more resistant than simple zinc chloride to leaching (losing soluble parts when water passes through). It gives equal protection against termites, and greater protection against decay fungi. Wood treated with water-soluble preservatives can be painted satisfactorily after it has been seasoned in order to remove the water added during the treatment.

Miscellaneous

Anti-Fog Preparation
(Stick)

	oz
Polyethylene glycol 4000	38.40
Polyethylene glycol 1540	25.60
Polyethylene glycol 500	64.00

Liquefy the ingredients by heat and mix thoroughly. Pour into suitable molds to form sticks.

Anti-Freeze

		oz
Propylene glycol		89.60
Water-free glycerin		38.40
Mix thoroughly		
% wt conc.	36	42
Freezing pt °C	–18	–23.5

Anhydrous Ammonia

Anhydrous ammonia, besides its primary use as a fertilizer, also acts as a fungicidal agent in the soil. It is usually marketed in liquefied form in iron cylinders.

Acids and Bases: pH Values

*p*H is the abbreviation for "Hydrogen Ion Concentration"; that is, the degree of acidity or alkalinity of a solution. It is measured on a scale of numbers ranging from 0 to 14. *p*H 7.0 is the neutral point; a solution of *p*H 7.0 is neither acid nor alkaline. The numbers from 7.0 to 1.0 denote acidity, the intensity increasing as the numbers decrease. Thus a solution of *p*H 3.8 is more acidic than one of *p*H 5.2. On the other hand, the numbers from 7.0 to 14.0 denote alkalinity, the alkalinity increasing as the numbers increase. Hence, a solution of *p*H 8.4 is slightly alkaline, whereas one of *p*H 9.2 is more alkaline.

These *p*H numbers present absolute and definite degrees of acidity or alkalinity. The values are logarithmic; thus an increase of one unit on the *p*H scale means a tenfold increase in the hydrogen ion concentration. An increase of two units on the *p*H scale means a hundred-fold increase.

The approximate *p*H values of some familiar chemical compounds are as follows:

Acids	*p*H Value	Bases	*p*H Value
Hydrochloric acid	1.0	Sodium bicarbonate	8.4
Sulfuric acid	1.2	Borax	9.2
Phosphoric acid	1.5	Ammonia	11.1
Sulfuric acid	1.5	Sodium carbonate	11.6
Acetic acid	2.9	Trisodium phosphate	12.0
Alum	3.2	Sodium metasilicate	12.2
Carbonic acid	3.8	Lime, saturated	12.3
Boric acid	5.2	Sodium hydroxide	13.0

Bell Metal

	parts
Copper, commercially pure	117
Tin	33

Melt together the metals, form and complete the bells by simple casting. This alloy is the most sonorous of all alloys. It has a low melting point, and a fine compact grain. Use about 0.1 more metal than the weight of the prospective bell in order to allow for waste during the melting and casting operations.

Beryllium

Beryllium, because of its resistance to corrosion, is becoming increasingly important for aircraft, missiles, and nuclear reactors. The purity of this metal is gradually being increased. Beryllium is very light, and has a melting point of 2340°F. (1280°C.). It is resistant to corrosion by carbon dioxide at high temperatures. Beryllium has a very low neutron-capture cross section, thereby making it a potent candidate for use in high-temperature gas-cooled reactors, as fuel cans, and other core components.

If beryllium were substituted for aluminum in the construction of airplanes, money could be saved by halving the weight of the planes and increasing their paying loads.

Borax

Use 0.2 to 5% of borax in most standard fertilizers.

Use borax to increase the efficiency of general weed killers.

Use borax for preserving timber, and for anti-freeze mixtures (as corrosion inhibitor).

Use borax for fire prevention by treating flammable materials with a solution of borax and boric acid.

Cerium Oxide

Cerium oxide is a remarkably efficient polishing agent for glass. It will remove nicks and scratches from lenses. It permits the production of distortion-free TV tubes, fine quality mirrors, and precision optical lenses.

Chlorine Sanitizing Agent

	lb
Trichloroisocyanuric acid	5.00
Sodium metasilicate, anhydrous	6.25
Sodium sulfate, anhydrous	7.50
Sodium tripolyphosphate, anhydrous	6.25

Mix thoroughly, and pack in dry, airtight containers.

The resultant compound is stable, and dissolves rapidly at room temperature to make a clear solution even in hard water. It makes its chlorine available rapidly, and is bactericidally effective against a broad variety of microorganisms. This sanitizing compound is very effective, and has a low toxicity to humans.

Corrosion Resistance of Titanium

Corrosive Medium	*Resistance of Titanium*
Aqua regia	Excellent
Chromic acid	Excellent to good
Hydrochloric acid	Good below 10%
Nitric acid	Excellent
Phosphoric acid	Poor
Sulfuric acid	Good below 5%
Aluminum chloride	Excellent to fair
Ammonium chloride	Excellent
Calcium chloride	Excellent
Chlorine water	Excellent
Cupric chloride	Excellent
Ferric chloride	Excellent
Sodium chloride	Excellent
Sodium hydroxide	Good below 50%

Cotton—Facts about It

Cotton is grown on about 900,000 farms in the southern part of the U.S.A. The size of the crop is about 15 million bales of cotton lint (each bale weighing about 500 pounds), and more than 6 million tons of cottonseed. After the cotton is harvested, it is hauled to the gins where the fibers are separated from the seed. These fibers are called lint. Most of the gins are equipped with devices for drying and cleaning the cottonseed and lint in order to preserve their quality.

The lint finds its way to the spinner, who shapes it into yarn. The seed finds its way to mills to be transformed into various products, such as cottonseed oil, meal, cake, hulls, and linters. There are about 1,000 cotton mills that manufacture raw cotton into cloth, cotton yarn, and thread. The accumulation of waste is sold for batting, wadding, and mattress felts.

The cottonseed crop in the U.S.A. is more than 6 million tons a year, most of which is sold to the cottonseed-processing mills. Cottonseed, after leaving the gins, still has some lint, and is therefore delinted immediately after it is cleaned. These fibers, when baled like cotton, are called cotton linters and are used for felts and waddings in upholstery for furniture and automobiles, mattresses, etc. Cotton linters are a source of cellulose which is used in the manufacture of rayon, cellophane, films, plastics, varnishes, and explosives.

After the crude cottonseed oil is refined, it is used chiefly in the manufacture of margarine, and as cooking and salad oils; or it is hydrogenated and sold as vegetable shortening.

Cottonseed cake is used chiefly for the feeding of livestock. If cottonseed cake is formed entirely from perfectly sound seed, it is made into a flour used for bread and cake to be eaten by persons that are not allowed to eat starches or sugar.

Cottonseed meal is valuable as a plant fertilizer.

Cottonseed hulls are used as a roughage feed, and as a source of chemical compounds, such as furfural. This compound, called artificial oil of ants is produced by distilling the hulls with dilute sulfuric acid; it is used in the manufacture of dyes.

Dishwashing Compound

Ethylene oxide condensate of an alkyl phenol	12¾	oz
Sodium tripolyphosphate	12	lb
Sodium metasilicate	18	lb
Borax	4	lb
Sodium carbonate, anhydrous, technical	5¼	lb

Reduce the ingredients to a powder and mix thoroughly.

Electroless Plating of Nickel

Electroless plating is a process for the deposition of nickel by chemical reduction in the absence of an electric current. Reduction of nickel salts by hypophosphite had been long known as a chemical reaction. The coatings contain about 7% of phosphorus, most likely in the form of finely dispersed phosphides. The coatings are slightly less magnetic, but are similar to electro-deposited nickel in resistance to rusting. Electroless plating has several advantages over electroplating:

1. The coating has a uniform thickness in recesses as well as on exposed surfaces.
2. Edges or points have no build-up of coating.
3. There is no need for electrical equipment.

In electroless plating, nickel can be put down directly upon surfaces that catalyze the reaction, for example, on aluminum, cobalt, copper, gold, iron, nickel, palladium, platinum, and silver. Graphite and silicon carbide, being semiconductors, may be electroless-plated by touching them with a piece of aluminum or steel to start the reaction. Ceramics, glass, and plastics, being nonconductors, may be electroless-plated after dipping them in a solution of palladium. Cadmium, lead and its alloys, manganese bronze, and silicon, cannot be electroless-plated.

The following baths may be used for electroless plating of nickel:

No. 1

	oz
Nickel chloride	4.0
Ammonium chloride	6.7
Sodium citrate	13.4
Sodium hypophosphite	1.3

*p*H ranges from 8 to 10.

No. 2

	oz
Nickel chloride	4.0
Sodium hydroxyacetate	6.7
Sodium hypophosphite	1.3

*p*H ranges from 4 to 4.5.

No. 3

	oz
Nickel chloride	4.0
Sodium citrate	2.0
Sodium acetate	0.7
Sodium hypophosphite	1.3

*p*H ranges from 4 to 4.5.

Dissolve all the ingredients in one gallon of water. Shake well until solution is complete.

The electroless plating operation is conducted at a temperature of 95°C. If the composition of the bath is kept constant, each bath will deposit nickel at a rate of about 0.0003 inch per hour.

Gems and Jewels

Gold: Pure gold, called 24 carat (K) gold, is much too soft to be used for jewelry, so it is made stronger by the addition of other metals. White gold is made by adding nickel and zinc. Pink- or rose-colored gold is made by adding brass and copper. Green-colored gold is made by adding silver to the gold.

Platinum and Palladium: These two metals, along with iridium, rhodium, and ruthenium, belong to the platinum group; all have a medium-brilliant grayish-white color. Platinum, which is most frequently used, is the most durable, and the most expensive.

Carat: This term (abbreviated, K) expresses the fineness of a gold alloy: maximum, 24 K. It is also a unit of weight; one carat equals 200 milligrams. One hundredth of a carat is termed a point.

Standard markings for gold jewelry are 10K, 14K, and 18K. The 18K is the most expensive.

The marking for platinum is "10% Irid. Plat."; for palladium, "pal."

Facet: A small plane surface of a cut gem.

Brilliant cut: The most popular cut for most of gem stones: it usually has 58 facets.

The price of stones is influenced by the color, size, cut, and degree of perfection. The most popular gems are listed in the following chart.

Gem	*Family*	*Most-prized Color*	*Clearness*	*Hardness*	*Price Range*
Alexandrite	Beryllium aluminate	Distinct color change, red to green	Transparent	Very hard	Very expensive
Amber	Fossil resin	Clear yellowish brown	Transparent to semi-translucent	Soft	Low
Amethyst	Quartz	Fairly deep purple, red flashes	Transparent	Relatively hard	Low to moderate
Aquamarine	Beryllium aluminum silicate	Deep clear blue	Transparent	Hard	Low to expensive
Bloodstone	Quartz	Dark green, many flecks	Opaque	Relatively hard	Moderate
Carnelian	Quartz	Reddish-brown	Translucent to semi-translucent	Relatively hard	Moderate
Cat's-eye (Oriental)	Beryllium aluminate	Honey color, sharp narrow eye	Translucent	Very hard	Very expensive
Citrine	Quartz	Light yellow-brown	Transparent	Relatively hard	Low
Coral	Organic source	Yellow-red	Translucent to opaque	Soft	Low
Diamond	Carbon	Blue-white	Transparent	Extraordinarily hard	Expensive to very expensive
Emerald	Beryllium aluminum silicate	Velvety grass-green	Clear to translucent	Hard	Expensive to very expensive
Jadeite	Chiefly sodium aluminum silicate	Emerald green	Semi-transparent to opaque	Relatively hard	Moderate to very expensive
Moonstone	Feldspar (alumino-silicate of potassium, sodium, calcium)	Bluish-white with moon effect	Semi-transparent to translucent	Relatively hard	Low to moderate
Opal	Hydrated silica	Black on white with play of color	Transparent to opaque	Relatively soft	Low to expensive
Pearl (Oriental)	Organic source	Depends on complexion of wearer	Translucent to opaque	Soft	Expensive
Peridot	Magnesium-iron silicate	Yellow-green	Transparent to translucent	Relatively hard	Moderate to expensive

Gem	Family	Most-prized Color	Clearness	Hardness	Price Range
Pyrope	Garnet group	Intense ruby-red	Transparent to translucent	Hard	Low to moderate
Ruby	Corundum (aluminum oxide)	Dark red, purple undertones	Semi-transparent to transparent	Extremely hard	Expensive to very expensive
Sapphire	Corundum (aluminum oxide)	Velvety corn-flower blue	Transparent, semi-transparent to translucent	Extremely hard	Expensive to very expensive
Sardonyx	Quartz	Alternate parallel bands of brown or red and white	Opaque	Relatively hard	Low to moderate
Spinel	Magnesium aluminate	Red	Transparent	Hard	Low to moderate
Topaz	Aluminum fluosilicate	Yellow-bronze	Transparent to translucent	Hard	Expensive
Tourmaline	Alumina and silica	Moss- or bottle-green	Transparent	Hard	Low to moderate
Turquoise	Hydrated aluminum phosphate	Sky-blue	Opaque	Relatively hard	Low to moderate
Zircon	Zirconium silicate	Deep blue	Transparent	Hard	Low to moderate

General Information

650 BTU are required to bake one pound of bread.

One cubic inch of water weighs 0.56 oz.

Germicide

Ortho-benzyl-para-chlorophenol is a safe germicide for soaps and cleansers. It mixes well with many cleaning compounds and soaps. It is effective against fungi at concentrations of 0.002%. Use this germicide in cleaners for hospitals, rest rooms, rug shampoos, scrub soaps, and dog soaps.

Glazes for Ceramics

No. 1: Boron Glaze

	parts
Calcium borate ($CaO \cdot B_2O_3 \cdot H_2O$)	12.0
Borax	3.0
Feldspar	15.0
Zinc oxide	3.0

No. 2: Titanium Glaze

	parts
Red lead (lead oxide)	100.0
Quartz	20.0
Kaolin	5.0
Zinc oxide	10.0
Titanium oxide	7.5

Both glazes mature at about 1750°F. The boron glaze is an opaque white glaze, while the titanium glaze is a light sandy color on a white body and an ivory color on a red body.

A clarifier suitable for both these glazes is as follows:

	parts
Lead oxide red	50.0
Quartz	37.5
Kaolin	5.0

Glycerin-Graphite Lubricant

	oz
Colloidal graphite	0.2
Glycerin, U.S.P.	49.8
Distilled water	50.0

or

	oz
* Concentrated dispersion of colloidal graphite	2.56
Glycerin, U.S.P.	61.44
Distilled water	64.00

* From Acheson Colloids Co., Port Huron, Mich.

Stir the graphite into the glycerin, then add the water and stir well. This lubricant penetrates tight-fitting parts and leaves a durable film of graphite on rubber surfaces.

Glycerin Viscosity

The viscosity of glycerin may be increased by adding to it "Kelube," a triisopropanolamine salt of alginic acid. Prepare smooth-flowing solutions of any desired viscosity in glycerin by varying the concentration of Kelube. Use this thickened glycerin as a lubricant for valves, in printing inks, and in the processing of textiles.

Honey as a Surgical Dressing

Pure honey is excellent for burns and many infected wounds. Apply the pure honey and cover with a dry gauze.

Johnson Grass in Cotton

Stoddard Solvent can be used for the control of Johnson grass in cotton. Use it as a spot-treatment in which the oil is directed at the crown of the plant. About five such spot-treatments are necessary in order to effect 98% control.

Metallic Sodium

The treatment of petroleum fractions with metallic sodium has various beneficial effects. Most of the sulfur compounds are eliminated, especially thiophenic sulfur (C_4H_4S), which is difficult to remove otherwise. Metallic sodium not only acts as a desulfurizer, but also improves the odor and color of the petroleum fraction, and reduces dissolved gum developers. This process has the advantage of producing an excellent product with little loss of volume. The metallic sodium can be procured as dispersions in inert hydrocarbon media or as coatings on inert solid particles.

Molasses

The term "molasses" refers to the following four by-products:

(1) Blackstrap molasses from the cane sugar industry; (2) beet molasses from the beet sugar industry; (3) hydrol from the corn milling industry, and (4) citrus molasses from the citrus fruit processing industry.

The major outlet for molasses has been industrial alcohol. Fairly large quantities are still being used for this purpose, but the competition of synthetic alcohol has reduced this market from 74% in 1944 to 17% in 1954.

The mixed-feed for the livestock industry is a good outlet for molasses. In 1947 about 528,000 tons of molasses (1 ton is 171 gallons) were used in mixed feeds.

Liquid molasses gives odor and taste to mixed feeds and also acts as a binder and dust settler. The quantity required to give these characteristics is estimated at 3–6% of molasses in the final feed. Most animals like the odor and taste that molasses imparts to feed, and they consume less palatable feeds in greater quantity when they are mixed with molasses. It prevents these feeds from sifting and blowing away. Liquid molasses adds moisture and thereby reduces the incidence of choking and coughing by livestock. It improves the appearance and feeling of feeds. Molasses also imparts other properties to feeds, such as improved digestibility and a mild laxative effect, and it helps to stabilize the feed mixture, to keep fine particles of vitamin and mineral mixtures evenly distributed while in storage or transit.

Molasses has approximately 70% of the carbohydrate value of yellow corn. Thus 143 lbs of molasses containing 48–52% sugar equal approximately 100 lbs of corn; or, 6.5 gallons of molasses (42° Bé.) equal approximately one bushel of corn.

Dried molasses products are made by drying molasses on an absorptive carrier, such as brewers' grains, corn oil and corn gluten meal, citrus meal, copra meal, grain bran and shorts, ground corncobs, bran and hulls, oat clippings, rice hulls, and bran. These dried products can be shipped, stored, and mixed as dry and granular ingredients of feed. These products have a much higher molasses content than the mixed feeds in which liquid molasses is used. The dried molasses products are intended as ingredients for further mixing.

As each of the carriers in the dried molasses products is a feed-mixing ingredient itself, it contributes food value to the product in the form of protein, fat, and carbohydrates. The feed value of dried molasses products on a per-pound basis is higher than that of the liquid molasses generally sold for livestock feed.

Beet sugar processors combine beet molasses with wet or dry beet pulp; and citrus processing plants mix citrus molasses with the citrus pulp. These products are used or fed directly without further mixing or dilution.

Mounting Medium for Microscopic Slides

Polyvinyl alcohol, high viscosity	0.25 oz
Acetone, 70%	0.83 oz
Glycerin	0.88 oz
Lactic acid	0.88 oz
Water	1.75 oz
Thymol	0.09 gm

Pass the polyvinyl alcohol through a No. 60 sieve, place it in a dry, glass-stoppered bottle, add the acetone, and shake well. Mix the glycerine and lactic acid with about 1 oz of water and add it to the acetone solution with constant shaking. Allow mixture to stand for 10–15 minutes, then add the remainder of the water, and the thymol. After further shaking, warm the bottle on a water bath at about 70°C. until solution is complete. This takes about 15 minutes.

The resulting mixture is a translucent, viscous, homogeneous liquid. This medium, when used to mount specimens on glass slides, is firm enough to handle within an hour of application. It is advisable to warm the mount over a low flame, thus reducing the setting time to about 5 minutes. This medium does not become brittle as other media do.

Odorless Firelighter

	parts by wt
Sawdust	15.0
Cork dust	15.0
Paraffin	24.0
Sugar	3.0
Potassium chlorate	3.0

Dissolve the sugar and potassium chlorate in the smallest amount of water, and mix thoroughly with the sawdust and cork dust. Place this mixture in a heated dough mixer, and pour in the melted paraffin. Keep stirring until a uniform mixture is obtained, and cast in blocks.

Paint Remover

	oz
Methylene chloride	49.92
Ethylene dichloride	48.00
Cellosolve (ethylene glycol monoethyl ether)	5.12
Methyl alcohol	8.32
Methylcellulose (medium viscosity)	2.56
Sodium petroleum sulfonate	6.40
Paraffin wax	3.84
Water	3.84

Mix the first six ingredients, then add the paraffin wax and shake well until solution is complete. Finally, add the water and shake well. This paint remover is not corrosive and it washes off easily under a stream of water. It meets the requirements of Air Force Specifications, 14119-B.

Pearl Dipping Solution

Nitrocellulose, high viscosity	1⅜	oz
Amyl acetate	15	oz
Pearl essence	½	oz
Dibutyl phthalate	24	min

Mix the nitrocellulose with about 11 oz of the amyl acetate. In a separate container mix the pearl essence with the remainder of the amyl acetate. Finally, mix the two solutions together, and add the dibutyl phthalate. Have the viscosity of this dipping solution from 80 to 90 seconds at 75°F., using a standard viscosity cup with ⅛ inch hole. Dip the articles to be coated into this solution, and allow them to dry from one to two hours. Three to four coatings are adequate. Have the articles thoroughly clean and smooth, and have the room used for drying dust-free, in a temperature range of 70–80°F.

Pearl essence is obtained principally from certain types of fish scales, such as sardine, herring, shad, pilchard, and bleak. The pearly appearance of the brilliant particles in the scales is due to tiny natural crystals of guanine, which are deposited in the thin tough layer of fatty tissue attached to the scales. The pearl essence is produced by removing the fatty tissue from the scales of the fish and separating the tiny fragile crystals of guanine from all foreign matter. Pearl essence is a suspension of the guanine crystals in a liquid such as amyl acetate, or acetone. Do not grind or violently mix the pearl essence with the lacquer as such treatment will damage the fragile crystals of guanine.

Pickling Bath for Metals

	oz
Renex 690 (polyoxyethylene nonyl phenol)	5.12
Phosphoric acid	16.65
Water	84.47
Kerosene	21.76

Mix the Renex with the acid and water and stir this mixture into the kerosene with rapid agitation. In practice, dilute this finished product with water, and apply it at a temperature of 185°F.

Use this pickling bath for removing scale or oxide from metals before finishing or plating.

Preserving Plants and Foliage

Preserve garden flowers, shrubbery, and tree foliage by placing mature specimens in a 50–50 mixture of glycerin and water for 3 weeks.

Flowers and foliage thus preserved will last indefinitely, and may be displayed either dry or in water.

Preserving Starfish

Place the starfish (or similar sea animal) in fresh water for six hours. Remove it to a solution of the following mixture:

Formaldehyde 40%	1 pt
Glycerin	8 oz
Water	9 pt

Mix well. Keep the starfish in this solution from 7 to 8 days, then dry it on a rack. Avoid direct sunlight.

Quaternary Ammonium Compound

N-Soya-N-ethyl morpholinium ethosulfate can serve as an antistatic, germicide, and a deodorizer. This compound is particularly effective in eliminating "hospital smell." It is recommended for use in hospital laboratories and washrooms, in dining rooms, and for the cleaning of floors, sickroom utensils, and refuse containers.

Radioactive Fallout

So-called radioactive fallout consists of atomized earth, building materials, rocks, and gases, sucked upward—sometimes to a height of 80,000 feet or more—and made radioactive by nuclear or thermonuclear explosions. These particles of matter in the air help form the mushroom cloud which is always seen with these explosions. These radioactive particles drop in the immediate area of the explosion, some may be carried by the upper winds for many miles. Sooner or later they do settle to earth, and this is called fallout.

Radioactive fallout created by explosions of atomic and hydrogen bombs is very likely to be highly concentrated. This fallout could settle anywhere, and as the upper winds could carry it to the remotest parts of the country, rural areas many miles away from the scene of the explosion may be endangered by it.

This addition of lime (calcium oxide) to the soil can reduce contamination of food crops by radioactive fallout. Plants grown in soil of high calcium content contain less strontium-90 than those grown in soil low in calcium content. Grass, on the other hand, shows a preference for strontium over calcium.

Removal of Carbon from Skin

The easiest way to remove carbon in the form of charcoal or coal from the skin is to first cover the hands with oil, then wash off with soap and water.

Sealing Agent for Laboratories

	oz
Soluble starch	2.90
Glycerin	7.40

Mix and heat until the solution becomes clear. The resultant "glycerite of starch" makes a good tight adhesive seal at room temperature, which can be removed easily by running water.

Shelters from Fallout

A frame house will give some protection from fallout. The danger from radiation might be cut by about one-half. On the floor, away from doors and windows, is about the best place to be.

A basement shelter will give even more protection. The radiation danger is reduced to about one-tenth.

An underground shelter with a covering of 3 feet of earth, and equipped with a door and air filter, will offer almost complete protection.

A storm cave or root cellar is almost ideal provided it is stocked with food, water, first-aid kits, blankets, fuel, lantern, etc.

Whether one is a city or country resident, one must prepare a shelter and stock it with a week's supply of food and water. It is essential that a radio, battery-operated, be kept in a safe place.

If one has been in a serious fallout area, all clothing must be destroyed and all exposed parts of the body must be thoroughly washed. If the contamination is not too serious, it may not be necessary to destroy the clothing, since it can be made safe by laundering or waiting for the radioactivity to decay.

Soap Bubble Solution

	oz
Soap flakes, fine	0.75
Glycerin	11.25
Water	15.00

Dissolve the soap in the water, add the glycerin and shake well. This solution will yield tough soap bubbles.

Solder for Stainless Steel

Soldering flux for stainless steel has a tendency to stand up in drops on the smooth surface of the metal. In order to overcome this tendency, add about 1/4 oz of glycerin to each 8 oz of the soldering flux.

Sterilizing of Water—Quick Method

To sterilize water quickly, add 2 drops of household bleach or tincture of iodine to each quart of water and allow it to stand for 30 minutes. The objectionable taste of bleach in the water can be overcome by pouring it from one glass to another a few times and allowing it to stand for a while. If these chemicals cannot be obtained, boil the water for 5 minutes or more.

Stiffener for Rayon

Soft, cold water	1 qt
Powdered gum arabic	2 oz

Dissolve the gum arabic in the water and heat the mixture until the gum is completely in solution. Mix one part of this solution with 5 or 10 parts of hot water, depending on the desired stiffness. Allow the solution to cool, then dip the piece of rayon (dress or other article) in it.

Stoddard Solvent for Weeds

Use Stoddard Solvent (cleaners' naphtha) as a selective spray for weeding carrots. Spray very young carrots with this oil; it will kill all the weeds without injuring the carrots.

Stop-Leak Preparations for Automobiles

No. 1

	oz
Soluble starch (Amylodextrin)	4.48
Asbestos	2.56
Wood flour	4.48
Water	107.52
Synthetic gum	1.28
Isopropyl alcohol	7.68

Mix the water with the starch, asbestos and wood flour. Dissolve the gum in the alcohol, and mix the two solutions thoroughly.

No. 2

	oz
Asbestos	2.56
Sodium silicate ($Na_2O{\cdot}3.5\ SiO_2$)	42.24
Water	83.20

Mix thoroughly.

These products can be used in water jackets and radiators.

Titanium

Titanium is never found in the pure state, but it occurs as an oxide in the ores, ilmenite ($FeTiO_3$), rutile (TiO_2), and titanite ($Ca\text{-}TiO_2\text{-}SiO_2$). The oxide is separated from its ore by treatment with potassium carbonate and aqueous hydrofluoric acid, which yields potassium fluotitanate. The fluotitanate is then extracted with hot water and decomposed with ammonia, and the resulting ammoniacal hydrated oxide is then ignited to yield titanium dioxide. The pure metal is obtained by treating the oxide with chlorine, which yields titanium tetrachloride, a volatile liquid; and then reducing this liquid with magnesium in a closed iron chamber to form metallic titanium. The metal, silver white in color, is melted and cast into ingots. Titanium is soluble in hot water, but insoluble in cold water. It melts at 3272°F., and boils at 5452°F. It has a specific gravity of 4.50.

The lightness and strength of titanium make it desirable for parts of jet engines and air frames that operate within a certain temperature range. Its properties may make it desirable for armour. The resistance of titanium to corrosion suggests its use on shipboard where contact with sea water is necessary. It is ideal for valves, salt-water piping, deck fittings, etc., as well as for equipment in the chemical industry where the resistance of titanium to certain acids and corrosive solutions (especially chlorides) makes it very attractive.

In overhauling engines, titanium parts show very little or no corrosion, whereas steel and aluminum parts are often badly corroded. The process of chemical machining, which is the removal of excess material by etching, is very promising. This development may go a long way toward solving the scrap-recovery problem, which is a big factor in the cost of using titanium.

Titanium is a metal valuable in national defense, and it is used in military aircraft. New processes, such as variations of the Kroll process, are being stimulated, and efforts are being made to intensify this work in order to lower the cost of sponge production, and effect greater recovery of scrap. The use of titanium will be increased if the cost of titanium mill products can be reduced.

Titanium is expected to supplant steel to a substantial degree in future aircraft (within certain temperature ranges) with a highly beneficial saving in weight.

Titanium is the metal of the future, and a "must." One pound of weight saved in an engine equals 4 pounds of weight saved in the frame structure for a bomber, or 2½ pounds saved in the frame structure of a fighter plane.

Uranium

Pure uranium consists of a mixture of atoms, 99.3% having a mass of 238, the other 0.7% having a mass of 235, i.e., a weight 235 times that of hydrogen. It is the 0.7% of those atoms of mass 235 which is the only naturally occurring fissionable material from which we at present know how to extract energy in a chain reaction. The remaining 99.3% uranium may be transformed into plutonium.

The energy that is eventually released in a reactor in the form of heat is of fantastic proportions. One pound of uranium of mass 235 releases energy equivalent to that obtained from burning 1,300 tons of coal, from 360,000 gallons of gasoline; and equivalent to a labor force of 57,000 men working 8 hours a day for one year.

Water Soluble Capsules

Prepare water soluble capsules from sodium cellulose sulfate films, they may be used as individual packages to contain bath salts, soap powders, etc. This compound can be obtained from the Tennessee Eastman Corporation.

White Soaps

It is essential that aluminum tanks are used in the manufacture of white soaps, and the pipe lines should be of some suitable material. Have all storage tanks and kettles ceramic lined. Check frequently all pipe lines for corrosive action.

Paints

Copper Color

A rich copper color can be produced by mixing a chrome yellow paint or enamel with a small quantity of burnt sienna color-in-oil.

House Paint

	oz
Basic white lead carbonate	4.48
Basic white lead sulfate	10.88
Zinc oxide	20.48
Titanium-magnesium mixture (titanium dioxide, 30, 70% magnesium silicate, 70)	28.16
Raw linseed oil	14.75
Bodied soybean oil	7.76
Bodied tung oil	1.94
Mineral spirits	6.12
Drier	5.43

The bodied tung oil used here has been thickened by heat. Unlike the raw tung oil, it dries in a clear, smooth film without wrinkling.
Total vehicle, 36%.
Percentage of drying oil in vehicle, 68%.
Percentage of thinner and drier, 32%.

Mix the oils with the thinner and drier, then stir in the four pigments.

Paints for the Exterior

No. 1: Cement Base

	lb
Portland cement	35.0
Hydrated magnesium lime	15.0
Water	q.s.

Tumble the dry powders in a pebble mill—without pebbles in the jar—for several hours. Stir about 7 lb of the mixed powder into 1 gallon of water. Stir a small portion of the water into the dry powder until a smooth paste has been formed, add the remainder of the water, and continue to stir until the resultant product is homogeneous. Use a stiff-bristled brush, and paint over damp surface. When the paint sets up, wet it down with water. Use two coats of cement-water paint, allowing 24 hours of drying time between coats. Store the dry powdered paint in moisture-proof containers.

No. 2: Oil Base

	lb
Pigment:	
White lead	39.00
Zinc oxide	16.38
Titanium dioxide	1.42
Silica and magnesium silicate	14.20
Vehicle:	
Pure linseed and Chinawood oil	17.11
Mineral spirits	7.54
Japan drier	4.35

Mix the pigments thoroughly with a small quantity of the oil in a mixing machine until a paste is formed. Finally, stir in the rest of the oil, mineral spirits, liquid drier, and coloring pigments if desired. Continue to mix until the product is uniform. Two coats are necessary for good coverage and durability. The first coat seals the surface to prevent "spotting" of the second coat. Allow 24 hours or more of drying time before applying the second coat. Use a 3-inch paint brush.

No. 3: Synthetic Rubber Base

	lb
Pigment:	
Titanium dioxide	16.72
Zinc oxide	7.60
Magnesium silicate	11.78
Kieselguhr	1.90
Vehicle:	
Rubber base solution, 28% solids	62.00

Prepare the vehicle by adding the synthetic rubber to treated drying oils, aromatic hydrocarbons, and coal tar thinners. Use the same method of mixing as for oil-base paints. Mix 1 pt of turpentine to 1 gallon of paint for the first coat. Allow 18 hours or more of drying time before applying the second coat.

No. 4: Whitewash

Casein	2½ lb
Trisodium phosphate	1½ lb
Lime paste	4 gal
Formaldehyde	1½ pt

Prepare the lime paste by mixing 25 lb of hydrated lime with 3 gallons of water. Dissolve the trisodium phosphate in ½ gallon of water. Soak the casein in 1 gallon of water for 2 hours, or until it is soft, add it to the first solution, and dissolve. Add the casein-trisoda solution to the lime paste, stirring continuously. Dissolve the formaldehyde in 1½ gallons of water, and just before use, add it slowly to the white mixture, stirring vigorously. Use two coats of whitewash. Dampen the walls with water before brushing on the first coat. Allow 24 hours of drying time between coats. Use a special whitewash brush.

The following paints for the exteror may be used on foundations, exterior walls, porches, and fences, but do not use them on surfaces that might be subject to abrasion.

Paints for Structural Steel

No. 1: Primer

Red lead paste (7% linseed oil)	50 lb
Leafed metallic lead paste	7½ lb
Raw linseed oil	1 gal
Drier	8 oz
Mineral spirits	12 oz

Second Coat

Red lead paste (7% linseed oil)	50 lb
Leafed metallic lead paste *	4½ lb
Raw linseed oil	6⅘ pt
Drier	8 oz
Turpentine	1¾ pt
Lampblack paste	enough to tint

* Leafed Metallic Lead Paste

The leafed metallic lead paste consists of

Flaked metallic lead	90%
Mineral spirits	9%
Stearic acid	1%

The sizes of the metallic constituents conform to the following requirements: Retained on:

100-mesh sieve	2%
200-mesh sieve	11%
325-mesh sieve	20%

Mix the leafed metallic lead paste thoroughly with one pint of linseed oil. Stir this mixture into the red lead paste, until the mixture is smooth and homogeneous. Finally, stir in the remainder of the raw linseed oil, drier, and thinner. Allow the finished paint to stand for 24 hours or more before using it.

The weight per gallon of this paint must not be less than 27 lb. The formulation described here meets the specifications of the California Highway Department.

Window Paint (Temporary)

The following formulation of a window paint will provide privacy without sacrificing any light:

	oz
Methylcellulose (400 or 1500 centipoises)	1.7
Mica, ground (325-mesh)	1.7
Glycerin	0.8
Water	37.5

Disperse the methylcellulose in 10 oz of water. Stir the ground mica into this dispersion, and add the glycerin. Finally, stir in the rest of the water. Apply this paint with a brush. Mica has good light transmission and extensive light scattering. When the paint is no longer needed, remove it with water.

Pharmaceutical and Proprietary Preparations

Acne Compact

	oz
Isopropyl stearate	40.96
Lecithin	1.28
Lanolin	3.84
Cetyl alcohol	2.56
Ceresin	5.12
Resorcinol	2.56
Sulfur	10.24
Titanium dioxide	53.76
Kaolin	7.68

Heat the first 7 components to 85°C. with constant stirring. Continue the stirring while adding the kaolin and titanium dioxide, and pour into molds to form compacts.

Anesthetic Cream for Burns

	oz
Vegetable oil	42.24
Anhydrous lanolin	38.40
Spermaceti	12.80
Isobutyl *p*-aminobenzoate	2.56
Water	32.00

Melt the fatty components and dissolve the aminobenzoate in them. Heat the water to the same temperature, and pour it, slowly but with thorough agitation, into the molten fats. Continue stirring until the mass is cold.

Perfume oil may be added if so desired.

Antibiotic Cream
(Germicidal)

	oz
Glyceryl monostearate	15.00
Spermaceti, U.S.P.	5.00
White mineral oil, heavy	4.00
Glycerin	6.00
n-Butyl-*p*-hydroxybenzoate (Butoben)	0.10
Dioctyl sodium sulfosuccinate (wetting agent)	0.02
Distilled water	69.88

Place the monostearate, spermaceti, mineral oil, glycerin, and Butoben in a suitable container, and heat to 75°C. Place the wetting agent in the water and heat to the same temperature. Pour the water solution into the melted fats, stirring at a medium rate of speed. Continue to stir until the cream is cold.

This cream, when combined with the proper amount of antibiotic, yields a product that is white and greaseless, with a soft, smooth texture. It does not stain clothing, and it washes off easily with water.

Anti-Dandruff Lotion

	oz
Isopropanol	64.00
Betanaphthol, U.S.P.	0.26
Salicylic acid, U.S.P.	0.26
Perfume oil	to suit
Water	64.00

Dissolve the betanaphthol, acid, and perfume oil in the isopropanol. Add the water and shake well. Allow the mixture to stand overnight, and filter if necessary. Do not use this lotion too frequently, as it has a tendency to dry the hair.

Antipruritic Lotion

(Anti-Itching)

	parts by wt
Menthol	0.3
Phenol	1.2
Coal tar solution, N.F. VI	8.0
Ethyl aminobenzoate, U.S.P. XI	8.0
Calamine lotion to make	120.0

Liquefy the first 4 ingredients by means of a slow heat. Heat the lotion to the same temperature and mix the two while constantly stirring until cool.

This lotion will alleviate the itch of eczema, poison ivy, insect bites, and the like.

Antiseptic

1–2% of *p*-chloro-*m*-xylenol is an excellent antiseptic in all applications of pharmacy and medicine.

Baby Lotion

		oz
1	Butyl stearate	19.20
	Span 60	3.84
	Hexachlorophene	0.39
2	Sucrose monopalmitate	4.80
	Methyl *p*-hydroxybenzoate	0.39
	Water	163.38

Mix the ingredients of (1) and heat to 75°C. Dissolve the monopalmitate and preservative in the water, and heat to 80°C. Stir (2) into (1), and continue to stir while cooling to room temperature. This lotion leaves an emollient, non-greasy, non-tacky film on the skin.

Baby Oil

No. 1

	oz
Acetylated monoglycerides from lard	38.40
Lanolin	12.80
Mineral oil	76.80

Mix and shake well. Filtration yields a bright clear solution.

No. 2

	oz
Acetylated lanolin	6.40
Mineral oil, 65/75 viscosity	121.60

Mix the acetylated lanolin with the mineral oil and heat slightly until clear.

For Baldness

The type of baldness known as Alopecia Areata can be greatly benefited by applications of benzyl benzoate.

Blackhead and Whitehead Lotion

	oz
Pepsin, of 4000 activity	1.28
Aluminum potassium sulfate, U.S.P.	2.56
Lactic acid, U.S.P.	1.28
Boric acid, U.S.P.	1.28
Distilled water	121.60

Mix and dissolve all ingredients in the water. Shake well, and allow solution to stand overnight. Filter if necessary.

Apply this lotion in the form of wet compresses, or dab it on with cotton. This lotion digests and dissolves blackheads and whiteheads. It serves remarkably to clarify the skin and give it a clean, fresh appearance.

Calamine Lotion

No. 1

Calamine, in fine powder	5.60 oz
Zinc oxide, in fine powder	5.60 oz
Sodium carboxymethylcellulose (medium viscosity)	1.50 oz
Dioctyl sodium sulfosuccinate	1.25 gm
Glycerin	2.00 oz
Distilled water	64.00 oz

Dissolve the carboxymethylcellulose in 40 oz of water and shake it well. Slowly add to this 19 oz of water, and the dioctyl sodium sulfosuccinate, previously dissolved in 5 oz of water. Rub the powders to a smooth paste with the glycerin plus about 3 oz of the carboxymethylcellulose solution, then add slowly the remainder of the solution with continuous trituration.

The resultant lotion pours easily from small dispensing bottles, it spreads smoothly on the skin, and dries to a flexible film. Liquefied phenol may be added if desired.

No. 2

Calamine	1.27 oz
Zinc oxide	1.27 oz
Polyvinyl alcohol (Elvanol 50–42: DuPont)	0.40 oz
Glycerin	3.65 dr
Water, q.s. to	15.25 oz

Rub the powders in a mortar, add the glycerin, then stir in the water in small portions to measure 15.25 oz.

No. 3: Improved

Calamine, in fine powder	10.72 oz
Zinc oxide, in fine powder	3.57 oz
Bentonite, in fine powder	2.15 oz
Sodium citrate	0.54 oz
Glycerin	3.38 oz
Liquefied phenol	2.71 dr
Distilled water	48.00 oz

Dissolve the sodium citrate in 35 oz of water, and stir in the fine powders. Add the liquefied phenol, then the glycerin, and the remainder of the water. Shake well.

The addition of sodium citrate renders the lotion readily pourable.

No. 4: Improved

Calamine, in fine powder	10.72 oz
Zinc oxide, in fine powder	3.57 oz
Sodium carboxymethyl cellulose	0.71 oz
Di-isopropyl naphthalene sulfonate	1.00 gm
Glycerin	3.38 oz
Liquefied phenol	2.71 dr
Distilled water	50.00 oz

Disperse the carboxymethylcellulose in about 4 oz of water at about 70°C. with constant stirring. Mix the naphthalene sulfonate with the fine powders, and stir in about 35 oz of water. Add the carboxymethylcellulose solution, then the liquefied phenol, glycerin, and the remainder of the water. Shake well. The carboxymethylcellulose and naphthalene sulfonate produce a product of greater suspensibility which leaves a very fine, adhesive film on application.

Chlorophyll Ointment

	oz
Stearic acid	28.0
Cetyl alcohol	6.0
Triethanolamine	1.6
Sodium lauryl sulfate	1.0
Glycerin	10.0
Sodium chlorophyllin	2.0
Distilled water	150.0

Melt the stearic acid and cetyl alcohol at 75°C. Dissolve the triethanolamine, sodium lauryl sulfate, and glycerin in the water, and pour this into the molten fats with vigorous stirring. Finally, incorporate the sodium chlorophyllin, previously dissolved in some of the water.

Cooling Emulsion

	oz
White mineral oil (65/75 viscosity)	12
Lanolin, anhydrous, U.S.P.	3
Trihydroxyethylamine oleate	6
Propylene glycol	3
Distilled water	96

Mix the first three ingredients and liquefy them by means of heat. Dissolve the propylene glycol in the water and heat to the same temperature. Mix the two solutions, and continue to stir until cold. Add some perfume oil if so desired.

Cooling Lotion for Sunburn

	oz
Zinc oxide, U.S.P.	18
Talcum powder	18
Bentonite *	6
Propylene glycol	6
Distilled water	72

* Colloidal native hydrated aluminum silicate.

Mix the propylene glycol with the water. Stir in the powdered ingredients and continue the agitation until the finished product is homogeneous. Add some perfume oil if so desired.

Cough Syrup for Children

	oz
Acetylsalicylic acid, U.S.P., powdered	1.5
Glycerin	45.0
Sodium citrate, U.S.P., powdered	3.0
Syrup of orange	15.0

Heat the glycerin to 70°C. and stir in the acetylsalicylic acid until solution is complete. Heat the syrup to 70°C. and stir in the citrate until solution is complete. Mix the two solutions and shake well. The dosage is about one teaspoon every 3 hours.

Dermatological Vehicle

Carbowax 4000	2	lb
Stearyl alcohol, U.S.P.	4	lb
Glycerin	3⅕	lb
Sodium lauryl sulfate	1⅘	oz
Water, distilled	9½	pt

Mix the Carbowax 4000 and stearyl alcohol together with the glycerin and heat to 60°C. Dissolve the sodium lauryl sulfate in the water and heat to the same temperature. Pour the hot water solution into the melted fats, with constant stirring. Allow the emulsion to cool while stirring slowly. This cream can be used as a base for various medicaments.

Diaper Rash Ointment

	oz
Balsam Peru, U.S.P. XI	1.0
Castor oil, U.S.P. XI	1.0
Petrolatum, white, U.S.P. XI	86.0
Boric acid, powdered, U.S.P. XI	2.0
Zinc oxide, U.S.P. XI	5.0
Zinc stearate, U.S.P. XI	5.0

Make an intimate mixture of the castor oil and the Peruvian balsam; stir this mixture into the petrolatum, mix thoroughly, and stir in the powdered components. Mix carefully, and put the mass through an ointment mill until it is perfectly smooth.

Diarrhea

Diarrhea is a condition that causes one to have too many bowel movements. The matter excreted may have blood in it. Much diarrhea is caused by bacteria. These organisms are so small that thousands of them can be carried on the foot of a fly. The flies get bacteria on their feet by walking in dirty places, and then wipe their feet on one's food and dishes.

Prevent diarrhea by keeping flies out of the house. Cover food, water, and dishes to keep flies away from them. Boil the water you use, because boiling water kills the bacteria that may be in the water. Use extreme care and cleanliness when touching food.

Diarrhea Mixture

Calcium carbonate, precipitated, U.S.P.	1 oz
Tincture of gambir	3 dr
Tincture of opium	30 min
Oil of cinnamon, U.S.P.	3 min
Distilled water, enough to make	7 oz

Mix the tinctures and dissolve the oil of cinnamon in the liquid. Stir in the carbonate, then the water, and shake well.

The dosage is 1 ounce.

Ear Drops

	oz
Antipyrene, U.S.P.	0.42
Benzocaine, U.S.P.	0.10
Glycerin, C.P.	7.50

Mix the two powders and dissolve them in the glycerin, previously heated. Filter through cotton.

Ephedrine Sulfate Jelly

Ephedrine sulfate, U.S.P.	154.25 gr
Sodium alginate	1.41 oz
Sodium benzoate	31.00 gr
Glycerin	3.53 oz
Methyl salicylate	0.10 cc
Eucalyptol	1.00 cc
Distilled water	28.75 oz

Rub the sodium alginate with the glycerin in a mortar until a smooth paste is obtained. Dissolve the ephedrine sulfate and sodium benzoate in the distilled water and add it in small portions to the sodium alginate-glycerin mixture, rubbing after each addition. Finally, stir in the methyl salicylate and eucalyptol, and allow the whole to stand for about 3 hours.

Foot Cream

	oz
Zinc undecylenate	30.0
Lanolin	30.0
Absorption base	37.5
Petrolatum	27.0
Undecylenic acid	3.0
Water	22.5
Perfume	to suit

Place the lanolin, absorption base, petrolatum, and undecylenic acid in a mixing kettle and heat to 55°C. Heat the water to the same temperature, and add it, a small amount at a time, to the molten fats, making sure that each portion added is emulsified. Maintain the temperature at 55°C. until all the water is added. Now stir in the powdered zinc undecylenate and the perfume, and continue to stir until cold.

Foot Powders

No. 1

	oz
Zinc peroxide	3.53
Sodium perborate	5.30
Boric acid	8.83
Bentonite	17.65

Mix the powders thoroughly. This foot powder is excellent for counteracting foul odor.

No. 2

Talcum powder	19¼ lb
Colloidal kaolin	5 lb
Methenamine, U.S.P., powdered	12 oz

Mix the powders thoroughly.

Methenamine is an antiseptic because it liberates formaldehyde in presence of free acid.

No. 3

Talcum powder	5 lb
Starch	11 oz
Aluminum potassium sulfate, exsiccated	1 oz
Zinc stearate	3 oz
Boric acid	6 oz
Salicylic acid	2 oz

Reduce all ingredients to a very fine powder and mix thoroughly.

No. 4

	lb
Salicylic acid	½
Boric acid	1½
Zinc stearate	¾
Aluminum potassium sulfate, exsiccated	¼
Starch	2½
Powdered talc	20

Mix the powders thoroughly.

For Fungus Infection

	oz
Silver nitrate	12.80
Ethyl alcohol	6.40
Water	108.80

Dissolve the nitrate in the water, add the alcohol, and shake well. Apply this lotion once, and then expose the lesions for a few minutes to direct sunlight.

For Gangrene

Tincture of benzoin is the most useful compound for the prevention of gangrene. Apply the tincture as a coating to the affected surface; it lasts for one or two days. Repeat the application if necessary.

Glycerite of Starch

	oz
Glycerin	89.60
Starch	12.80
Water	25.60

Make a homogeneous paste of the starch and water and add it slowly to the glycerin. Mix thoroughly, and heat to 150°C. with constant stirring. Remove from the fire when the mass is translucent. Pack in tightly sealed containers.

Hydrocortisone Ointment

	oz
Sesame oil	15.00
Glyceryl monostearate (Aldo 33)	3.75
Cetyl alcohol, pure	11.20
Polyoxyethylene (40) stearate (Myrj 52)	3.75
Glycerin	18.60
Water, distilled	22.75
Hydrocortisone, U.S.P., microfine	0.75

Melt the first three ingredients at 70°C. Add Myrj 52 and maintain the temperature at 70°C. Mix the glycerin with the water and heat, in a separate container, at 75°C. Add the hydrocortisone to the aqueous glycerin solution and stir rapidly until a uniform slurry is obtained. Incorporate this slurry into the melted mixture and stir rapidly to form an emulsion. Continue stirring until the emulsion gradually cools and thickens into a smooth, uniform ointment. This ointment is neither too drying, nor too greasy.

Hydrocortisone has been found particularly effective for the following skin conditions:

Contact dermatitis, dermatitis of eyelids, chronic dermatitis of hands or feet, drug eruptions, eczema of nipples and areolae, psoriasiform (the formation of scaly patches) dermatitis, and stasis (stagnation of the blood) dermatitis.

The beneficial effects of hydrocortisone usually appear within one or two days after treatment. Relief from burning, itching, or stinging is rapid, and improvement is apparent within 24 to 48 hours. Erythema (abnormal redness of the skin) subsides quickly, and the pain is relieved.

Hydrophilic Ointment Base

		by wt
1	White petrolatum	4.82 oz
	Cetyl alcohol	1.25 oz
	White beeswax	0.72 oz
	Stearyl alcohol	0.54 oz
	Glycerin	1.45 oz
2	Distilled water	9.00 oz
	Sodium lauryl sulfate	0.20 oz
	Zephiran chloride * 12.5%	5.00 min

* Zephiran chloride is a mixture of high molecular weight alkyl dimethylbenzyl ammonium chlorides. It is a cationic detergent, and germicide of high bactericidal and bacteriostatic potency. It can be obtained from Winthrop-Stearns, Inc., New York 18, N. Y.

Heat (1) to 80°C. Heat (2) to the same temperature. Pour the oily mixture into the aqueous solution, slowly with constant stirring. Pour into suitable containers at 40°C.

This ointment base has good stability, and is compatible with moderately acid and alkaline substances. It is comparatively greaseless, and is easily rinsed off with water. It does not interfere with the efficacy of any therapeutic agent.

Industrial Barrier Cream

No. 1

	oz
Stearic acid	3.00
Phenol	0.75
Chlorocresol	0.30
Powdered hard soap	18.00
Glycerin	9.00
Sodium chloride	1.50
Distilled water	82.95
Sterilized kaolin (China clay)	30.00
Bentonite (a colloidal native hydrated aluminum silicate)	4.50

Heat the stearic acid together with the phenol and chlorocresol at about 55–60°C. Mix the soap, glycerin, and sodium chloride in with the water and heat at about 65–70°C. Pour the water solution into the stearic acid mixture, while stirring briskly. Finally, stir in the kaolin and the bentonite, and continue stirring until the mass is cold. This cream is an oil- and solvent-barrier and is excellent for the prevention of contact dermatitis (inflammation of the skin).

No. 2

		oz
1	Stearic acid	3.84
	Glycerin	11.52
	Chlorocresol	0.38
	Phenol	0.96
2	Powdered soap	23.04
	Sodium chloride	1.92
	Distilled water	106.17
3	Sterilized kaolin	38.40
	Bentonite	5.76

Mix (1) and heat to about 75°C. Mix (2) and heat to the same temperature. Pour (2) into (1) slowly, with constant stirring. Finally, add (3), with constant stirring, and continue mixing until the mass is homogeneous and of proper consistency. This cream will prevent contact dermatitis.

Iodine Solution
(Improved)

	oz
Iodine	2.56
Sodium iodide	3.07
Propylene glycol	32.00
Distilled water	90.37

Mix and shake well until solution is complete. This solution does not irritate the skin, and it has a high bactericidal efficiency. The iodine content of this solution is equivalent to that in the present official tincture of iodine.

Lotion Vehicle for Dermatological Medications
No. 1

	oz
Cetyl alcohol	3.75
Paraffin wax	0.25
Sodium lauryl sulfate	1.25
Glycerin	11.83
Water to make	236.00

Melt the wax and cetyl alcohol at 80°C. Dissolve the lauryl sulfate in a mixture of the glycerin and 50 oz of water and heat to 80°C. Add the water solution to the molten fats slowly, stirring constantly until an emulsion forms. Continue to stir and add sufficient water to make 236 oz.

No. 2

	oz
Cetyl alcohol	1.33
Paraffin wax	0.10
Glycerin	4.23
Sodium lauryl sulfate	0.44
Water, distilled	78.00

Melt the cetyl alcohol and wax at about 80°C. Mix the glycerin with the water and dissolve the sodium lauryl sulfate in this. Heat the water solution to about 80°C., and pour it slowly into the molten fats, stirring constantly until the emulsion forms. Continue to stir until cold.

Lotions for Furunculosis
(Boils)

Tetracycline	74	gr
Glycerin, U.S.P.	1¾	oz
Zinc oxide, U.S.P.	1¼	oz
Talc	1¼	oz
Bentonite	⅞	oz
Water, distilled, q.s.	16	oz

Dissolve the tetracycline in some of the water mixed with the glycerin, and stir in the powdered zinc oxide, talc, and bentonite. Shake well and add enough water to measure 16 ounces. Most patients using this lotion can carry on their normal activities with greater ease.

Lice Infestation

Three varieties of lice—the head louse, the body louse, and the crab louse—infest the human body. One of the most common predisposing causes of infestation is lack of personal cleanliness.

The lice themselves seldom cause serious trouble, but the scratching which they induce very often results in skin lesions and infections.

The head louse infests the hair of the head and causes itching and irritation of the scalp. The body louse dwells in the seams of clothing; its bites are irritating and cause severe itching. The crab louse usually fastens itself to the short hairs of the genital region, and severe itching is the characteristic symptom. All these species live on the blood of man.

Hair Wash for Lice and Nits

Quassia, powdered	6	oz
Acetic acid	2	dr
Salicylic acid	47	gr
Glycerin	1	oz
Spirit of camphor	80	min
Spirit of rosemary	80	min
Specially denatured alcohol	3	oz
Rose water	4	oz
Distilled water, enough to make	67	oz

Boil the powdered quassia in 3 pts of water for 15 minutes. When cold, strain and add to this strained solution the glycerin, acids, and rose water. Dissolve the camphor and rosemary spirits in the alcohol and add it to the water solution. Shake well and add enough distilled water to make 67 ounces. Allow solution to stand overnight, then filter.

Disinfect thoroughly all clothing worn by the person. This can be accomplished by steaming under pressure, boiling, ironing with a hot iron, or dipping in gasoline or naphtha. After all lice and nits have been destroyed, use extreme care and cleanliness to prevent recurrence.

Menthol Lotion

Menthol	18.52 gr
Hexachlorophene	9.26 gr
Alcohol or isopropanol	7.00 oz
Glycerin	2.00 oz
Water	11.00 oz

Dissolve the menthol and hexachlorophene in the alcohol, add the glycerin, and stir in the water with vigorous shaking. Allow the mixture to stand overnight, and filter if necessary. Use this lotion as a relief in itching conditions.

Ointment Base, Washable

No. 1

	oz
Carbowax compound 4000	21.0
Stearyl alcohol	39.0
Glycerin	30.0
Sodium lauryl sulfate	1.0
Water	90.0

Melt and mix thoroughly, continue stirring until cold.

This ointment will make an excellent vehicle for a great variety of medicaments. The consistency of this ointment may be varied by increasing or decreasing the amount of water. This washable ointment base is superior to the U.S.P. Hydrophilic Ointment.

No. 2

	oz
Petrolatum	12.00
* Ceramol	6.00
Cetyl alcohol	1.00
Stearyl alcohol	1.00
Propylene glycol	4.00
Distilled water	37.75

* Brand name of Lanette Wax SX.

Melt the petrolatum, Ceramol, and alcohols together and keep the mixture at about 65°C. Mix the propylene glycol with the water and heat to the same temperature. Stir the water solution slowly into the melted fats. When emulsification is complete, continue the stirring slowly until cold.

No. 3

	oz
Stearyl alcohol	32.000
White petrolatum	32.000
Propylene glycol	15.360
Polyoxyethylene (40) stearate	6.400
Methyl *p*-hydroxy benzoate	0.032
Propyl *p*-hydroxy benzoate	0.019
Distilled water	42.240

Heat the petrolatum and stearyl alcohol at 75°C. Mix the other ingredients with the water and heat to the same temperature. Pour the oily mixture slowly into the aqueous solution, and continue to stir until cold. This ointment base has good stability and it is superior to the U.S.P. XIV product; it is an excellent vehicle for a great variety of medicaments. The propylene glycol—besides being a humectant—acts as an accessory preservative in the base, thus fortifying the *p*-hydroxy benzoates.

Paste for Acid Burns

	oz
Carbowax 4000	82.2
Glycerin, U.S.P.	27.0
Procaine hydrochloride, powdered, U.S.P.	1.8
Magnesium sulfate, powdered, U.S.P.	30.0
Magnesium oxide, powdered, U.S.P.	9.0

Mix the first three components and heat gently until all are liquefied. Remove the heat and allow the mixture to cool somewhat; then stir in the magnesium sulfate and oxide. Continue to mix until a smooth paste is obtained.

This paste is especially recommended for burns from hydrofluoric acid. Wash the burned area freely with water for several hours, then apply the paste as a wet dressing.

Poison Ivy Ointment

	oz
Carbowax 4000	21.0
Stearyl alcohol	39.0
Glycerin	30.0
Sodium lauryl sulfate	1.0
Water	90.0
Zirconium oxide	10.0

Melt and mix the first 5 ingredients thoroughly. Stir in the zirconium oxide, and continue to stir until the mass is cold. The consistency of this ointment may be varied by increasing or decreasing the amount of water.

This ointment, if applied immediately, will prevent the development of irritation from poison ivy. If the poisoning is allowed to develop, this ointment will promptly clear up the irritation.

Protective Cream

(Poison Ivy–Poison Oak)

	oz
Glyceryl monostearate (Aldo 28)	7.50
Lanolin alcohol	4.50
Triethanolamine ricinoleate	0.75
Glycerin	4.50
Distilled water	50.85
Methanol	4.50
Oleyl alcohol, N.F.	2.25
Chlorocresol	0.15
Zirconium oxide (this can be varied)	3.00

Melt the first 3 ingredients. Dissolve the glycerin in the water and heat, in a separate container, to the same temperature. Pour the water solution slowly into the oily mixture with constant stirring. While it is cooling, stir in the methanol, oleyl alcohol, and chlorocresol. Finally, stir in the zirconium oxide, and continue stirring until the mass is cold.

Safflower Oil

The safflower plant is being grown in California, Oregon, and western Nebraska. The safflower oil derived from this plant contains about 80% of linoleic acid, as compared with corn, soybean, and cottonseed oils which contain only about 45% of linoleic acid. One or two tablespoons a day of this oil will keep the cholesterol level in a person's blood from rising.

Safflower oil tastes like cream; it can be mixed with coffee, and fruit juices, or used as a salad dressing.

Styptic Pencils

	oz
Ammonium chloride, U.S.P.	8.0
Cupric sulfate, U.S.P.	8.0
Zinc sulfate, U.S.P.	8.0
Ferric sulfate	8.0
Potassium alum, U.S.P.	101.0

Liquefy the ingredients by means of a slow heat, and pour into molds.

Tooth Paste

No. 1

	oz
Glycerite of starch	64.0
Sodium sulforicinoleate	12.8
Kaolin, N.F.	51.2
Flavor, color, and water	to suit

Mix the glycerite of starch with the sodium sulforicinoleate and stir in the kaolin. Add enough water and color to yield a product of the proper consistency; then stir in the flavor and mix all thoroughly. Sodium sulforicinoleate has the quality of removing scale from teeth.

No. 2

	oz
Dicalcium phosphate (dental grade)	60.00
Calcium carbonate, precipitated, U.S.P.	13.50
Tertiary magnesium phosphate	1.50
Sodium lauryl sulfate (foaming agent)	2.50
Flavor	q.s.
Glycerin	22.50
Sorbo syrup	22.50
Water, distilled	24.00
Saccharin, U.S.P. (sweetener)	0.15
Ethyl *p*-hydroxybenzoate (preservative)	0.15
Irish moss extractives (stabilizer)	2.00

Mix the water with the glycerin, sorbo syrup, preservative, sweetener and stabilizer, and heat slowly to effect complete solution. Stir in the foaming agent, polishing powders and flavor, and render the finished product homogeneous by means of a mixing-milling deaeration process.

For Warts

Mix and melt about equal parts of oxycholesterol and petrolatum to form an ointment base. When cool, incorporate in it 3 or 4% of formalin.

Warts, Removal of

It has been established that methionine (a natural or synthetic amino acid containing sulfur) can be used for the treatment of warts. It is administered orally to patients with warts at the rate of 1 to 2 grams per day. The warts usually disappear within ten days after treatment begins.

Stain Removers

Blood Stains

Blood stains cannot always be identified by sight, because numerous other stains have the same appearance. In case of doubt, apply a few drops of peroxide to the stain. If the stain is blood, there will be effervescence.

For Catsup, Chili Sauce, Mustard, Relish

To remove these stains from tablecloths, first sponge the spots with clear cold water, then rub them with glycerin, and allow this to remain for about 30 minutes. Finally, wash in warm soapy water to which a little ammonia 28% has been added.

Remove grass stains by the same method.

Dry Cleaning Agent

Glycerin	8.0 oz
Glacial acetic acid	2.0 oz
Methyl alcohol	2.0 oz
Lactic acid	2.0 oz
Amyl acetate	2.0 oz
Hydrofluoric acid, dilute	5–6 drops
Butyl alcohol	q.s.
Oleic acid	1.0 oz

Mix the first five ingredients thoroughly and add the hydrofluoric acid. Next add enough butyl alcohol to obtain a clear solution. Finally, add the oleic acid, and allow the mixture to stand overnight to effect complete solution of the oleic acid.

This preparation is safe to use on rayon, silk, and cotton fabrics. It will remove tannin stains caused by coffee, tea, coca-cola, beer, and other soft drinks. It will be difficult to remove a tannin stain if it is well oxidized. The mixture is also useful in removing many fruit, ink and dye stains; it is reasonably safe on most dyed fabrics.

For Dye-Stains

To remove dye stains from the hands, use a strong solution of potassium permanganate, then follow this with a solution of either sodium bisulfite or oxalic acid. The skin will become brown from the permanganate solution, but the final washing will remove all traces of the brown together with the dye-stains.

For Fruit Stains

Sponge the stains with cool water, and rub lightly with glycerin. Allow it to remain for several hours. Apply several drops of white vinegar, allow this to stand a few minutes, then rinse. Finally, launder in warm suds.

Glycerin As Stain Remover

To remove tea, coffee and fruit stains from practically any material rub glycerin into the stain, leave the material overnight, and flush this out with warm, soapy water the following morning. The most obstinate stain will disappear with this treatment, provided the material has not been dry-cleaned or the stain has not been oxidized.

To remove a long-set fruit stain from linen, moisten the stain with glycerin, put it aside for an hour; then stretch the material tightly and pour boiling water through the stain. Rinse thoroughly, and dry.

To remove milk stains, mix one part of glycerin with three parts of water in a shallow dish, resting the stained part in this and rub it gently. Leave it for 15 minutes and then rinse thoroughly.

To remove scorch marks from woolens, apply glycerin to the mark, allow the material to soak for several hours; then flush it out with soap and water and rinse thoroughly.

For Ink Stains (Sticks)

No. 1

	lb
Polyethylene glycol 4000	10.0
Triethanolamine	3.6
Oxalic acid	3.1

Melt the glycol 4000, stir in the triethanolamine and oxalic acid, and continue the stirring until a clear solution is formed. When the mixture becomes fairly viscous, pour into molds.

No. 2

	lb
Polyethylene glycol 4000	14.0
Sodium bisulfite, powdered	5.0
Carbitol solvent	1.0

Melt the glycol 4000, add the Carbitol, and stir in the powdered bisulfite. Continue the stirring until the mixture becomes fairly viscous, then pour into molds.

These water-soluble sticks will remove ink stains from fabrics.

For Potassium Permanganate

To remove from the skin the brown discoloration caused by potassium permanganate, apply vinegar, lemon juice, or a 1% solution of oxalic acid.

To remove such stains from a basin or dish, fill it with warm water, and add 1 teaspoon of oxalic acid crystals for every 2 quarts of water. Allow the dish or basin to stand for 15 minutes, then rinse it.

Rust Removal from Cement

	oz
Sodium citrate	5.0
Glycerin	30.0
Water	30.0
Calcium carbonate, prepared, powdered	q.s.

Mix the glycerin with the water and dissolve the sodium citrate in it. Stir in enough of the calcium carbonate to form a heavy paste. Spread a thick coating of this paste on the stained area and let it dry. Repeat the treatment if necessary. Allow a week or more for complete removal from badly stained areas.

For Tobacco Stains

	oz
Hydrochloric acid, C.P.	0.5
Glycerin	12.5
Rose water	113.0

Mix the glycerin with the rose water, add the acid, and shake well. Exercise great care in handling the acid. Saturate a piece of cotton with this solution and rub it gently over the stained area. Repeat the process if necessary until the desired results are obtained. The glycerin helps to whiten the skin and leaves it soft and smooth.

Veterinary Preparations

Acute Dermatitis (Inflammation of Skin)

	oz
Tincture of iodine, 7%	3.0
Glycerin	9.0

Mix and shake well.

Acute Eczema

No. 1

Methylene blue or Gentian violet	0.5 oz
Specially denatured alcohol	16.0 oz

Dissolve the crystals in the alcohol and shake well.

No. 2

	oz
Bismuth subnitrate	4.50
Zinc oxide	4.50
Glycerin	1.50
Corn starch	1.50
Water	30.00

Mix the glycerin with the water and stir in the powdered ingredients.

In cases of itching without any visible eruption, use the following lotion:

	oz
Talcum powder	6.0
Zinc oxidc	6.0
Glycerin	4.0
Specially denatured alcohol, 50% enough to make	40.0

Mix the glycerin with the dilute alcohol, and stir in the powders.

Dog Shampoo

Soft soap	8½	oz
Glycerin	2½	oz
Water	24	oz
Thymol	⅜	oz
Eucalyptus oil	2	dr
Specially denatured alcohol	2	oz

Mix the water with the glycerin and dissolve the soap in it. Dissolve the oil and the thymol in the alcohol. Slowly pour the alcoholic solution into the soap solution and shake well.

Bronchial Asthma

	oz
Belladonna tincture	1.0
Licorice fluid extract	4.0

Glycerin	5.0
Potassium iodide	1.0
Water	13.0

Dissolve the iodide in the water. Stir in the glycerin, then the tincture and the fluidextract, and mix thoroughly. The dosage is one teaspoon every four hours.

Ear Mange (Scabby Eruption)

No. 1

	oz
Balsam of Peru	4.0
Glycerin	4.0

No. 2

Tincture of iodine	1.0
Glycerin	9.0

Mix the ingredients thoroughly. Cleanse the ear by sponging with dilute alcohol. When dry, apply the medication.

Lotion for Alopecia (Loss of Hair)

Mercuric chloride	175.0 gr
Glycerin	4.0 oz
Specially denatured alcohol, 50%	20.0 oz

Dissolve the mercuric chloride in the diluted alcohol, add the glycerin and shake well.

Lotion for Seborrhea *

	oz
Salicylic acid	0.5
Glycerin	1.5
Specially denatured alcohol	29.0

*Seborrhea is an excessive discharge from the sebaceous glands, which forms an oily coating or crust on the skin.

Dissolve the acid in the alcohol, add the glycerin, and shake well.

Stimulating Liniment

No. 1

Tincture of iodine, 7%	12.0 oz
Turpentine oil	3.0 oz
Glycerin	3.0 oz
Croton oil	25.0 min

Mix the iodine with the glycerin, then add the croton oil and turpentine oil, and mix well. Apply daily without any covering.

No. 2

	oz
Tincture of iodine, 7%	9.0
Spirit of camphor (1 oz camphor in 9 oz alcohol)	9.0
Glycerin	9.0
Isopropyl alcohol	23.0

Mix thoroughly. Apply to affected surface, and rub well. Cover with cotton and bandage.

Tests: Various

Colorimetric Determination of Uranium in Phosphate Rock and Carnotite

1. Weigh 10 g of sample (100-mesh or finer), and transfer it to a 250 cc beaker. Add 50 cc of nitric acid (2 parts acid to 3 parts water), and digest on a steam bath for 30 minutes. Filter through a No. 42 Whatman filter paper, and wash the filter paper and residue with 50 cc of warm nitric acid (2 parts acid to 3 parts of water). Prepare a 50% solution of aluminum nitrate by dissolving 250 g of aluminum nitrate in 250 cc of nitric acid (2:3) and dilute this to 500 cc with nitric acid (2:3). Add 20 cc of this solution to the filtrate and washings. Retain the filtrate.

2. Place the filter paper and residue in a platinum crucible and ignite it until the filter paper is completely destroyed. Cool the residue, moisten it with 5 drops of sulfuric acid (1 part acid to 1 part water), and place it on a hot plate at a low heat. Fill the crucible ⅔ full of hydrofluoric acid, 48%, and evaporate to dryness. Fuse the residue with 3 g of potassium persulfate and cool the melt. Dissolve the melt in 50 cc of 30% nitric acid (3 parts acid to 7 parts water), and mix with the retained filtrate. Dilute the mixed solutions with 30% nitric acid to a volume of 200 cc.

3. Transfer 50 cc of the 200 cc solution of this sample to a 125 cc separatory funnel, and add 50 cc of a mixture of tributyl phosphate and methyl isobutyl ketone (1 part tributyl phosphate to 1 part methyl isobutyl ketone). Shake the contents vigorously for about 30 seconds, allow the phases to separate, then draw off and discard the lower layer (water). Again add 50 cc of 30% nitric acid to the separatory funnel, shake the contents vigorously for about 30 seconds; then allow the phases to separate and draw off and discard the lower (water) as before. Repeat the washings with 30% nitric acid four more times.

4. Remove the uranium from the tributyl phosphate by adding 20 cc of a mixture of ammonium acetate and ammonium fluoride solution to the

separatory funnel.* Shake the contents vigorously for about 15 seconds, allow the phases to separate, then draw off the water, and pour the solution into a 150 cc beaker. Repeat this last operation twice.

5. Transfer the solution from the 150 cc beaker to a 250 cc separatory funnel. Wash the beaker with two 10 cc portions of water, and add the washings to the separatory funnel. Add exactly 25.0 cc of 1% 8-hydroxyquinoline in chloroform (5 g of 8-hydroxyquinoline in 500 cc of chloroform) to the separatory funnel. Shake the contents vigorously for 30 seconds, and allow the phases to separate.

6. Place a 12.5 cm folded filter paper (Reeve Angel, No. 812) in the mouth of a 100 cc beaker, and filter the chloroform-8-hydroxyquinoline extract through this folded filter paper. Transfer this filtered extract to a 5-cm cell. Read the percentage transmitted with a Beckman spectrophotometer against a reference solution of 1% 8-hydroxyquinoline in chloroform (obtain a standard transmittancy-concentration curve by running a known amount of uranium through the entire procedure), using a wave length of 470 millimicrons and a slit 0.04 mm wide. Determine the amount of U_3O_8 in the sample by comparing the transmittancy of the sample with the standard curve. Read the amount of U_3O_8 in the sample from the curve and calculate the percent of U_3O_8 in the original sample. Use a factor of 0.8480 to convert U_3O_8 to the uranium content. Analyze a blank simultaneously with the samples to enable you to apply a correction for the presence of uranium in the reagents.

The nitric acid dissolves any lead or other metals, thus preventing any damage to the platinum crucible used for the potassium persulfate fusion. The aluminum nitrate is used to complex the phosphate ion. The tributyl phosphate-methyl isobutyl ketone is used for the purpose of extracting the uranium from the nitric acid solution. The ketone is used for the purpose of obtaining rapid phase-separation of the tributyl phosphate from the acid solution. The nitric acid solution washes out impurities from the phosphate-ketone extract. The acetate-fluoride solution removes the uranium from the phosphate-ketone extract. The ammonium fluoride prevents the interference from traces of thorium in the color development of phosphate-ketone extract. The acetate-fluoride solution removes the

* To prepare this solution, dissolve 125 g of ammonium acetate and 1 g of ammonium fluoride in 500 cc of water. With a *p*H meter adjust the *p*H of the solution to 7.6 with ammonium hydroxide.

To Detect Uranium

All uranium minerals emit rays, called radiations, that can easily be detected by radiometric measuring devices. The uranium radiations are usually differentiated as alpha, beta, and gamma rays.

ALPHA RAYS: These rays carry considerable energy but they have very little penetrating power. Most alpha rays will be stopped by a thin sheet of paper.

BETA RAYS: The penetrating power of beta rays is much greater than that of alpha rays. They can penetrate thin glass, about 1 foot of air, and a few millimeters of rock.

GAMMA RAYS: These rays have a much higher velocity than either alpha or beta. The gamma particles derived from uranium decay can penetrate 3 inches of lead, 1 foot of rock, 2½ feet of metal, or several hundred feet of air. Most field counters are in reality gamma-ray detectors.

Geiger Counter

The essential part of this counter is the Geiger tube, an ionization tube made of metal or glass. Its length varies from 4 inches to several feet; its diameter varies from less than 1 inch to several inches. The Geiger tube is usually filled with argon gas, but helium or krypton gas may be used instead. The Geiger counter operates thus: a high voltage from portable dry cell batteries is applied between a thin metal wire, usually made of tungsten and running the length of the tube (positive electrode), and the wall of the tube (negative electrode). When this tube is brought near a source of radioactivity, it is continuously struck by radioactive particles. The walls of the tube normally repulse the alpha particles unless thin-walled mica windows are provided that will admit some alpha particles. Beta-gamma counters with glass 0.005 to 0.007 inch thick in the sensitive area admit only the most energetic of the beta rays. Gamma rays, being the most penetrating, pass through the outer wall of the metal or glass tube. About 0.5 percent of the gamma rays remain within the tube and react with molecules of the enclosed gas to produce electrons. These negatively charged particles are attracted toward the positively charged center-wire, thus creating an electrical impulse that is recorded in the flash of a neon light, the motion of a needle on a meter, or a light, sharp sound in headphones.

Scintillation Counter

This device depends upon the ability of gamma rays to produce tiny flecks of light (scintillations) in sodium iodide crystals, rather than upon their ionizing effect upon gases contained in Geiger tubes. Scintillation counters consist of two fundamental parts:

(1) The crystals (potassium iodide, sodium iodide, or stilbene) which convert the radiation into visible light; and

(2) A photoelectric cell with a meter circuit to record the scintillations. The sensitivity of this instrument depends upon the size of the crystals, which may vary from 0.5 to 5 inches in cross section. The scintillation counter is much more sensitive than the Geiger counter, as the crystal reacts with greater efficiency, and therefore responds to a much larger proportion of the gamma rays. Scintillation may be produced by as much as 50 percent of the gamma rays that strike the crystal, whereas Geiger tubes may react to only 0.5 percent of the gamma rays. The scintillation counter may approach 100 percent efficiency if large, thalium-activated, sodium iodide crystals are used. Because of this greater sensitivity car-borne and air-borne prospectors employ the scintillation counter successfully.

Two B batteries are necessary to furnish 700 to 1500 volts in order to operate most Geiger or scintillation counters. Transistors may be employed, thus eliminating part of the excessive bulk and weight. Too much vibration should be avoided, as they may cause filaments to short-circuit internally and burn out the tube.

Most counters are affected by slight radiations from extraneous sources, such as cosmic rays, and rocks that contain small quantities of radioactive material. This accidental radioactivity is called "background count."

In order to calibrate the counter, the background count should be taken at a place in which no radioactive substances are present. The uranium content of a sample can be estimated fairly accurately by checking it with a standard sample of known uranium content.

Standard uranium samples can be obtained from the National Bureau of Standards, U.S. Dept. of Commerce, Washington 25, D.C.

Gravimetric Determination of Thorium in Monazite Sand of North and South Carolina

The sample of sand is treated with hydrofluoric acid in order to remove the silica and to aid in decomposing it. If the sample contains much silica, this treatment should be repeated. The residue is fused with dried potassium acid fluoride, and great care must be exercised throughout the fusion because the material tends to foam, creep, and sputter. Water is used to loosen the fusion, hydrofluoric acid is added, the mixture is digested, and all the insoluble fluorides are removed by filtration.

This step removes the following soluble fluorides: Aluminum, beryllium, columbium, iron, tantalum, titanium, and zirconium.

Fuming sulfuric acid converts the insoluble fluorides into sulfates. This treatment usually makes all the material soluble, but if some insoluble material should remain, the addition of ammonium hydroxide and sodium metabisulfite will dissolve it. The sulfate solution is neutralized with ammonium hydroxide, and sodium metabisulfite crystals are added to bring about the reduction of cerium. If cerium is present, the solution will be yellow; the addition of metabisulfite will render it colorless unless iron is present. Ammonium hydroxide is added to the solution, forming a precipitate of insoluble hydroxides. Thus the sample is freed from calcium, magnesium, and the alkali elements.

If many oxides other than thoria and rare earth are present, it is best to remove the iron by extraction with ether. The ammonium hydroxide precipitate is dissolved in hydrochloric acid (1 part acid to 1 part water), then cooled and shaken with ether. The ammonium hydroxide precipitate is dissolved in hydrochloric acid, and amonium hydroxide is added until a faint turbidity or precipitate is formed. This precipitate is dissolved by adding just enough hydrochloric acid. A few sodium metabisulfite crystals are added, and precipitation is effected by adding a hexamine solution.

In order to effect complete separation of the thorium from the rare earths several precipitations are necessary. It is advisable to place a pad of macerated filter paper in the apex of the filter paper when filtering all precipitations encountered here. The filtrate is tested for complete precipitation by adding 1 cc of hexamine solution. The filtrate is tested for complete removal of rare earths by making it strongly ammoniacal, whereupon the rare earth hydroxides will precipitate. The last hexamine precipitate is dissolved in hydrochloric acid and evaporated to dryness. The oxalic acid precipitates the thorium as the oxalate. This final step removes from the thorium any traces of titanium or zirconium that may have been retained with the insoluble fluorides.

This gravimetric method for the determination of thorium in monazite sand, based on the work of A. M. Ismail and H. F. Harwood is as follows:

1. Weigh 10 g of the sample, transfer it to a 30 cc platinum crucible, and moisten it with a little water. Add 20 cc of hydrofluoric acid, 48%, and evaporate it to dryness on a steam bath. If the sample contains much silica, repeat this treatment. Add 8 g of potassium acid fluoride (KF·HF, Harshaw Chem. Co.) that has been dried in a desiccator, and cover the crucible. Place the covered crucible over a very low flame and use extreme care in driving off any moisture and reaction gases. Gradually increase the flame until the molten mass becomes clear over the full flame of a Meeker burner, and carefully whirl the clear melt in order to mix well. Cool while whirling in order to form a thin coating on the sides of the crucible.

Transfer the melt from the crucible to a large platinum dish by means of hot water from a wash bottle. Use a platinum rod to break up the melt, add 100 cc of water and 25 cc of hydrofluoric acid, 48%, and digest on a steam bath for 15 minutes. Dilute with water to a volume of 200 cc, and digest on the steam bath for one hour. Cool, and filter through a No. 42 Whatman filter. Wash the insoluble fluorides a few times with dilute hydrofluoric acid (add 1 part hydrofluoric acid to 7 parts of water) and then once with distilled water.

Transfer the filter paper and precipitate to a small platinum dish, and ignite it at 500°C. Cool, add 5 cc of nitric acid and 10 cc of sulfuric acid, and use extreme care in heating it on the hot plate until fumes of sulfur trioxide are evolved. Cool, and wash down the sides of the dish with cool water. Fume again, cool, and wash down the sides twice more. Pour 200 cc of cold distilled water into a 600 cc beaker, and transfer all the material from the platinum dish to it by means of cool water from a wash bottle. Stir well, and add 10 cc of nitric acid and 10 cc of hydrochloric acid. Set it on a hot plate to boil until the solution is complete.

2. Neutralize the clear solution with ammonium hydroxide, and add 0.3 g of sodium metabisulfite crystals to reduce the cerium (from yellow to colorless). Make the solution ammoniacal with a 10% excess of ammonium hydroxide, and allow the solution to cool and the precipitate to settle. Filter through a No. 40 Whatman filter paper, and wash the precipitate with a 2% ammonium chloride solution in ammonium hydroxide solution (dissolve 2 g of ammonium chloride in a solution composed of 90 cc of water and 10 cc of ammonium hydroxide). Dissolve the precipitate with hot hydrochloric acid (1 part acid to 2 parts water) into the original beaker. Add ammonium hydroxide (1 part ammonium hydroxide to 1 part water) until the solution is faintly turbid. Add 3–4 drops of

hydrochloric acid (1 part acid to 1 part water), and dilute the solution to 200 cc. Add enough ammonium chloride to make a 5% solution of the salt, then add a few crystals of sodium metabisulfite. Stir well, and warm the solution to 70°C.

3. Add slowly a 2% hexamine solution (dissolve 2 g of hexamine in 100 cc of water) until the solution becomes turbid. Add 4 cc more of the hexamine solution, and stir well. Heat to not over 75°C., and allow the precipitate to settle. Add 1 cc more of hexamine solution, stir well, and allow to settle. Filter through a No. 40 Whatman filter paper, and wash the precipitate with a 5% ammonium chloride solution (5 g ammonium chloride in 100 cc water, and add 2 drops of ammonium hydroxide to neutralize this solution). Test the filtrate with 1 cc of hexamine solution in order to complete precipitation. Dissolve the precipitate with hot hydrochloric acid (1 part of acid to 2 parts water) in a 250 cc beaker, and wash the filter paper with hot 5% hydrochloric acid (5 parts of acid to 95 parts water). Repeat the precipitation with hexamine twice, test the filtrate with 1 cc hexamine solution, then test filtrate with an excess of ammonium hydroxide. Finally place the solution on a steam bath and evaporate to dryness.

4. Pour 25 cc of 10% oxalic acid solution (10 g oxalic acid in 100 cc water) onto the residue, stir and dilute to a volume of 100 cc. Cover the beaker, and boil the solution gently for several minutes. Again adjust the solution to a volume of 100 cc, and allow it to stand overnight. Filter through a No. 42 Whatman filter paper, and wash the precipitate with a 2% oxalic acid solution (2 g oxalic acid in 100 cc water). Ignite at 1000°C. to constant weight, and cool in a desiccator. Weigh as thorium oxide (ThO_2), and make the calculations as follows:

$$\frac{\text{Weight of thorium oxide}}{\text{Weight of sample taken}} \times 100 = \begin{array}{l}\text{percent of thorium}\\ \text{oxide in the sample.}\end{array}$$

To Detect Ethyl Alcohol

Trace amounts of ethyl alcohol in liquids that are free from water can be detected by the following method:

The ethyl alcohol is first oxidized to acetaldehyde, and the latter is then identified by the reaction with nitroprusside. As little as 3 millionths of a gram of ethyl alcohol in one drop of benzene-alcohol mixture can be easily detected.

Place two to three drops of the sample in a very small test tube and drop several centigrams of hot copper wire or black copper oxide into the tube. Moisten a disc of filter paper with one drop of a freshly made reagent (equal volumes 5% sodium nitroferricyanide solution and 20% aqueous morpholine solution) and place it over the top of the test tube. A deep-to-light blue stain appears immediately on the paper if ethyl alcohol is present.

Hydrogen Peroxide in Milk

Dissolve 1 g of vanadic acid in 100 g of dilute sulfuric acid (when diluting, add the acid to the water, and handle it with caution). Add 10 drops of the diluted sulfuric acid to 10 cc of the milk. The appearance of a red color will indicate the presence of hydrogen peroxide. Heating the milk will not affect this test.

To Determine Moisture and Fat in Cocoa

Have the cocoa press cake samples finely grated and mixed with pre-dried sand. Determine its moisture by drying for 2 hours at 220°F. Determine its fat by allowing the dried sample to stand overnight in trichloroethylene, or by heating in trichloroethylene with reflux for about 15 minutes. Filter the solution through a sintered glass crucible. Wash the residue 2 or 3 times with trichloroethylene. Dry for 1½ hours at 220°F., cool, and weigh. This method is an indirect one in which the defatted, dry residue is weighed instead of the separated fat.

To Detect Peroxides in Organic Liquids

Make an acidified solution of ferrous thiocyanate by dissolving ferrous sulfate and potassium thiocyanate in distilled water that contains a little sulfuric acid. Render this pink solution colorless immediately before use by treating it with a small amount of zinc dust. Shake the organic liquid to be treated with a few cubic centimeters of the reagent in a stoppered flask just large enough to hold the liquids. An intense red color will appear if the liquid contains a large amount of peroxides; a faint pink color, if only a very small amount of peroxides is present. If the reagent remains colorless, one may infer that the solvent under test is completely free of peroxides.

As a reagent, this ferrous thiocyanate solution is far superior to the potassium iodide and starch solution.

To Determine Rubber Content of Plant Specimens

Make a 3-hour extraction of a 5 g ground sample with acetone, followed by a 3-hour extraction with benzene. After drying, weigh the benzene extract direct as rubber. In order to ensure complete extraction, increase the length of the extraction period. Add 1 per cent of trichloroacetic acid to the benzene in order to speed up the solution of the rubber.

Appendix A: Weights and Measures; Conversion Tables

UNITED STATES MEASURES AND WEIGHTS

Linear Measure

12 inches (in)	= 1 foot (ft)
3 feet	= 1 yard (yd)
5½ yards	= 1 rod (rd) = 16½ feet
40 rods	= 1 furlong (fur) = 220 yards = 660 feet
8 furlongs	= 1 statute mile (mi) = 1760 yards = 5280 feet
1 international nautical mile	= 6076.10333 feet = 1852 meters

Area Measure

144 square inches (sq in)	= 1 square foot (sq ft)
9 square feet	= 1 square yard (sq yd)
30¼ square yards	= 1 square rod (rd) = 272¼ square feet
160 square rods	= 1 acre = 4840 square yards = 43560 sq ft
640 acres	= 1 square mile (sq mi)
1 mile square	= 1 section of land
6 miles square	= 1 township—36 sections—36 square miles

Cubic Measure

1728 cubic inches (cu in)	= 1 cubic foot (cu ft)
27 cubic feet	= 1 cubic yard (cu yd)

Dry Measure

2 pints (pt)	= 1 quart (qt) = 67.2006 cubic inches
8 quarts	= 1 peck (pk) = 537.605 cubic inches = 16 pints
4 pecks	= 1 bushel (bu) = 2150.42 cubic inches = 32 quarts

Liquid Measure

4 gills (gi)	= 1 pint (pt) = 28.875 cubic inches
2 pints	= 1 quart (qt) = 57.75 cubic inches
4 quarts	= 1 gallon (gal) = 231 cubic inches = 8 pints = 32 gills

Surveyors Chain Measure

7.92 inches (in)	= 1 link (li)
100 links	= 1 chain (ch) = 4 rods = 66 feet
80 chains	= 1 statute mile (mi) = 320 rods = 5280 feet

Apothecaries Liquid Measure

60 minims (min)	= 1 fluid dram (fl dr) = 0.2256 cubic inch
8 fluid drams	= 1 fluid ounce (fl oz) = 1.8047 cubic inches
16 fluid ounces	= 1 pint (pt) = 28.875 cubic inches = 128 fluid drams
2 pints	= 1 quart (qt) = 57.75 cubic inches = 32 fl ozs = 256 fl dr
4 quarts	= 1 gallon (gal) = 231 cubic inches = 128 fl ozs = 1024 fl drs

Apothecaries Weight

(The "grain" is the same in avoirdupois, troy, and apothecaries weight.)

20 grains	= 1 scruple (S ap)
3 scruples	= 1 dram ap (dr ap) = 60 grains
8 drams ap	= 1 ounce ap (oz ap) = 24 scruples = 480 grains
12 ounces ap	= 1 pound ap (lb ap) = 96 drams ap = 288 scruples = 5760 grains

Avoirdupois (avdp) Weight

27 11/32 grains	= 1 dram (dr)
16 drams	= 1 ounce (oz) 437.5 grains
16 ounces	= 1 pound (lb) = 256 drs = 7000 gr
100 pounds	= 1 hundred weight (cwt)
20 hundred weight	= 1 ton = 2000 pounds

In "gross" or "long" measure, the following values are recognized:

112 pounds	= 1 long hundredweight
20 gross or long hundred weights	= 1 long ton = 2240 pounds

Troy Weight

24 grains	= 1 pennyweight (dwt)
20 pennyweights	= 1 ounce troy (oz t) = 480 grains
12 ounces troy	= 1 pound (lb t) = 240 pennyweights = 5760 grains

Metric Measures and Weights

Designations of multiples and subdivisions of any unit may be arrived at by joining together the name of the unit with the following prefixes:

deka, 10,
hecto, 100,
kilo, 1000,
deci, 0.1,
centi, 0.01,
milli, 0.001.

When it is necessary to provide for multiples larger than 1000 and for subdivisions smaller than one-thousandth, the following prefixes are used:
myria, 10,000,
mega, 1,000,000,
micro, one-millionth.

Linear Measure

10 millimeters (mm)	= 1 centimeter (cm)
10 centimeters	= 1 decimeter = 100 millimeters
10 decimeters (dm)	= 1 meter (m) = 1000 millimeters
10 meters	= 1 dekameter (dkm)
10 dekameters	= 1 hectometer (hm) = 100 meters
10 hectometers	= 1 kilometer (km) = 1000 meters

Area Measure

100 square millimeters (mm^2)	= 1 square centimeter (cm^2)
10,000 sq centimeters	= 1 sq meter (m^2) = 1,000,000 sq millimeters
100 square meters	= 1 are (a)
100 ares	= 1 hectare (ha) = 10,000 square meters
100 hectares	= 1 sq kilometer (km^2) = 1,000,000 sq m

Cubic Measure

1000 cubic millimeters (mm^3)	= 1 cubic centimeter (cm^3)
1000 cubic centimeters	= 1 cubic decimeter (dm^3) = 1,000,000 cubic mm
1000 cubic decimeters	= 1 cubic meter (m^3) = 1 stere = 1,000,000 cubic centimeters = 1,000,000,000 cubic millimeters

Volume Measure

10 milliliters (ml)	= 1 centiliter (cl)
10 centiliters	= 1 deciliter (dl) = 100 milliliters
10 deciliters	= 1 liter = 1000 milliliters
10 liters	= 1 dekaliter (dkl)
10 dekaliters	= 1 hectoliter (hl) = 100 liters
10 hectoliters	= 1 kiloliter (kl) = 1000 liters

The liter is defined as the volume occupied, under standard conditions, by a quantity of pure water having a mass of one kilogram. This volume is very nearly equal to 1000 cubic centimeters or one cubic decimeter; the actual metric equivalent is, 1 liter = 1000.028 cubic centimeters.

Weight Measure

10 milligrams (mg)	= 1 centigram (cg)
10 centigrams	= 1 decigram (dg) = 100 milligrams
10 decigrams	= 1 gram (g) = 1000 milligrams
10 grams	= 1 dekagram (dkg)
10 dekagrams	= 1 hectogram (hg) = 100 grams
10 hectograms	= 1 kilogram (kg) = 1000 grams
1000 kilograms	= 1 metric ton

TABLE OF EQUIVALENTS

Length

1 angstrom (Å) (A unit of measurement of the wave length of electromagnetic radiations) equivalent to:	0.1 millimicron 0.0001 micron 0.0000001 millimeter 0.000000004 inch
1 cable length	120 fathoms 720 feet 219.456 meters
1 centimeter	0.3937 inch
1 chain (ch) (surveyors)	66 feet 20.117 meters
1 chain (engineers)	100 feet 30.48 meters
1 decimeter (dm)	3.937 inches
1 dekameter (dkm)	32.808 feet
1 fathom	6 feet 1.829 meters
1 foot (ft)	0.305 meter
1 furlong (fur)	10 chains (surveyors) 660 feet 220 yards ⅛ statute mile 201.168 meters
1 hand (not in current use in the U.S.A.)	4 inches
1 inch (in)	2.540 centimeters
1 kilometer (km)	0.624 mile
1 league (land)	3 statute miles 4828 kilometers
1 link (li) (surveyors)	7.92 inches 0.201 meters
1 link (engineers)	1 foot 0.305 meter
1 meter (m)	39.37 inches 1.094 yards
1 micron (μ) (the Greek letter Mu)	0.001 millimeter 0.00003937 inch

1 mil	0.001 inch 0.0254 millimeter
1 mile (mi) (statute or land)	5280 feet 1.609 kilometers
1 mile (nautical, international)	1.852 kilometers 1.151 statute miles 0.999 U.S. nautical miles
1 millimeter (mm)	0.03937 inch
1 millimicron (mμ)	0.001 micron 0.00000003937 inch
1 point (typography)	0.013837 inch 1/72 inch (approximately) 0.351 millimeter
1 rod (rd)	16.5 feet 5.5 yards 5.029 meters
1 yard (yd)	0.914 meter

Surface Areas

1 acre	43,560 square feet 4840 square yards 0.405 hectare
1 are	119.596 square yards 0.025 acre
1 hectare	2.471 acres
1 square centimeter (cm^2)	0.155 square inch
1 square decimeter (dm^2)	15.500 square inches
1 square foot (sq ft)	929.034 square centimeter
1 square inch (sq in)	6.452 square centimeters
1 square kilometer (km^2)	247.104 acres 0.386 square mile
1 square meter (m^2)	1.196 square yards 10.764 square feet
1 square mile (sq mi)	259.00 hectares
1 square millimeter (mm^2)	0.002 square inch
1 square rod (sq rd)	25.293 square meters
1 square yard (sq yd)	0.836 square meter

Volumes

1 barrel (bbl), liquid	31 to 42 gallons
1 barrel (bbl), dry commodities such as fruits, vegetables, etc.	7056 cubic inches 105 dry quarts 3.281 bushels

1 barrel, standard, cranberry	5826 cubic inches 86.703 dry quarts 2.709 bushels
1 bushel (bu) (U.S.)	2150.42 cubic inches 35.238 liters
1 bushel, British Imperial	1.032 U.S. bushels 2219.36 cubic inches
1 cord (cd) (firewood)	128 cubic feet
1 cubic centimeter (cm^3)	0.061 cubic inch
1 cubic decimeter (dm^3)	61.023 cubic inches
1 cubic foot (cu ft)	7.481 gallons 28.317 cubic decimeters
1 cubic inch (cu in)	0.554 fluid ounce 4.433 fluid drams 16.387 cubic centimeters
1 cubic meter (m^3)	1.308 cubic yards
1 cubic yard (cu yd)	0.765 cubic meter
1 cup, measuring	8 fluid ounces ½ liquid pint
1 dram, fluid (fl dr) U.S.	⅛ fluid ounce 0.226 cubic inch 3.697 milliliters 1.041 British fluid drams
1 drachm, fluid (fl dr) British	0.961 U.S. fluid dram 0.217 cubic inch 3.552 milliliters
1 dekaliter (dkl)	2.642 gallons 1.135 pecks
1 gallon (gal) U.S.	231 cubic inches 3.785 liters 0.833 British gallon 128 U.S. fluid ounces
1 gallon (British Imperial)	277.42 cubic inches 1.201 U.S. gallons 4.546 liters 160 British fluid ounces
1 gill (gi)	7.219 cubic inches 4 fluid ounces 0.118 liter

1 hectoliter (hl)	26.418 gallons 2.838 bushels
1 liter	1.057 liquid quarts 0.908 dry quart 61.025 cubic inches
1 milliliter (ml)	0.271 fluid dram 16.231 minims 0.061 cubic inch
1 ounce, fluid (fl oz) U.S.	1.805 cubic inches 29.573 milliliters 1.041 British fluid ounces
1 ounce, fluid, British	0.961 U.S. fluid ounce 1.734 cubic inches 28.412 milliliters
1 peck (pk)	8.810 liters 33.600 cubic inches
1 pint (pt), dry	0.551 liter 28.875 cubic inches
1 pint (pt), liquid	0.473 liters 67.201 cubic inches
1 quart (qt), dry (U.S.)	1.101 liters 0.969 British quart 57.75 cubic inches
1 quart (qt), liquid (U.S.)	0.946 liter 0.833 British quart 69.354 cubic inches
1 quart (qt) (British)	1.032 U.S. dry quarts 1.201 U.S. liquid quarts
1 tablespoon	3 teaspoons 4 fluid drams ½ fluid ounce
1 teaspoon	⅓ tablespoon 1⅓ fluid drams
1 water ton (English)	270.91 U.S. gallons 224 British Imperial gallons

Weights

1 assay ton (AT)	29.167 grams
1 carat (C)	200 milligrams 3.086 grains

1 dram, apothecaries (dr ap)	60 grains 3.888 grams
1 dram, avoirdupois (dr avdp)	27.344 grains 1.772 grams
1 grain	64.799 milligrams
1 gram (g)	15.432 grains 0.035 ounce, avoirdupois
1 hundredweight, gross (gross cwt)	112 pounds 50.802 kilograms
1 hundredweight, net (net cwt)	100 pounds 45.359 kilograms
1 kilogram (kg)	2.205 pounds
1 microgram (μg)	0.000001 gram
1 milligram (mg)	0.015 grain
1 ounce, avoirdupois (oz avdp)	437.5 grains 0.911 troy ounce 28.350 grams
1 ounce, apothecaries or troy (oz ap)	1.097 avdp ounces 31.103 grams
1 pennyweight (dwt)	1.555 grams
1 point	0.01 carat 2 milligrams
1 pound, avoirdupois (lb avdp)	7000 grains 1.215 apothecaries pounds 453.592 grams
1 pound, apothecaries (lb ap)	5760 grains 0.823 avoirdupois pound 373.242 grams
1 scruple (S ap)	20 grains 1.296 grams
1 ton, long	2240 pounds 1.12 short tons 1.016 metric tons
1 ton, short	2000 pounds 0.893 long ton 0.907 metric ton
1 ton (t) metric	2204.622 pounds 0.984 long ton 1.102 short tons

Interrelation of Units of Measurement

Units of Length

Units	*Inches*	*Links*	*Feet*	*Yards*	*Rods*	*Chains*	*Miles*	*Centimeters*	*Meters*
1 inch	1	0.126263	0.0833333	0.0277778	0.00505051	0.00126263	0.000015783	2.540005	0.02540005
1 link	7.92	1	0.66	0.22	0.04	0.01	0.000125	20.11684	0.2011684
1 foot	12	1.515152	1	0.333333	0.0606061	0.0151515	0.0001894	30.48006	0.3048006
1 yard	36	4.54545	3	1	0.181818	0.0454545	0.0005682	91.44018	0.9144018
1 rod	198	25	16.5	5.5	1	0.25	0.003125	502.9210	5.029210
1 chain	792	100	66	22	4	1	0.0125	2011.684	20.11684
1 mile	63,360	8000	5280	1760	320	80	1	160,934.72	1609.3472
1 centi	0.3937	0.049709	0.0328083	0.0109361	0.0019884	0.0004971	0.00000622	1	0.01
1 meter	39.37	4.970960	3.280833	1.0936111	0.1988384	0.0497096	0.00062137	100	1

Units of Area

Units	*Acres*	*Square Miles*	*Sq Centi*	*Square Meters*	*Hectares*
1 sq inch	0.00000015942	0.00000000025	6.451626	0.0006451626	0.000000064516
1 sq link	0.00001	0.00000001563	404.6873	0.04046873	0.00000404687
1 sq foot	0.0000229568	0.00000003587	929.0341	0.09290341	0.00000929034
1 sq yard	0.000206612	0.00000032283	8361.307	0.8361307	0.0000836131
1 sq rod	0.00625	0.00000976563	252,929.5	25.29295	0.002529295
1 sq chain	0.1	0.00015625	4,046,873	404.6873	0.0404687
1 acre	1	0.0015625	40,468,726	4046.873	0.404687
1 sq mile	640	1	25,899,984,703	2,589,998	258.9998
1 sq centi	0.000000025	0.00000000004	1	0.0001	0.00000001
1 sq meter	0.000247104	0.00000038610	10,000	1	0.0001
1 hectare	2.47104	0.003861006	100,000,000	10,000	1

Units of Area

Units	*Square Inches*	*Square Links*	*Square Feet*	*Square Yards*	*Square Rods*	*Square Chains*
1 sq inch	1	0.0159423	0.006944	0.000771605	0.0000255076	0.00000159423
1 sq link	62.7264	1	0.4356	0.0484	0.0016	0.0001
1 sq foot	144	2.295684	1	0.1111111	0.00367309	0.000229568
1 sq yard	1296	20.6612	9	1	0.03305785	0.00206612
1 sq rod	39204	625	272.25	30.25	1	0.0625
1 sq chain	627,264	10,000	4356	484	16	1
1 acre	6,272,640	100,000	43560	4840	160	10
1 sq mile	4,014,489,600	64,000,000	27,878,400	3,097,600	102,400	6400
1 sq centimeter	0.15499969	0.00247104	0.001076387	0.0001195985	0.00000395367	0.000000247104
1 sq meter	1549.9960	24.7104	10.76387	1.195985	0.0395367	0.00247104
1 hectare	15,499,969	247104	107,638.7	11,959.85	395.367	24.7104

Units of Volume

Units	*Cubic Inches*	*Cubic Feet*	*Cubic Yards*	*Cubic Centimeters*	*Cubic Decimeters*	*Cubic Meters*
1 cu inch	1	0.000578704	0.000021434	16.387162	0.01638716	0.00001638716
1 cu foot	1728	1	0.0370370	28317.016	28.317016	0.028317016
1 cu yard	46,656	27	1	764559.4	764.5594	0.7645594
1 cu centimeter	0.06102338	0.0000353145	0.000001308	1	0.001	0.000001
1 cu decimeter	61.02338	0.03531445	0.001307943	1000	1	0.001
1 cu meter	61023.38	35.31445	1.3079428	1,000,000	1000	1

Units of Liquid Measure

Units	*Minims*	*Fluid Drams*	*Fluid Ounces*	*Gills*	*Liquid Pints*	*Liquid Quarts*	*Gallons*	*Milli-liters*	*Liters*	*Cubic Inches*	*Cubic Feet*
1 minim	1	0.01667	0.002083	0.000521	0.000130	0.000065	0.000016	0.061610	0.000061	0.003759	0.0000022
1 fl dr	60	1	0.125	0.03125	0.007813	0.003906	0.000976	3.69661	0.003697	0.225586	0.0001306
1 fl oz	480	8	1	0.25	0.0625	0.03125	0.007813	29.5729	0.029573	1.80469	0.0010444
1 gill	1920	32	4	1	0.25	0.125	0.03125	118.292	0.118292	7.21875	0.0041775
1 lq pt	7680	128	16	4	1	0.5	0.125	473.166	0.473166	28.875	0.0167101
1 lq qt	15,360	256	32	8	2	1	0.25	946.332	0.946332	57.75	0.0334201
1 gal	61,440	1024	128	32	8	4	1	3785.329	3.785329	231	0.1336806
1 ml	16.2311	0.270518	0.033815	0.008454	0.002113	0.001057	0.000264	1	0.001	0.061025	0.0000353
1 liter	16,231.1	270.518	33.8148	8.45369	2.11342	1.05671	0.264178	1000	1	61.0251	0.0353154
1 cu in	265.974	4.43290	0.554113	0.138528	0.03463	0.01732	0.004329	16.3867	0.01638	1	0.000579
1 cu ft	459,603.1	7660.052	957.5065	239.3766	59.84416	29.9221	7.480519	28,316.22	28.31622	1728	1

Units of Dry Measure

Units	*Dry Pints*	*Dry Quarts*	*Pecks*	*Bushels*	*Liters*	*Dekaliters*	*Cubic Inches*	*Cubic Feet*
1 dry pint	1	0.5	0.0625	0.015625	0.550598	0.0550598	33.600313	0.01944463
1 dry quart	2	1	0.125	0.03125	1.101197	0.1101197	67.200625	0.03888925
1 peck	16	8	1	0.25	8.80957	0.880957	537.605	0.311114
1 bushel	64	32	4	1	35.2383	3.52383	2150.42	1.244456
1 liter	1.81621	0.908103	0.113513	0.028378	1	0.1	61.0251	0.0353154
1 dekaliter	18.1621	9.08103	1.13513	0.28378	10	1	610.251	0.353154
1 cubic inch	0.0297616	0.0148808	0.001860	0.00046503	0.016387	0.0016387	1	0.0005787037
1 cubic foot	51.428093	25.714047	3.2142558	0.80356395	28.31622	2.831622	1728	1

Units of Weight Not Greater than Pounds and Kilograms

Units	Grains	Apoth Scruples	Penny-weights	Avdp Drams	Apoth Drams	Avdp Ounces	Troy or Apoth Ounces	Apoth or Troy Pounds	Avdp Pounds	Milligrams	Grams
1 grain	1	0.05	0.041667	0.036571	0.016667	0.002286	0.00208	0.000174	0.000143	64.79892	0.064799
1 apoth scruple	20	1	0.833333	0.731429	0.33333	0.045714	0.041667	0.003472	0.002857	1295.978	1.295978
1 pennyweight	24	1.2	1	0.877714	0.4	0.05486	0.05	0.004167	0.003429	1555.174	1.555174
1 avdp dram	27.34375	1.367187	1.139323	1	0.455729	0.0625	0.056966	0.004747	0.003906	1771.845	1.771845
1 apoth dram	60	3	2.5	2.194286	1	0.137143	0.125	0.01042	0.008571	3887.935	3.887935
1 avdp ounce	437.5	21.875	18.22917	16	7.29167	1	0.911458	0.075955	0.0625	28,349.53	28.34953
1 ap or troy ounce	480	24	20	17.55428	8	1.097143	1	0.083333	0.068571	31,103.48	31.10348
1 ap or troy pound	5760	288	240	210.6514	96	13.16571	12	1	0.822857	373,241.8	373.2418
1 avdp pound	7000	350	291.6667	256	116.6667	16	14.58333	1.215278	1	453,592.4	453.5924
1 milligram	0.015432	0.000772	0.000643	0.000564	0.000257	0.000035	0.000032	0.000003	0.000002	1	0.001
1 gram	15.4324	0.771618	0.643015	0.564383	0.257206	0.035274	0.032151	0.002679	0.002205	1000	1
1 kilogram	15,432.86	771.6178	643.0149	564.3833	257.2059	35.27396	32.15074	2.679229	2.204622	1,000,000	1000

Units of Weight Not Less Than Avoirdupois Ounces

Units	Avoirdupois Ounces	Avoirdupois Pounds	Short Hundred Weights	Short Tons	Long Tons	Kilograms	Metric Tons
1 avoirdupois ounce	1	0.0625	0.000625	0.00003125	0.00002790	0.02834953	0.00002834953
1 avoirdupois pound	16	1	0.01	0.0005	0.00044643	0.45359243	0.0004535924
1 short hundred weight	1600	100	1	0.05	0.04164286	45.359243	0.045359243
1 short ton	32,000	2000	20	1	0.8928571	907.18486	0.90718486
1 long ton	35,840	2240	22.4	1.12	1	1016.0470	1.01604704
1 kilogram	35.273957	2.20462234	0.022046	0.001102311	0.0009842	1	0.001
1 metric ton	35,273.957	2204.62234	22.04622	1.1023112	0.9842064	1000	1

Temperature Conversion Tables

°F.	°C.	°F.	°C.	°F.	°C.	°F.	°C.	°F.	°C.
–40	–40.0	9	–12.8	58	14.4	107	41.7	156	68.9
–39	–39.4	10	–12.2	59	15.0	108	42.2	157	69.4
–38	–38.9	11	–11.7	60	15.6	109	42.8	158	70.0
–37	–38.3	12	–11.1	61	16.1	110	43.3	159	70.6
–36	–37.8	13	–10.6	62	16.7	111	43.9	160	71.1
–35	–37.2	14	–10.0	63	17.2	112	44.4	161	71.7
–34	–36.7	15	–9.4	64	17.8	113	45.0	162	72.2
–33	–36.1	16	–8.9	65	18.3	114	45.6	163	72.8
–32	–35.6	17	–8.3	66	18.9	115	46.1	164	73.3
–31	–35.0	18	–7.8	67	19.4	116	46.7	165	73.9
–30	–34.4	19	–7.2	68	20.0	117	47.2	166	74.4
–29	–33.9	20	–6.7	69	20.6	118	47.8	167	75.0
–28	–33.3	21	–6.1	70	21.1	119	48.3	168	75.6
–27	–32.8	22	–5.6	71	21.7	120	48.9	169	76.1
–26	–32.2	23	–5.0	72	22.2	121	49.4	170	76.7
–25	–31.7	24	–4.4	73	22.8	122	50.0	171	77.2
–24	–31.1	25	–3.9	74	23.3	123	50.6	172	77.8
–23	–30.6	26	–3.3	75	23.9	124	51.1	173	78.3
–22	–30.0	27	–2.8	76	24.4	125	51.7	174	78.9
–21	–29.4	28	–2.2	77	25.0	126	52.2	175	79.4
–20	–28.9	29	–1.7	78	25.6	127	52.8	176	80.0
–19	–28.3	30	–1.1	79	26.1	128	53.3	177	80.6
–18	–27.8	31	–0.6	80	26.7	129	53.9	178	81.1
–17	–27.2	32	0.0	81	27.2	130	54.4	179	81.7
–16	–26.7	33	0.6	82	27.8	131	55.0	180	82.2
–15	–26.1	34	1.1	83	28.3	132	55.6	181	82.8
–14	–25.6	35	1.7	84	28.9	133	56.1	182	83.3
–13	–25.0	36	2.2	85	29.4	134	56.7	183	83.9
–12	–24.4	37	2.8	86	30.0	135	57.2	184	84.4
–11	–23.9	38	3.3	87	30.6	136	57.8	185	85.0
–10	–23.3	39	3.9	88	31.1	137	58.3	186	85.6
–9	–22.8	40	4.4	89	31.7	138	58.9	187	86.1
–8	–22.2	41	5.0	90	32.2	139	59.4	188	86.7
–7	–21.7	42	5.6	91	32.8	140	60.0	189	87.2
–6	–21.1	43	6.1	92	33.3	141	60.6	190	87.8
–5	–20.6	44	6.7	93	33.9	142	61.1	191	88.3
–4	–20.0	45	7.2	94	34.4	143	61.7	192	88.9
–3	–19.4	46	7.8	95	35.0	144	62.2	193	89.4
–2	–18.9	47	8.3	96	35.6	145	62.8	194	90.0
–1	–18.3	48	8.9	97	36.1	146	63.3	195	90.6
0	–17.8	49	9.4	98	36.7	147	63.9	196	91.1
1	–17.2	50	10.0	99	37.2	148	64.4	197	91.7
2	–16.7	51	10.6	100	37.8	149	65.0	198	92.2
3	–16.1	52	11.1	101	38.3	150	65.6	199	92.8
4	–15.6	53	11.7	102	38.9	151	66.1	200	93.3
5	–15.0	54	12.2	103	39.4	152	66.7	201	93.9
6	–14.4	55	12.8	104	40.0	153	67.2	202	94.4
7	–13.9	56	13.3	105	40.6	154	67.8	203	95.0
8	–13.3	57	13.9	106	41.1	155	68.3	204	95.6

Temperature Conversion Tables (Con.)

°F.	°C.	°F.	°C.	°F.	°C.	°F.	°C.	°F.	°C.
205	96.1	254	123.3	303	150.6	352	177.8	401	205.0
206	96.7	255	123.9	304	151.1	353	178.3	402	205.6
207	97.2	256	124.4	305	151.7	354	178.9	403	206.1
208	97.8	257	125.0	306	152.2	355	179.4	404	206.7
209	98.3	258	125.6	307	152.8	356	180.0	405	207.2
210	98.9	259	126.1	308	153.3	357	180.6	406	207.8
211	99.4	260	126.7	309	153.9	358	181.1	407	208.3
212	100.0	261	127.2	310	154.4	359	181.7	408	208.9
213	100.6	262	127.8	311	155.0	360	182.2	409	209.4
214	101.1	263	128.3	312	155.6	361	182.8	410	210.0
215	101.7	264	128.9	313	156.1	362	183.3	411	210.6
216	102.2	265	129.4	314	156.7	363	183.9	412	211.1
217	102.8	266	130.0	315	157.2	364	184.4	413	211.7
218	103.3	267	130.6	316	157.8	365	185.0	414	212.2
219	103.9	268	131.1	317	158.3	366	185.6	415	212.8
220	104.4	269	131.7	318	158.9	367	186.1	416	213.3
221	105.0	270	132.2	319	159.4	368	186.7	417	213.9
222	105.6	271	132.8	320	160.0	369	187.2	418	214.4
223	106.1	272	133.3	321	160.6	370	187.8	419	215.0
224	106.7	273	133.9	322	161.1	371	188.3	420	215.6
225	107.2	274	134.4	323	161.7	372	188.9	421	216.1
226	107.8	275	135.0	324	162.2	373	189.4	422	216.7
227	108.3	276	135.6	325	162.8	374	190.0	423	217.2
228	108.9	277	136.1	326	163.3	375	190.6	424	217.8
229	109.4	278	136.7	327	163.9	376	191.1	425	218.3
230	110.0	279	137.2	328	164.4	377	191.7	426	218.9
231	110.6	280	137.8	329	165.0	378	192.2	427	219.4
232	111.1	281	138.3	330	165.6	379	192.8	428	220.0
233	111.7	282	138.9	331	166.1	380	193.3	429	220.6
234	112.2	283	139.4	332	166.7	381	193.9	430	221.1
235	112.8	284	140.0	333	167.2	382	194.4	431	221.7
236	113.3	285	140.6	334	167.8	383	195.0	432	222.2
237	113.9	286	141.1	335	168.3	384	195.6	433	222.8
238	114.4	287	141.7	336	168.9	385	196.1	434	223.3
239	115.0	288	142.2	337	169.4	386	196.7	435	223.9
240	115.6	289	142.8	338	170.0	387	197.2	436	224.4
241	116.1	290	143.3	339	170.6	388	197.8	437	225.0
242	116.7	291	143.9	340	171.1	389	198.3	438	225.6
243	117.2	292	144.4	341	171.7	390	198.9	439	226.1
244	117.8	293	145.0	342	172.2	391	199.4	440	226.7
245	118.3	294	145.6	343	172.8	392	200.0	441	227.2
246	118.9	295	146.1	344	173.3	393	200.6	442	227.8
247	119.4	296	146.7	345	173.9	394	201.1	443	228.3
248	120.0	297	147.2	346	174.4	395	201.7	444	228.9
249	120.6	298	147.8	347	175.0	396	202.2	445	229.4
250	121.1	299	148.3	348	175.6	397	202.8	446	230.0
251	121.7	300	148.9	349	176.1	398	203.3	447	230.6
252	122.2	301	149.4	350	176.7	399	203.9	448	231.1
253	122.8	302	150.0	351	177.2	400	204.4	449	231.7

Temperature Conversion Tables (Con.)

°F.	°C.	°F.	°C.	°F.	°C.	°F.	°C.	°F.	°C.
450	232.2	460	237.8	470	243.3	480	248.9	490	254.4
451	232.8	461	238.3	471	243.9	481	249.4	491	255.0
452	233.3	462	238.9	472	244.4	482	250.0	492	255.6
453	233.9	463	239.4	473	245.0	483	250.6	493	256.1
454	234.4	464	240.0	474	245.6	484	251.1	494	256.7
455	235.0	465	240.6	475	246.1	485	251.7	495	257.2
456	235.6	466	241.1	476	246.7	486	252.2	496	257.8
457	236.1	467	241.7	477	247.2	487	252.8	497	258.3
458	236.7	468	242.2	478	247.8	488	253.3	498	258.9
459	237.2	469	242.8	479	248.3	489	253.9	499	259.4

Measure of Contents of 55-gallon Drums

Use these tables for purposes of general inventory where and when it is desired to make approximate measurements. Insert an ordinary yardstick through the bunghole, and note the number of wet inches shown on the stick. Locate this number on the table under column marked Wet Inches. The gallons of liquid in the drum will be found opposite this number under the temperature at which the measurement was taken.

These tables were calculated for 95% (190 proof) alcohol in standard drums, but they can be used for approximate gaging of other liquids.

Drum Horizontal

Wet Inches	*70°F.*	*60°F.*	*50°F.*	*40°F.*	*30°F.*	*20°F.*	*10°F.*
20	54.3	54.7	55.0	55.3	55.6	55.9	
19	52.1	52.5	52.7	53.1	53.3	53.7	54.0
18	49.7	50.0	50.3	50.6	50.9	51.2	51.5
17	47.1	47.4	47.6	47.9	48.2	48.5	48.8
16	44.3	44.5	44.8	45.1	45.3	45.6	45.9
15	41.2	41.5	41.7	42.0	42.2	42.5	42.7
14	38.1	38.4	38.6	38.8	39.0	39.2	39.5
13	34.9	35.1	35.3	35.5	35.7	36.0	36.2
12	31.6	31.8	32.0	32.2	32.4	32.5	32.7
11	28.3	28.4	28.6	28.8	29.0	29.1	29.3
10	25.0	25.1	25.3	25.4	25.6	25.7	25.8
9	21.6	21.8	21.9	22.0	22.2	22.3	22.4
8	18.4	18.5	18.6	18.7	18.9	19.0	19.1
7	15.3	15.4	15.5	15.6	15.7	15.8	15.8
6	12.3	12.3	12.4	12.5	12.6	12.6	12.7
5	9.5	9.5	9.6	9.6	9.7	9.7	9.8
4	6.8	6.8	6.9	7.0	7.0	7.1	7.1
3	4.4	4.5	4.5	4.5	4.5	4.6	4.6
2	2.4	2.4	2.4	2.5	2.5	2.5	2.5
1	0.8	0.8	0.8	0.8	0.8	0.8	0.8

Measure of Contents of 55-gallon Drums (Con.)

Drum Vertical

Wet Inches	*70°F.*	*60°F.*	*50°F.*	*40°F.*	*30°F.*	*20°F.*	*10°F.*
31	53.5	53.8					
30	51.7	52.0	52.3	52.6	52.9	53.3	53.6
29	50.1	50.3	50.6	50.9	51.2	51.5	51.8
28	48.3	48.6	48.9	49.2	49.4	49.7	50.0
27	46.6	46.9	47.1	47.4	47.7	48.0	48.3
26	44.9	45.1	45.4	45.7	45.9	46.2	46.5
25	43.2	43.4	43.7	43.9	44.1	44.5	44.7
24	41.5	41.7	41.9	42.2	42.4	42.7	42.9
23	39.6	39.9	40.1	40.4	40.6	40.8	41.1
22	37.9	38.2	38.4	38.6	38.8	39.1	39.3
21	36.2	36.4	36.7	36.9	37.1	37.3	37.5
20	34.5	34.7	34.9	35.1	35.3	35.5	35.8
19	32.8	33.0	33.2	33.4	33.6	33.8	34.0
18	31.1	31.3	31.5	31.7	31.8	32.0	32.2
17	29.4	29.6	29.7	29.9	30.1	30.3	30.4
16	27.6	27.7	27.9	28.1	28.3	28.4	28.5
15	26.0	26.1	26.3	26.4	26.6	26.7	26.8
14	24.2	24.3	24.4	24.6	24.7	24.9	25.0
13	22.4	22.6	22.7	22.8	23.0	23.1	23.2
12	20.7	20.8	20.9	21.1	21.2	21.4	21.5
11	19.0	19.1	19.2	19.4	19.5	19.6	19.7
10	17.2	17.3	17.4	17.5	17.6	17.7	17.8
9	15.5	15.6	15.7	15.8	15.9	16.0	16.0
8	13.8	13.9	14.0	14.0	14.1	14.2	14.3
7	12.1	12.1	12.2	12.3	12.4	12.4	12.5
6	10.4	10.4	10.5	10.5	10.6	10.7	10.7
5	8.7	8.7	8.8	8.8	8.9	8.9	9.0
4	6.9	7.0	7.0	7.1	7.1	7.2	7.2
3	5.1	5.2	5.2	5.2	5.3	5.3	5.3
2	3.4	3.4	3.4	3.5	3.5	3.5	3.5
1	1.7	1.7	1.7	1.7	1.7	1.8	1.8

Appendix B: Composition of Foods

Compositions of Foods, 3⅓ Oz, Edible Portion

Food	Water Pct	Food Energy Cal	Protein Gm	Fat Gm	Carbohydrate Gm	Ash Gm	Calcium Mg	Phosphorus Mg	Iron Mg	Vitamin A IU	Thiamin Mg	Riboflavin Mg	Niacin Mg	Ascorbic Acid Mg
Almonds, dried, unblanched	4.7	597	18.6	54.1	19.6	3.0	254	475	4.4		0.25	0.67	4.6	
Apple, raw	84.1	58	0.3	0.4	14.9	0.3	6	10	0.3	90	0.04	0.03	0.2	5
Apple butter	53.1	184	0.4	0.8	45.4	0.3	14	21	0.6		0.01	0.02	0.2	2
Apple juice	85.9	50	0.1		13.8	0.3	6	10	0.5	40	0.02	0.03		1
Applesauce, canned, sweetened	79.8	72	0.2	0.1	19.7	0.2	4	8	0.4	30	0.02	0.01		1
Apricots, raw	85.4	51	1.0	0.1	12.9	0.6	16	23	0.5	2790	0.03	0.05	0.8	7
Apricots, dried, sulfured	24.0	262	5.2	0.4	66.9	3.5	86	119	4.9	7430	0.01	0.16	3.3	12
Apricots, dried, cooked, sweetened	65.8	123	1.5	0.1	31.6	1.0	24	34	1.4	2110		0.04	0.9	3
Asparagus, raw	93.0	21	2.2	0.2	3.9	0.7	21	62	0.9	1000	0.16	0.19	1.4	33
Asparagus, cooked	92.5	20	2.4	0.2	3.6	1.3	19	53	1.0	1040	0.13	0.17	1.2	23
Asparagus, frozen	93.0	21	2.2	0.2	3.9	0.7	21	62	0.9	850	0.14	0.15	1.2	21
Avocados, raw	65.4	245	1.7	26.4	5.1	1.4	10	38	0.6	290	0.06	0.13	1.1	16
Bacon, medium fat, raw	20.0	630	9.1	65.0	1.1	4.3	13	108	0.8		0.38	0.12	1.9	
Bacon, medium fat, fried	13.0	607	25.0	55.0	1.0	6.0	25	255	3.3		0.48	0.31	4.8	
Bacon, Canadian, raw	56.0	231	22.1	15.0	0.3	6.2	13	210	3.3		0.91	0.25	5.2	
Bananas, raw	74.8	88	1.2	0.2	23.0	0.8	8	28	0.6	430	0.04	0.05	0.7	10
Barley, pearled, light, dry	11.1	349	8.2	1.0	78.8	0.9	16	189	2.0		0.12	0.08	3.1	
Beans, red kidney, raw	12.2	336	23.1	1.7	59.4	3.6	163	437	6.9		0.57	0.22	2.5	2
Beans, red kidney, canned or cooked	76.0	90	5.7	0.4	16.4	1.5	40	124	1.9		0.05	0.05	0.8	
Beans, lima, immature seeds, raw	66.5	128	7.5	0.8	23.5	1.7	63	158	2.3	280	0.21	0.11	1.4	32
Beans, lima, immature seeds, cooked	74.9	95	5.0	0.4	18.3	1.4	29	77	1.7	290	0.14	0.09	1.1	15
Beans, lima, immature seeds, canned	80.9	71	3.8	0.3	13.5	1.5	27	73	1.7	130	0.04	0.04	0.5	8
Beans, lima, immature seeds, frozen	71.6	109	6.4	0.7	19.9	1.4	53	134	1.9	220	0.10	0.07	0.8	17
Beans, green, raw	88.9	35	2.4	0.2	7.7	0.8	65	44	1.1	630	0.08	0.11	0.5	19
Beans, green, cooked, little water, short time	92.5	22	1.4	0.2	4.7	1.2	36	23	0.7	660	0.07	0.10	0.5	14
Beans, green, canned	93.5	18	1.0	0.1	4.2	1.2	27	19	1.4	410	0.03	0.04	0.3	4
Beans, green, frozen	88.9	35	2.4	0.2	7.7	0.8	65	44	1.1	450	0.07	0.10	0.6	11
Beans, wax or yellow, canned	93.5	18	1.0	0.1	4.2	1.2	27	19	1.4	100	0.03	0.04	0.3	4
Beans, wax or yellow, raw	88.9	35	2.4	0.2	7.7	0.8	65	44	1.1	150	0.08	0.11	0.5	19
Beef cuts, medium fat:														
Chuck, cooked	51.0	309	26.0	22.0		0.7	11	117	3.1		0.05	0.20	4.1	
Flank, cooked	51.0	314	25.0	23.0		0.6	11	117	3.0		0.05	0.20	4.1	
Porterhouse, cooked	49.0	342	23.0	27.0		1.1	11	170	3.0		0.06	0.18	4.7	
Rib roast, cooked	51.0	319	24.0	24.0		1.2	10	185	3.0		0.06	0.18	4.3	
Round, cooked	59.0	233	27.0	13.0		1.3	11	224	3.4		0.08	0.22	5.5	
Rump, cooked	46.0	378	21.0	32.0		0.5	8	85	2.5		0.04	0.15	3.1	
Sirloin, cooked	54.0	297	23.0	22.0		1.1	10	175	2.9		0.06	0.19	4.8	

Compositions of Foods, 3⅓ Oz, Edible Portion

Food	Water Pct	Food Energy Cal	Protein Gm	Fat Gm	Carbohydrate Gm	Ash Gm	Calcium Mg	Phosphorus Mg	Iron Mg	Vitamin A IU	Thiamin Mg	Riboflavin Mg	Niacin Mg	Ascorbic Acid Mg
Beef, dried or chipped	47.7	203	34.3	6.3		11.6	20	404	5.1		0.07?	0.32?	3.8?	
Beer (4% alcohol)	90.2	48	0.6		4.4	0.2	4	26				0.03	0.2	
Beets, common red, raw	87.6	42	1.6	0.1	9.6	1.1	27	43	1.0	20	0.02	0.05	0.4	10
Beets, commond red, cooked	88.3	41	1.0	0.1	9.8	0.8	21	31	0.7	20	0.02	0.04	0.3	7
Blackberries, raw	84.8	57	1.2	1.0	12.5	0.5	32	32	0.9	200	0.04	0.04	0.4	21
Blackberries, canned, water packed	88.7	43	0.9	0.7	9.4	0.3	18	19	0.7?	180	0.01	0.02	0.2	6
Blueberries, raw	83.4	61	0.6	0.6	15.1	0.3	16	13	0.8	280	0.02?	0.02?	0.3?	16
Blueberries, canned, water packed	90.0	37	0.4	0.4	9.0	0.2	11	6	0.5?	40	0.01	0.01	0.2	13
Blueberries, frozen, without sugar	83.4	61	0.6	0.6	15.1	0.3	16	13	0.8	240	0.02?	0.02?	0.3?	14
Bluefish, cooked, baked	69.2	155	27.4	4.2		1.9	23	293	0.7		0.12	0.11	2.2	
Bouillon cubes	5.0	48	6.0?	2.5		68.0						1.80	25.6	
Brains, all kinds, raw	78.9	125	10.4	8.6	0.8	1.4	16	330	3.6		0.23	2.6	4.4	18
Bran, breakfast cereal	2.6	242	12.0	3.4	74.2	7.8	94	1312	10.3		0.37	0.39	19.2	
Brazil nuts	5.3	646	14.4	65.9	11.0	3.4	186	693	3.4		0.86			
Bread, whole wheat	36.6	240	9.3	2.6	49.0	2.5	96	263	2.2		0.30	0.13	3.0	
Bread, whole wheat, toasted	26.0	280	10.9	3.0	57.2	2.9	112	307	2.6		0.28	0.15	3.5	
Broccoli, flower stalks, cooked	89.9	29	3.3	0.2	5.5	1.1	130	76	1.3	3400	0.07	0.15	0.8	74
Brussels sporuts, cooked	84.9	47	4.4	0.5	8.9	1.3	34	78	1.3	400	0.04	0.12	0.5	47
Brussels sprouts, frozen	84.9	47	4.4	0.5	8.9	1.3	34	78	1.3	340	0.05	0.14	0.6	63
Buckwheat flour, dark	12.0	347	11.7	2.5	72.0	1.8	33	347	2.8		0.58	0.15	2.9	
Butter	15.5	716	0.6	81.0	0.4	2.5	20	16		3300		0.01	0.1	
Cabbage, raw	92.4	24	1.4	0.2	5.3	0.8	46	31	0.5	80	0.06	0.05	0.3	50
Cabbage, cooked	92.4	24	1.4	0.2	5.3	0.8	46	31	0.5	90	0.05	0.05	0.3	31 or 19 †
Cabbage, celery or Chinese, raw	95.4	14	1.2	0.3	2.4	0.7	43	41	0.9	260	0.03	0.04	0.4	31
Cabbage, celery or Chinese, cooked	95.4	14	1.2	0.3	2.4	0.7	43	41	0.9	260	0.02	0.03	0.3	22
Cantaloups, raw	94.0	20	0.6	0.2	4.6	0.6	17	16	0.4	3420	0.05	0.04	0.5	33
Carrots, raw	88.2	42	1.2	0.3	9.3	1.0	39	37	0.8	12000	0.06	0.06	0.5	
Carrots, cooked	91.5	30	0.6	0.5	6.4	1.0	26	26	0.6	12500	0.05	0.05	0.4	4
Cashew nuts, roasted	3.6	578	18.5	48.2	27.0	2.7	46	428	5.0		0.63	0.19	2.1	
Cauliflower, raw	91.7	25	2.4	0.2	4.9	0.8	22	72	1.1	90	0.11	0.10	0.6	69
Cauliflower, cooked	91.7	25	2.4	0.2	4.9	0.8	22	72	1.1	90	0.06	0.08	0.5	28
Celery, raw	93.7	18	1.3	0.2	3.7	1.1	50	40	0.5		0.05	0.04	0.4	7
Chard, leaves and stalks, raw	91.8	21	1.4	0.2	4.4	2.2	105 *	36	2.5	2800	0.06	0.07	0.4	38
Chard, leaves and stalks, cooked	91.8	21	1.4	0.2	4.4	2.2	105 *	36	2.5	3110	0.04	0.06	0.4	17
Chard, leaves only, raw	91.0	27	2.6	0.4	4.8	1.2	105 *	36	2.5	8720	0.06	0.18	0.4	38

* Contains oxalic acid.

† Depending on the amount of water and length of time.

Compositions of Foods, 3⅓ Oz, Edible Portion

Food	Water Pct	Food Energy Cal	Protein Gm	Fat Gm	Carbohydrate Gm	Ash Gm	Calcium Mg	Phosphorus Mg	Iron Mg	Vitamin A IU	Thiamin Mg	Riboflavin Mg	Niacin Mg	Ascorbic Acid Mg
Chard, leaves only, cooked	91.0	27	2.6	0.4	4.8	1.2	105 *	36	2.5	9690	0.04	0.16	0.3	17
Cheese, cheddar	37.0	398	25.0	32.2	2.1	3.7	725	495	1.0	1400	0.02	0.42		
Cheese, cottage, from skim milk	76.5	95	19.5	0.5	2.0	1.5	96	189	0.3	20?	0.02	0.31	0.1?	
Cheese, Limburger	45.0	345	21.2	28.0	2.2	3.6	590	393	0.6	1280	0.08	0.50	0.2	
Cheese, Swiss	39.0	370	27.5	28.0	1.7	3.8	925	563	0.9	1450	0.01	0.40?	0.1?	
Cherries, raw	83.0	61	1.1	0.5	14.8	0.6	18	20	0.4	620	0.05	0.06	0.4	8
Chicken, canned, boned, meat only	61.9	199	29.8	8.0		2.4	14	148	1.8		0.04	0.16	6.4	
Coconut, fresh, meat	46.9	359	3.4	34.7	14.0	1.0	21	98	2.0		0.10	0.01	0.2	2
Collards, raw	86.6	40	3.9	0.6	7.2	1.7	249	58	1.6	6870	0.11	0.27	2.0?	100
Collards, cooked	86.6	40	3.9	0.6	7.2	1.7	249	58	1.6	7630	0.08	0.24	1.7?	44–33 †
Corn, sweet, yellow, raw	73.9	92	3.7	1.2	20.5	0.7	9	120	0.5	390	0.15	0.12	1.7	12
Corn, sweet, yellow, cooked	75.5	85	2.7	0.7	20.2	0.9	5	52	0.6	390	0.11	0.10	1.4	8
Cranberries, raw	87.4	48	0.4	0.7	11.3	0.2	14	11	0.6	40	0.03?	0.02?	0.1	12
Cress, garden, raw	87.2	41	4.2	1.4	5.3	1.9	211	38?	2.9?	2970	0.11	0.17	1.0	87
Cress, garden, cooked	87.2	41	4.2	1.4	5.3	1.9	211	38?	2.9?	3300	0.07	0.15	0.8	39–29 †
Cress, water, leaves and stalks, raw	93.6	18	1.7	0.3	3.3	1.1	195	46	2.0	4720	0.08	0.16	0.8	77
Cucumbers, raw, pared	96.1	12	0.7	0.1	2.7	0.4	10	21	0.3		0.03	0.04	0.2	8
Cucumbers, raw, unpared	96.1	12	0.7	0.1	2.7	0.4	10	21	1.2	260	0.03	0.04	0.2	8
Currants, red, raw	84.4	55	1.2	0.2	13.6	0.6	36	33	0.9	120	0.04			36
Dandelion greens, raw	85.8	44	2.7	0.7	8.8	2.0	187	70	3.1	13650	0.19	0.14	0.8?	36
Dandelion greens, cooked	85.8	44	2.7	0.7	8.8	2.0	187	70	3.1	15170	0.13	0.12	0.7?	16
Dates, "fresh" and dried	20.0	284	2.2	0.6	75.4	1.8	72	60	2.1	60	0.09	0.10	2.2	
Doughnuts, cake type	18.7	425	6.6	21.0	52.7	1.0	73	286	0.7?	140	0.16	0.13	1.2	
Eels, raw	71.6	162	18.6	9.1		1.0	18	202	0.7	1800	0.28	0.37	1.4	
Eggplant, raw	92.7	24	1.1	0.2	5.5	0.5	15	37	0.4	30	0.04	0.05	0.6	5
Eggs, raw, whole	74.0	162	12.8	11.5	0.7	1.0	54	210	2.7	1140	0.10	0.29	0.1	
Eggs, raw, white	87.8	50	10.8		0.8	0.6	6	17	0.2			0.26	0.1?	
Eggs, raw, yolk	49.4	361	16.3	31.9	0.7	1.7	147	586	7.2	3210	0.27	0.35		
Eggs, hard cooked	74.0	162	12.8	11.5	0.7	1.0	54	210	2.7	1140	0.08	0.27	0.1	
Eggs, poached	73.7	160	12.7	11.4	0.6	1.5	54	210	2.7	1130	0.08	0.24	0.1	
Eggs, dried, whole	5.0	592	46.8	42.0	2.5	3.6	190	767	8.8	3740	0.34	1.06	0.2	
Endive, raw	93.3	20	1.6	0.2	4.0	0.9	79	56	1.7	3000	0.07	0.12	0.4	11
Figs, raw	78.0	79	1.4	0.4	19.6	0.6	54	32	0.6	80	0.06	0.05	0.5	2
Figs, dried	24.0	270	4.0	1.2	68.4	2.4	186	111	3.0	80	0.16	0.12	1.7	
Flounder, raw	82.7	68	14.9	0.5		1.3	61	195	0.8		0.06	0.05	1.7	
Fruit cocktail, canned	80.6	70	0.4	0.2	18.6	0.3	9	12	0.4	160	0.01	0.01	0.4	2

* Contains oxalic acid

† Depending on the amount of water and length of time.

Compositions of Foods, 3⅓ Oz, Edible Portion

Food	Water Pct	Food Energy Cal	Protein Gm	Fat Gm	Carbohydrate Gm	Ash Gm	Calcium Mg	Phosphorus Mg	Iron Mg	Vitamin A IU	Thiamin Mg	Riboflavin Mg	Niacin Mg	Ascorbic Acid Mg
Gooseberries, raw	88.9	39	0.8	0.2	9.7	0.4	22	28	0.5	290				33
Grapefruit, raw	88.8	40	0.5	0.2	10.1	0.4	22	18	0.2		0.04	0.02	0.2	40
Grapes, raw	81.9	70	1.4	1.4	14.9	0.4	17	21	0.6	80	0.06	0.04	0.2	4
Guavas, common, raw	80.6	70	1.0	0.6	17.1	0.7	30	29	0.7	250	0.07	0.04	1.2	302
Haddock, raw	80.7	79	18.2	0.1		1.4	23	197	0.7		0.05	0.08	2.4	
Haddock, cooked, fried	66.9	158	18.7	5.5	7.0	1.9	18	182	0.6		0.04	0.09	2.6	
Halibut, raw	75.4	126	18.6	5.2		1.0	13	211	0.7	440	0.07	0.06	9.2	
Halibut, cooked, broiled	64.2	182	26.2	7.8		1.9	14	267	0.8		0.06	0.07	10.5	
Heart, beef, raw	77.6	108	16.9	3.7	0.7	1.1	9	203	4.6	30	0.58	0.89	7.8	6
Heart, chicken, raw	69.6	157	20.5	7.0	1.6	1.3	23	142	1.7	30	0.12	0.91	5.2	6
Herring, Atlantic, raw	67.2	191	18.3	12.5		2.7		256	1.1	110	0.02	0.15	3.4	
Herring, lake, raw	74.0	140	18.5	6.8		1.1	12	152	0.5	100?	0.09	0.09	3.1	
Honey, strained or extracted	20.0	294	0.3		79.5	0.2	5	16	0.9			0.04	0.2	4
Honeydew melon, raw	90.5	32	0.5		8.5	0.5	17?	16?	0.4?	40	0.05	0.03	0.2	23
Ice cream, plain	62.1	207	4.0	12.5	20.6	0.8	123	99	0.1	520	0.04	0.19	0.1	1
Kale, raw	86.6	40	3.9	0.6	7.2	1.7	225	62	2.2	7540	0.10	0.26	2.0	115
Kale, cooked	86.6	40	3.9	0.6	7.2	1.7	225	62	2.2	8380	0.07	0.23	1.7	51
Kidneys, raw, beef	74.9	141	15.0	8.1	0.9	1.1	9	221	7.9	1150	0.37	2.55	6.4	13
Kohlrabi, raw	90.1	30	2.1	0.1	6.7	1.0	46	50	0.6		0.06	0.05	0.2	61
Kohlrabi, cooked	90.1	30	2.1	0.1	6.7	1.0	46	50	0.6		0.04	0.04	0.2	37
Lamb, rib chop, cooked	40.0	418	24.0	35.0		1.2	11	200	3.0		0.14	0.26	5.6	
Lamb, shoulder, roast, cooked	50.0	342	21.0	28.0		1.0	9	188	2.6		0.12	0.22	4.6	
Lamb, leg roast, cooked	56.0	274	24.0	19.0		1.1	10	257	3.1		0.14	0.25	5.1	
Lemons	89.3	32	0.9	0.6	8.7	0.5	40	22	0.6		0.04		0.1	50
Lentils, dry, whole	11.2	337	25.0	1.0	59.5	3.3	59	423	7.4	570	0.56	0.24	2.2	5
Lettuce, raw, headed	94.8	15	1.2	0.2	2.9	0.9	22	25	0.5	540	0.04	0.08	0.2	8
Lettuce, raw, all other	94.8	15	1.2	0.2	2.9	0.9	62	20	1.1	1620	0.04	0.08	0.2	18
Limes	86.0	37	0.8	0.1	12.3	0.8	40?	22?	0.6?		0.04		0.1	27
Liver, beef, cooked, fried	57.2	208	23.6	7.7	9.7	1.8	8	486	7.8	53500	0.26	3.96	14.8	31
Liver, calf, raw	70.8	141	19.0	4.9	4.0	1.3	6	343	10.6	22500	0.21	3.12	16.1	36
Liver, chicken, raw	69.6	141	22.1	4.0	2.6	1.7	16	240	7.4	32200	0.20	2.46	11.8	20
Loganberries, raw	82.9	62	1.0	0.6	15.0	0.5	35	19	1.2	200?	0.03?	0.07?	0.3?	24
Mackerel, raw, common, Atlantic	68.1	188	18.7	12.0		1.2	5	239	1.0	450?	0.15	0.35	8.4	
Mangos, raw	81.4	66	0.7	0.2	17.2	0.5	9	13	0.2	6350	0.06	0.06	0.9	41
Milk, cow, whole	87.0	68	3.5	3.9	4.9	0.7	118	93	0.1	160?	0.04	0.17	0.1	1
Milk, cow, nonfat	90.5	36	3.5	0.1	5.1	0.8	123	97	0.1		0.04	0.18	0.1	1
Milk, cow, canned, evaporated, unsweetened	73.7	138	7.0	7.9	9.9	1.5	243	195	0.2	400	0.05	0.36	0.2	1

Compositions of Foods, 3⅓ Oz, Edible Portion

Food	Water Pct	Food Energy Cal	Protein Gm	Fat Gm	Carbohydrate Gm	Ash Gm	Calcium Mg	Phosphorus Mg	Iron Mg	Vitamin A IU	Thiamin Mg	Riboflavin Mg	Niacin Mg	Ascorbic Acid Mg
Milk, goat	87.4	67	3.3	4.0	4.6	0.7	129	106	0.1	160?	0.04	0.11	0.3	1
Molasses, cane, blackstrap	24.0	213			55.0	0.5?	579	85	11.3		0.28	0.25	2.1	
Mung bean sprouts, raw	92.4	23	2.9	0.2	4.1	0.4	29	59	0.8	10	0.07	0.09	0.5	15
Mushrooms, raw	91.1	16	2.4	0.3	4.0	1.1	9	115	1.0		0.10	0.44	4.9	5
Mustard greens, raw	92.2	22	2.3	0.3	4.0	1.2	220	38	2.9	6460	0.09	0.20	0.8	102
Mustard greens, cooked	92.2	22	2.3	0.3	4.0	1.2	220	38	2.9	7180	0.06	0.18	0.7	45
Oatmeal, cooked	84.8	63	2.3	1.2	11.0	0.7	9	67	0.7		0.10	0.02	0.2	
Okra, raw	89.8	32	1.8	0.2	7.4	0.8	82	62	0.7	740	0.08	0.07	1.1	30
Okra, cooked	89.8	32	1.8	0.2	7.4	0.8	82	62	0.7	740	0.06	0.06	0.8	20
Olives, pickled, green	75.2	132	1.5	13.5	4.0	5.8	87	17	1.6	300				
Olives, pickled, ripe, Mission	71.8	191	1.8	21.0	2.6	2.8	87	17	1.6	60				
Onions, mature, raw	87.5	45	1.4	0.2	10.3	0.6	32	44	0.5	50	0.03	0.04	0.2	9
Onions, mature, cooked	89.5	38	1.0	0.2	8.7	0.6	32	44	0.5	50	0.02	0.03	0.2	6
Onions, young, green	87.6	45	1.0	0.2	10.6	0.6	135	24	0.9	50?	0.03?	0.04?	0.2?	24
Oranges	87.2	45	0.9	0.2	11.2	0.5	33	23	0.4	190?	0.08	0.03	0.2	49
Oysters, meat only, raw	80.5	84	9.8	2.1	5.6	2.0	94	143	5.6	320	0.15	0.20	1.2	
Papayas, raw	88.7	39	0.6	0.1	10.0	0.6	20	16	0.3	1750	0.03	0.04	0.3	56
Parsley, common, raw	83.9	50	3.7	1.0	9.0	2.4	193*	84	4.3	8230	0.11	0.28	1.4	193
Parsnips, raw	78.6	78	1.5	0.5	18.2	1.2	57	80	0.7		0.08	0.12	0.2	18
Parsnips, cooked	83.5	60	1.0	0.5	13.9	1.1	57	80	0.7		0.06	0.10	0.2	12
Peaches, raw	86.9	46	0.5	0.1	12.0	0.5	8	22	0.6	880	0.02	0.05	0.9	8
Peanuts, roasted, shelled	2.6	559	26.9	44.2	23.6	2.7	74	393	1.9		0.30	0.13	16.2	
Peanut butter	1.7	576	26.1	47.8	21.0	3.4	74	393	1.9		0.12	0.13	16.2	
Pears, raw	82.7	63	0.7	0.4	15.8	0.4	13	16	0.3	20	0.02	0.04	0.1	4
Peas, green, immature, raw	74.3	98	6.7	0.4	17.7	0.9	22	122	1.9	680	0.34	0.16	2.7	26
Peas, green, immature, cooked	81.7	70	4.9	0.4	12.1	0.9	22	122	1.9	720	0.25	0.14	2.3	15
Peas, mature dry seeds, entire seeds	11.6	339	23.8	1.4	60.2	3.0	57	388	4.7	370	0.77	0.28	3.1	2
Peas, split	10.0	344	24.5	1.9	61.7	2.8	33	268	5.1	370	0.77	0.28	3.1	2
Pecans	3.0	696	9.4	73.0	13.0	1.6	74	324	2.4	50	0.72	0.11	0.9	2
Peppers, green, raw	92.4	25	1.2	0.2	5.7	0.5	11	25	0.4	630	0.04	0.07	0.4	120
Peppers, cooked, parboiled then baked	91.9	26	1.3	0.2	6.0	0.6	11	25	0.4	740	0.04	0.07	0.4	99
Persimmons, raw	78.2	78	0.8	0.4	20.0	0.6	6	26	0.3	2710	0.05	0.05		11
Pickles, dill, cucumber	93.2	11	0.7	0.2	2.1	3.8	25	20	1.2	310		0.06		6
Pies, apple	47.8	246	2.1	9.5	39.5	1.1	7	24	0.4	160	0.03	0.02	0.2	1
Pies, cherry	46.2	253	2.4	9.8	40.4	1.2	10	27	0.4	380	0.03	0.02	0.2	1
Pies, coconut custard	58.5	204	5.2	8.7	26.3	1.3	125	116	1.2	230	0.05	0.16	0.3	
Pies, lemon meringue	47.4	252	3.6	10.1	37.4	1.5	20	51	0.5	170	0.03	0.08	0.2	1

* Contains oxalic acid.

Compositions of Foods, 3⅓ Oz, Edible Portion

Food	Water Pct	Food Energy Cal	Protein Gm	Fat Gm	Carbohydrate Gm	Ash Gm	Calcium Mg	Phosphorus Mg	Iron Mg	Vitamin A IU	Thiamin Mg	Riboflavin Mg	Niacin Mg	Ascorbic Acid Mg
Pies, pumpkin	58.9	202	4.2	9.6	25.8	1.5	54	81	0.8	1910	0.03	0.12	0.3	
Pimientos, canned	92.4	27	0.9	0.5	5.8	0.4	7	17	1.5	2300	0.02	0.06	0.4	95
Pineapple, raw	85.3	52	0.4	0.2	13.7	0.4	16	11	0.3	130	0.08	0.02	0.2	24
Pineapple, canned	78.0	78	0.4	0.1	21.1	0.4	29	7	0.6	80	0.07	0.02	0.2	9
Pineapple juice, canned	86.2	49	0.3	0.1	13.0	0.4	15	8	0.5	80	0.05	0.02	0.2	9
Plums, raw	85.7	50	0.7	0.2	12.9	0.5	17	20	0.5	350	0.06	0.04	0.5	5
Pork, fresh, ham, cooked	42.0	400	24.0	33.0		1.2	11	238	3.1		0.53	0.24	4.7	
Pork chops, cooked	50.0	333	23.0	26.0		1.2	11	235	3.0		0.83	0.24	5.0	
Pork, cured, ham, smoked, cooked	39.0	397	23.0	33.0	0.4	5.4	10	166	2.9		0.54	0.21	4.2	
Pork, cured, boiled ham	47.8	302	22.8	22.7		6.7	9	92	2.7		1.01	0.26	5.1	
Potatoes, baked	73.8	98	2.4	0.1	22.5	1.2	13	66	0.8	20	0.11	0.05	1.4	17
Potatoes, boiled, unpeeled	77.8	83	2.0	0.1	19.1	1.0	11	56	0.7	20	0.10	0.04	1.2	15
Potatoes, boiled, peeled before cooking	77.8	83	2.0	0.1	19.1	1.0	11	56	0.7	20	0.09	0.03	1.0	14
Potato flour	7.0	357	7.1	0.7	82.2	3.0	25	88	4.0	40	0.30	0.11	4.5	23
Prunes, dried, unsulfured, raw	24.0	268	2.3	0.6	71.0	2.1	54	85	3.9	1890	0.10	0.16	1.7	3
Radishes, raw	93.6	20	1.2	0.1	4.2	1.0	37	31	1.0	30	0.03	0.02	0.3	24
Raisins, unsulfured, dried	24.0	268	2.3	0.5	71.2	2.0	78	129	3.3	50	0.15	0.08	0.5	
Raspberries, black, raw	80.6	74	1.5	1.6	15.7	0.6	40	37	0.9		0.02	0.07?	0.3?	24?
Raspberries, red, raw	84.1	57	1.2	0.4	13.8	0.5	40	37	0.9	130	0.02	0.07?	0.3?	24
Rhubarb, stems only, cooked, sugar added	62.9	141	0.4	0.1	36.0	0.6	41 *	20	0.4	20	0.01		0.1	6
Rice, brown, raw	12.0	360	7.5	1.7	77.7	1.1	39	303	2.0		0.32	0.05	4.6	
Rutabagas, raw	89.1	38	1.1	0.1	8.9	0.8	55	41	0.4	330	0.07	0.08	0.9	36
Rutabagas, cooked	90.8	32	0.8	0.1	7.5	0.8	55	41	0.4	350	0.05	0.07	0.7	21
Rye flour, light	11.0	356	9.4	1.0	77.9	0.7	22	185	1.1		0.15	0.07	0.6	
Rye flour, dark	11.0	318	16.3	2.6	68.1	2.0	54	536?	4.5		0.61	0.22	2.7	
Salmon, Pacific, broiled or baked	64.5	170	28.0	5.6	0.2	1.7		417?	1.2?		0.10	0.28	8.1	
Salmon, canned, king (including bones)	64.7	203	19.7	13.2		2.4	154	289	0.9	230	0.03	0.14	7.3	
Salmon, canned, pink (including bones)	70.0	143	20.5	6.2		2.6	187	286	0.8	70	0.03	0.18	8.0	
Salmon, canned, red (including bones)	67.2	173	20.2	9.6		3.0	259	344	1.2	230	0.04	0.16	7.3	
Sardines, Atlantic, canned in oil	47.1	338	21.1	27.0	1.0	3.9	354	434	3.5		0.01	0.14	3.9	
Sardines, pilchards, Pacific, canned	65.2	200	17.7	13.5	0.7	2.9	381?	168?	4.1	30?	0.01	0.30?	7.4?	
Sauerkraut, canned	93.2	16	1.1	0.2	3.4	2.1	36	18	0.5	30	0.03	0.06	0.1	16
Sausage, frankfurter, cooked	62.0	248	14.0	20.0	0.2	2.0	6	49	1.2		0.16	0.18	2.5	
Sausage, liverwurst	59.0	263	16.7	20.6	1.5	2.2	9	238	5.4	5750	0.17	1.12	4.6	
Scallops, raw (edible muscle)	80.3	78	14.8	0.1	3.4	1.4	26	208	1.8		0.04	0.10	1.4	
Shad, American, raw	70.2	168	18.7	9.8		1.4		260	0.5		0.15	0.24	8.4?	

* Contains oxalic acid.

Compositions of Foods, 3⅓ Oz, Edible Portion

Food	Water Pct	Food Energy Cal	Protein Gm	Fat Gm	Carbohydrate Gm	Ash Gm	Calcium Mg	Phosphorus Mg	Iron Mg	Vitamin A IU	Thiamin Mg	Riboflavin Mg	Niacin Mg	Ascorbic Acid Mg
Shrimp, canned, dry pack	66.2	127	26.8	1.4		5.8	115	263	3.1	60	0.01	0.03	2.2	
Soup, canned, bean, condensed	64.7	154	6.9	4.1	23.6	0.7	75	82	2.2		0.08	0.08	0.7	
Soup, canned, pea, condensed	72.4	114	5.2	1.6	20.4	0.4	26	80	1.2	360?	0.14	0.06	1.0	3
Soup, canned tomato, condensed	81.4	74	1.8	1.8	14.6	0.4	21	31	0.7	1000?	0.02	0.08	0.6	7
Soup, canned, vegetable, condensed	83.2	65	3.3	1.4	11.5	0.5	26	40	0.6		0.04	0.06	0.9	6
Soybeans, whole, mature, dried	7.5	331	34.9	18.1	34.8	4.7	227	586	8.0	110	1.07	0.31	2.3	
Soybean flour, low fat	11.0	228	44.7	1.1	37.7	5.5	265	626	13.0	70	1.10	0.35	2.9	
Soybean flour, full fat	9.0	347	35.9	20.6	29.9	4.6	195	553	12.1	140	0.77	0.28	2.2	
Soybean sprouts, raw	86.3	46	6.2	1.4	5.3	0.8	48	67	1.0	180	0.23	0.20	0.8	13
Spaghetti, cooked	60.6	149	5.1	0.6	30.2	3.5	9	65	0.6		0.02	0.02	0.5	
Spaghetti, enriched, cooked	60.6	149	5.1	0.6	30.2	3.5	9	65	1.1		0.17	0.10	1.4	
Spinach, raw	92.7	20	2.3	0.3	3.2	1.5	81*	55	3.0	9420	0.11	0.20	0.6	59
Spinach, cooked	90.8	26	3.1	0.6	3.6	1.9	124*	33	2.0	11780	0.08	0.20	0.6	30
Spinach, frozen	92.7	20	2.3	0.3	3.2	1.5	81*	55	3.0	6820	0.07	0.17	0.5	38
Squash, summer, cooked	95.0	16	0.6	0.1	3.9	0.4	15	15	0.4	260	0.04	0.07	0.6	11
Squash, winter, baked	85.7	47	1.9	0.4	11.0	1.0	24	35	0.8	6190	0.05	0.15	0.6	7
Squash, winter, boiled	88.6	38	1.5	0.3	8.8	0.8	19	28	0.6	4950	0.04	0.10	0.4	5
Strawberries, raw	89.9	37	0.8	0.5	8.3	0.5	28	27	0.8	60	0.03	0.07	0.3	60
Sugar, dark brown	3.0	370			99.5	1.2	76	37	2.6					
Sweet potatoes, baked, yellow	61.1	152	2.2	0.9	34.4	1.4	37	60	0.9	9510	0.10	0.06	0.8	23
Sweet potatoes, yellow, boiled	68.5	123	1.8	0.7	27.9	1.1	30	49	0.7	7700	0.09	0.05	0.6	20
Swordfish, cooked, broiled	64.8	178	27.4	6.8		1.7	20	251	1.1	2300	0.05	0.06	10.3	
Tangerines	87.3	44	0.8	0.3	10.9	0.7	33?	23?	0.4?	420?	0.07	0.03?	0.2?	31
Tomatoes, raw	94.1	20	1.0	0.3	4.0	0.6	11	27	0.6	1100	0.06	0.04	0.5	23
Tomato juice, canned	93.5	21	1.0	0.2	4.3	1.0	7?	15?	0.4?	1050	0.05	0.03	0.8	16
Tomato catsup	69.5	98	2.0	0.4	24.5	3.6	12	18	0.8	1880?	0.09	0.07	2.2	11
Tomato flakes	3.0	340	10.8	3.3	76.7	6.2	119	293	6.5	3720	0.65	0.43	6.5	114
Tongue, beef, raw	68.0	207	16.4	15.0	0.4	0.9	9	187	2.8		0.12	0.29	5.0	
Tortillas, made from yellow corn	41.9	211	5.8	2.8	48.6	0.9	111	184	2.2	210	0.19	0.06	1.0	
Tuna fish, canned	52.5	290	23.8	20.9		2.3	7	294	1.2	220?	0.04	0.10	10.8	
Turkey, raw	58.3	268	20.1	20.2		1.0	23	320	3.8		0.09	0.14	8.0	
Turnips, raw	90.9	32	1.1	0.2	7.1	0.7	40	34	0.5		0.05	0.07	0.5	28
Turnips, cooked	92.3	27	0.8	0.2	6.0	0.7	40	34	0.5		0.04	0.06	0.4	18
Turnip greens, raw	89.5	30	2.9	0.4	5.4	1.8	259	50	2.4	9540	0.09	0.46	0.8	136
Turnip greens, cooked	89.5	30	2.9	0.4	5.4	1.8	259	50	2.4	10600	0.06	0.41–0.36 †	0.7	60–45 †

* Contains oxalic acid.

† Depending on the amount of water and length of time.

Compositions of Foods, 3⅓ Oz, Edible Portion

Food	*Water Pct*	*Food Energy Cal*	*Protein Gm*	*Fat Gm*	*Carbohydrate Gm*	*Ash Gm*	*Calcium Mg*	*Phosphorus Mg*	*Iron Mg*	*Vitamin A IU*	*Thiamin Mg*	*Riboflavin Mg*	*Niacin Mg*	*Ascorbic Acid Mg*
Veal, cutlet, cooked	60.0	219	28.0	11.0		1.4	12	258	3.5		0.08	0.28	6.1	
Veal, shoulder roast, boned, cooked	59.0	228	28.0	12.0		1.4	12	258	3.6		0.13	0.31	7.9	
Vinegar		12			5.?	0.3	7	10	0.5					
Walnuts	3.3	654	15.0	64.4	15.6	1.7	83	380	2.1	30	0.48	0.13	1.2	3
Watermelons	92.1	28	0.5	0.2	6.9	0.3	7	12	0.2	590	0.05	0.05	0.2	6
Wheat, whole grain, hard	13.0	330	14.0	2.2	69.1	1.7	36	383	3.1		0.57	0.12	4.3	
Wheat flour, whole	12.0	333	13.3	2.0	71.0	1.7	41	372	3.3		0.55	0.12	4.3	
Wheat products, germ	11.0	361	25.2	10.0	49.5	4.3	84	1096	8.1		2.05	0.80	4.6	
Wheat, shredded, plain	5.6	360	10.1	2.5	80.1	1.7	47	360	3.5		0.22	0.12	4.4	
Whey, dried	6.2	344	12.5	1.2	72.4	7.7	679	576		50	0.49	2.50	0.8	
Wild rice, parched, raw	8.5	364	14.1	0.7	75.3	1.4	19	339			0.45	0.63	6.2	
Yeast, compressed, baker's	70.9	86	10.6?	0.4	13.0	2.4	25	605	4.9		0.45	2.07	28.2	
Yeast, dried, brewer's	7.0	273	36.9?	1.6	37.4	7.9	106	1893	18.2		9.69	5.45	36.2	

Appendix C: Atomic Weights: Bibliography: Suppliers

INTERNATIONAL ATOMIC WEIGHTS, 1955

	Symbol	*Atomic Number*	*Atomic Weight*		*Symbol*	*Atomic Number*	*Atomic Weight*
Actinium	Ac	89	227	Gadolinium	Gd	64	157.26
Aluminum	Al	13	26.98	Gallium	Ga	31	69.72
Americium	Am	95	243	Germanium	Ge	32	72.60
Antimony	Sb	51	121.76	Gold	Au	79	197.00
Argon	A	18	39.944	Hafnium	Hf	72	178.50
Arsenic	As	33	74.91	Helium	He	2	4.003
Astatine	At	85	210	Holmium	Ho	67	164.94
Barium	Ba	56	137.36	Hydrogen	H	1	1.0080
Berkelium	Bk	97	249	Indium	In	49	114.82
Beryllium	Be	4	9.013	Iodine	I	53	126.91
Bismuth	Bi	83	209.00	Iridium	Ir	77	192.20
Boron	B	5	10.82	Iron	Fe	26	55.85
Bromine	Br	35	79.916	Krypton	Kr	36	83.80
Cadmium	Cd	48	112.41	Lanthanum	La	57	138.92
Calcium	Ca	20	40.08	Lead	Pb	82	207.21
Californium	Cf	98	249.00	Lithium	Li	3	6.940
Carbon	C	6	12.011	Lutetium	Lu	71	174.99
Cerium	Ce	58	140.13	Magnesium	Mg	12	24.32
Cesium	Cs	55	132.91	Manganese	Mn	25	54.94
Chlorine	Cl	17	35.457	Mendelevium	Mv	101	256.00
Chromium	Cr	24	52.01	Mercury	Hg	80	200.61
Cobalt	Co	27	58.94	Molybdenum	Mo	42	95.95
Copper	Cu	29	63.54	Neodymium	Nd	60	144.27
Curium	Cm	96	245	Neptunium	Np	93	237.00
Dysprosium	Dy	66	162.51	Neon	Ne	10	20.183
Erbium	Er	68	167.27	Nickel	Ni	28	58.71
Europium	Eu	63	152	Niobium	Nb	41	92.91
Fluorine	F	9	19	Nitrogen	N	7	14.008
Francium	Fr	87	223	Osmium	Os	76	190.20

INTERNATIONAL ATOMIC WEIGHTS, 1955 (Con.)

	Symbol	*Atomic Number*	*Atomic Weight*
Oxygen	O	8	16
Palladium	Pd	46	106.4
Phosphorus	P	15	30.975
Platinum	Pt	78	195.09
Plutonium	Pu	94	242.00
Potassium	K	19	39.100
Praseodymium	Pr	59	140.92
Promethium	Pm	61	145
Protactinium	Pa	91	231
Radium	Ra	88	226.05
Radon	Rn	86	222
Rhenium	Re	75	186.22
Rhodium	Rh	45	102.91
Rubidium	Rb	37	85.48
Ruthenium	Ru	44	101.10
Samarium	Sm	62	150.35
Scandium	Sc	21	44.96
Selenium	Se	34	78.96
Silicon	Si	14	28.09
Silver	Ag	47	107.880
Sodium	Na	11	22.991
Strontium	Sr	38	87.63
Sulfur	S	16	32.066
Tantalum	Ta	73	180.95
Technetium	Tc	43	99
Tellurium	Te	52	127.61
Terbium	Tb	65	158.93
Thallium	Tl	81	204.39
Thorium	Th	90	232.05
Thulium	Tm	69	168.94
Tin	Sn	50	118.70
Titanium	Ti	22	47.90
Tungsten	W	74	183.86
Uranium	U	92	238.07
Vanadium	V	23	50.95
Xenon	Xe	54	131.30
Ytterbium	Yb	70	173.04
Yttrium	Y	39	88.92
Zinc	Zn	30	65.38
Zirconium	Zr	40	91.22

BIBLIOGRAPHY

Acta Metallurgica
Agricultural Chemicals
A.M.A. Arch. Dermatol.
Am. Acad. Arts
Am. Chemist
Am. Druggist
Am. Ink Maker
Am. J. Med. Sci.
Am. J. Phar.
Am. J. Sci.
Am. Paint and Varnish Mfrs. Assoc.
Am. Perfumer
Am. Scientist
Analytical Chemistry
Bakers Digest
Bakers Weekly
Baking Industry
British Bee Journal
British Chem. Abstracts
Bull. Am. Soc. of Hospital Pharmacists
Bur. of Standards J. Research
Ceramic Industry
Chem. Abstracts
Chemical Eng. News
Chemist and Druggist (England)
Chemistry and Industry (England)
Chemical Engineering
Chemical and Met. Eng.
Chem. Eng. Progress
Chem. Revs.
Drug and Allied Industries
Drug and Cosmetic Industry
Drug Topics
Eng. Mining J.

Farben-Ztg. (Germany)
Food Engineering
Food Industries
Food Research
Food Technology
Ice Cream Trade Journal
Ice Cream Review, The
Ind. Chemist
Ind. Eng. Chem.
J. Agr. Research
J. Am. Chem. Soc.
J. Am. Pharm. Assoc.
J.A.M.A.
J. Applied Chem.
J. Assoc. Official Agr. Chem.
J. of the Chem. Soc. (England)
J. of the Am. Oil Chemists
J. Oil and Fat Ind.
J. Florida Med. Assoc.
J. Proc. Oil Technol. Assoc. (India)
Manufacturing Chemist (England)
Manufacturing Confectioner
Metals & Alloys
Metal Industry (England)
New Jersey Journal of Pharm.
Oil Paint and Drug Reporter
Pacific Drug Review
Paint Manufacture (Brit.)
Paint, Oil and Chem. Review
Perfumery Essent. Oil Record (England)
Proc. Am. Pharm. Assoc.
Proc. Oil Tech. Assoc.
Power
Schimmel Briefs (Germany)
Science
Schweiz, Apoth. Ztg.
Soap, Perfumery and Cosmetics
Soap and Sanitary Chemicals
The American Bottler
The Industrial Chemist (England)
The Lancet
The Laundry Manager
The Merck Index
The Merck Report
The Pharmaceutical Journal
U.S. Dept. of Agric. Publications
U.S. Dept. of Commerce Publications
Veterinary Medicine

SOURCES OF SUPPLY

Abrasives

Charles B. Chrystal Co., Inc., 53 Park Place, New York 7, N.Y.
Industrial Minerals & Chemicals Co., 836 Gilman St., Berkeley 10, Calif.
Tamms Silica Co., 228 N. LaSalle St., Chicago 1, Ill.

Absorption Bases and Lanolin Products

Robinson Wagner Co., Inc., 110 E. 42nd St., New York 17, N.Y.
Pfaltz & Bauer, Inc., Empire State Bldg., New York 1, N.Y.

Acetylated Lanolin Alcohols

American Cholesterol Products, Inc., Milltown, N.J.

Acetylated Monoglycerides from Lard

Distillation Products Industries, Division of Eastman Kodak Co.

Acids and Basic Industrial Chemicals

General Chemical Div. Allied Chemical and Dye Corp., 40 Rector St., New York, N.Y.

Harshaw Chemical Co., Cleveland, Ohio

Philipp Brothers Chemicals, Inc., 37 Wall St., New York 5, N.Y.

Acryloid B 66

Rohm & Haas Company, Washington Square, Philadelphia 5, Penna.

Albatex

Whittaker, Clarke & Daniels, Inc., 100 Church St., New York 8, N.Y.

Alcohols

U.S. Industrial Chemicals, Inc., 120 Broadway, New York 5, N.Y.

Alcosolve 2

London Solvents Ltd., London, England

Alkyl Aryl Sodium Sulfonates

Aceto Chemical Co., Inc., 40–40 Lawrence St., Flushing 54, N.Y.

Allantoin

Schuylkill Chemical Co., 2346 Sedgley Ave., Philadelphia, Pa.

Allyl Cyclohexane-Propionate

Bush Aromatics, 629 Grove St., Jersey City 2, N.J.

Aluminum Chlorhydroxide Complex

Reheis Company, Inc., Berkeley Heights, N.J.

Ambreine

Givaudan-Delawanna, Inc., 321 W. 44th St., New York 18, N.Y.

Amerchol L-101 & Modulan

American Cholesterol Products, Inc., Milltown, N.J.

Aminomethyl-Propanol

Commercial Solvents Corp., 260 Madison Ave., New York 17, N.Y.

Ammonium, Calcium, Potassium, and Sodium Chemicals

Mathieson Chemical Corp., Baltimore 3, Md.
Niagara Alkali Co., New York 17, N.Y.
Solvay Process Division Allied Chemical and Dye Corp., 61 Broadway, New York 6, N.Y.

Aniline Dyes, Certified Food and Cosmetic Colors

National Aniline Division Allied Chemical and Dye Corp., New York 6, N.Y.

H. Kohnstamm & Co., Inc., 161 Ave. of Americas, New York 11, N.Y.

Leeben Chemical Co., Inc., 103 Lafayette, New York 12, N.Y.

Arlacel 83

Atlas Powder Company, Wilmington 99, Delaware

Arochlor 1254 & 5460

Monsanto Chemical Co., P.O. Box 478, St. Louis, Missouri

Aroma Benzoin Siam

Stafford Allen & Sons, Ltd., Wharf Road, London, England

Astrotone

E. I. du Pont de Nemours & Co., Wilmington, Delaware

Auranthiol 100%

F. Ritter & Co., Los Angeles 27, California

Bentonite

American Colloid Co., Merchandise Mart Plaza, Chicago, Ill.

Borax and Boric Acid

Pacific Coast Borax Co., 100 Park Ave., New York, N.Y.

Brewers Yeast

Anheuser-Busch, Inc., St. Louis 18, Mo.

Butoben

Merck & Company, Rahway, N.J.

Butoxy-Polyoxypropylene Glycol

Colgate-Palmolive Company, 105 Hudson St., Jersey City 2, N.J.

Butylated Hydroxyanisole (BHA)

Eastman Chemical Products, Inc., Kingsport, Tenn.

Calcium Cyclamate

Chas. Pfizer & Co., Inc., 630 Flushing Ave., Brooklyn 6, N.Y.

Carbitol Solvent

Carbide and Carbon Chemicals Co., 30 E. 42nd St., New York 17, N.Y.

Carbowax 4000

Glyco Products Co., Inc., Empire State Bldg., New York 1, N.Y.

Carbowax Compound 4000
Carbowax Polyethylene Glycol 1500

Carbide and Carbon Chemicals Co., 30 E. 42nd St., New York 17, N.Y.

Ceramol

Aceto Chemical Co., Inc., 40–40 Lawrence St., Flushing, N.Y.

Cerium Oxide

Lindsay Chemical Co., 268 Ann St., West Chicago, Illinois

Cetyl Alcohol

Aceto Chemical Co., Inc., 40–40 Lawrence St., Flushing, N.Y.
Givaudan-Delawanna, Inc., 330 W. 42nd St., New York 18, N.Y.

Chlordane

S. B. Penick & Co., 100 Church Street, New York 8, N.Y.

Chlordane and DDT

Prentiss Drug and Chemical Co., Inc., 110 William St., New York 38, N.Y.

Chlorhydrol

Reheis Co., Inc., Berkeley Heights, N.J.

Chlorophyll Water-Soluble

National Alfalfa Dehydrating & Milling Co., Lamar, Colorado

Chocolate Base

The Nestle Company, Inc., 2 William Street, White Plains, N.Y.

Chocolate Liquor

Blumenthal Bros. Chocolate Co., Margaret and James Sts., Philadelphia 37, Pa.

Citronellyl Oxyacetaldehyde

Verona Chemical Co., 26 Verona Ave., Newark 4, N.J.

Citrus Pectin, Rapid-Set or Slow-Set

California Fruit Growers Exchange, Ontario, Calif.

Civettiane

Perfumery Associates, Inc., 135 Fifth Ave., New York 10, N.Y.

Civettine

Firmenich & Cie., 250 W. 18th St., New York 11, N.Y.

Cobee 92 Coconut Fat

E. F. Drew & Company, Boonton, N.J.

Coconut Diethanolamide

Stepan Chemical Co., 20 N. Wacker Drive, Chicago 6, Illinois

Coconut Fatty Acids

A. Gross & Company, 295 Madison Ave., New York 17, N.Y.

Corn-Oil Lecithin

The Arthur Rude Co., San Francisco 11, Calif.

Corn Starch & Corn Syrup

Penick & Ford, Ltd., Inc., 420 Lexington Ave., New York 17, N.Y.

Corn Syrup Powdered

Clinton Corn Processing Co., Clinton, Iowa

Corn Syrup Powdered (Frodex)

American Maize Products Co., 250 Park Ave., New York 17, N.Y.

Corn Syrup Solids

The Hubinger Company, Keokuk, Iowa

Corn Sugar

Clinton Foods, Inc., Clinton, Iowa

Cosmetic and Pharmaceutical Chemicals

Fine Organics, Inc., New York 3, N.Y.
Eastman Chemical Products, Inc., Kingsport, Tenn.
Heyden Newport Chemical Corp., 342 Madison Ave., New York 17, N.Y.

Cosmetic Preservatives

Goldschmidt Chemical Corp., 153 Waverly Place, New York 14, N.Y.

Crodacol "O" Deodorized

Croda, Inc., 15 East 26th St., New York 10, N.Y.

Crude Drugs, Gums, etc.

S. B. Penick & Co., 100 Church St., New York 8, N.Y.
Peek & Velsor, Inc., 100 Gold St., New York, N.Y.

Crystal O Castor Oil

The Baker Castor Oil Co., 120 Broadway, New York 5, N.Y.

"Cumin" Ketone

Verona Chemical Co., 26 Verona Ave., Newark, N.J.

Deltyl Extra

Givaudan-Delawanna, Inc., New York, N.Y.

Dieldrin

Shell Chemical Corp., 460 Park Ave., New York 22, N.Y.

Diethyl Toluamide, Meta

Montrose Chemical Co., 120 Lister Ave., Newark 5, N.J.

Digalloyl Trioleate

Firmenich, Inc., 250 West 18th St., New York 11, N.Y.

Dioctyl Sodium Sulfosuccinate

American Cyanamid, 30 Rockefeller Plaza, New York 20, N.Y.

Dodecyl Benzene Sulfonate

Pilot Chemical Co., 215 W. 7th St., Los Angeles, Calif.

Edible Safflower Oil

Welch, Holme & Clark Company, Inc., No. 1 Hudson St., New York 13, N.Y

Emcol MAS

Witco Chemical Co., Inc., 122 E. 42nd St., New York 17, N.Y.

Emulsifiers

Atlas Powder Company, Wilmington 99, Delaware

Emulsifying Type Shortening

Armour & Company, Chicago 9, Illinois
Swift & Company, Chicago 9, Illinois

Essential Oils and Aromatic Chemicals

Dodge & Olcott, Inc., 180 Varick St., New York 14, N.Y.
Florsynth Laboratories, Inc., New York 61, N.Y.
Fritzsche Bros. Inc., 76 Ninth Ave., New York 11, N.Y.
Givaudan-Delawanna, Inc., 321 W. 44th St., New York 18, N.Y.
S. B. Penick & Company, 100 Church St., New York 8, N.Y.
Ungerer & Co., 161 Sixth Ave., New York 11, N.Y.

Esters and Chlorinated Products

Glyco Products Co., 417 Fifth Ave., New York, N.Y.

Ethanolamide of Coconut Fatty Acids

Stepan Chemical Co., 20 N. Wacker Drive, Chicago 6, Illinois

Ethoxylan & Ethoxylan 50 & 100

N. I. Malmstrom & Company, 147 Lombardy St., Brooklyn 22, N.Y.

Ethyl Decylate

F. Ritter & Co., Los Angeles 27, California

Eutanol G

Fallek Products Co., 165 Broadway, New York 6, N.Y.

Exaltolide

Firmenich & Cie, 250 W. 18th St., New York 11, N.Y.

Fatty Acids

Armour Chemical Division, 1353 West 31st St., Chicago 9, Illinois
Vegetable Oil Products Co., Inc., 401 Canal Ave., Wilmington, Calif.

Fatty Acids and Derivatives

Emery Industries, Inc., Carew Tower, Cincinnati 2, Ohio
E. F. Drew & Co. Inc., New York 10, N.Y.

Filtrosol A

Schimmel & Co., Inc., 601 West 26th St., New York 1, N.Y.

Fine Chemicals

Merck & Co. Inc., Rahway, N.J.
Seydel Chemical Co., Jersey City 2, N.J.
Shulton Fine Chemicals Division, 630 Fifth Ave., New York 20, N.Y.

Freon Propellents

E. I. duPont de Nemours & Co., Inc., Freon Division 134, Wilmington 98, Delaware

G-2162

Atlas Powder Co., Wilmington 99, Delaware

Glucose and Caramel

Union Sales Corp., Columbus, Ind.

Glucose Oxidase

Fermco Chemicals, Inc., 4941 So. Racine Ave., Chicago 9, Illinois

Glyceryl Monostearate (Aldo 28)

Glyco Chemicals Div., Chas. L. Huisking & Co., Inc., 417 Fifth Ave., New York 16, N.Y.

Glyceryl Monostearate

The North-Western Chemical Co., 120 Aurora St., West Chicago, Illinois

Gums

Paul A. Dunkell & Co., Inc., 26 Journal Sq., Jersey City 6, N.J.
Thurston & Bradich, 286 Spring St., New York 13, N.Y.

Hoop Cheese

Purity Mfg. Co., 4151 Knopp, Cattaraugus, N.Y.

Hyamine

Rohm & Haas Company, Washington Square, Philadelphia 5, Penna.

Hydratropyl Alcohol

Verona Chemical Co., 26 Verona Ave., Newark 4, N.J.

Hydrocortisone U.S.P. Microfine

Merck & Co., Inc., Rahway, N.J.

Ice Cream Stabilizer

Kelco Company, 120 Broadway, New York 5, N.Y.

Insecticide Chemicals

Prentiss Drug & Chem. Co., Inc., 110 William St., New York 38, N.Y.
S. B. Penick & Company, 100 Church St., New York 8, N.Y.

Invert Sugar

The National Sugar Refining Co., New York, N.Y. or Philadelphia, Pa.

Irish Moss Extractive

S. B. Penick & Company, 100 Church St., New York 8, N.Y.

Iso-Bergamate

Dragoco Inc., 432 Fourth Ave., New York 16, N.Y.

Isopropyl Linoleate

Van Dyk & Co., Inc., Main & William Sts., Belleville 9, N.J.

Isopropyl Palmitate

Givaudan-Delawanna, Inc., 321 West 44th St., New York 36, N.Y.

Jasmia A

Fritzsche Bros., Inc., 76 Ninth Ave., New York 11, N.Y.

Kelcoloid

Kelco Co., 120 Broadway, New York 5, N.Y.

Kieselguhr

Johns-Manville, P.O. Box 60, New York 16, N.Y.

Lampblack Paste

Columbian Carbon Co., 380 Madison Ave., New York 17, N.Y.

Lanfrax

Malmstrom Chemical Corp., 259 Parkhurst St., Newark 5, N.J.

Lanogene

Robinson Wagner Co., Inc., 110 E. 42nd St., New York 17, N.Y.

Lanolin

Robinson Wagner Co., Inc., 110 E. 42nd St., New York 17, N.Y.

Lanolin Alcohol

Croda Inc., 51 Madison Ave., New York 10, N.Y.

Lantrol

Malmstrom Chemical Corp., 259 Parkhurst St., Newark 5, N.J.

Lauric Acid

Aceto Chemical Co., Inc., 40–40 Lawrence St., Flushing 54, N.Y.

Lauric Diethanolamide (Ninol AA-62 Extra)

The Stepan Chemical Co., 20 N. Wacker Drive, Chicago 6, Illinois

Lauric Ethanol

Jefferson Chemical Co., Inc., 1121 Walker Ave., Houston 2, Texas

Lauryl Sulfate of Triethanolamine

The Stepan Chemical Co., 20 N. Wacker Drive, Chicago 6, Illinois

Lemon Juice, Powdered

Bordens Foods Company, 350 Madison Ave., New York 17, N.Y.

Liquid Lanolin

Croda, Inc., 15 East 26th St., New York 10, N.Y.

Liquid Sugar

Refined Syrups & Sugars, Inc., Yonkers 1, N.Y.

Low Molecular Weight Polyethylene

Semet-Solvay Petrochemical Division, Allied Chemical & Dye Corp., New York, N.Y.

L-Lysine Monohydrochloride

E. I. duPont de Nemours & Company, Wilmington, Delaware

Magnesium Silicate (Asbestine)

International Talc Co., Inc., 90 West St., New York 6, N.Y.

Menthanyl Acetate

Givaudan-Delawanna, Inc., 321 W. 44th St., New York 36, N.Y.

Methionine Metallic Sodium

U.S. Industrial Chemical Co., 99 Park Ave., New York 16, N.Y.

Methyl Para-hydroxybenzoate

Chemo Puro Mfg. Corp., 26–32 Skillman Ave., Long Island City 1, N.Y.

Micro-Cel

Johns-Manville, Box 60, New York 16, N.Y.

Minerals, Colors, Pigments, and Chemicals

Whittaker, Clark & Daniels, 100 Church St., New York 8, N.Y.

Miranol "MM"

The Miranol Chemical Co., Inc., 277 Coit St., Irvington, N.J.

Mono Sodium Glutamate

International Minerals & Chem. Corp., Chicago 6, Ill.

Morpholine

Carbide and Carbon Chemicals Co., 30 East 42nd St., New York 17, N.Y.

Muguet Aldehyde

Van Ameringen-Haebler, Inc., 521 West 57th St., New York 19, N.Y.

Muguet Fleur

Givaudan-Delawanna, Inc., 321 W. 44th St., New York 36, N.Y.

Myristic Acid

Aceto Chemical Co., Inc., 40–40 Lawrence St., Flushing 54, N.Y.

Myrj 52

Atlas Powder Company, Wilmington 99, Delaware

Nekal BX

General Aniline & Film Corp., 435 Hudson St., New York 14, N.Y.

Ninol AA62

Stepan Chemical Company, 20 N. Wacker Drive, Chicago 6, Ill.

Non-Fat Dry Milk Solids

American Dry Milk Institute, Inc., 221 N. LaSalle St., Chicago 1, Ill.

Nulomaline

American Molasses Co., 120 Wall St., New York 5, N.Y.

Octadienol 1473

Polak's Frutal Works, Middletown, N.Y.

Oleic Acid

Emery Industries, Inc., Carew Tower, Cincinnati 2, Ohio

Oleic Monoethanolamine

Carbide and Carbon Chemicals Co., 30 E. 42nd St., New York 17, N.Y.

Oleyl Alcohol, N.F.

Aceto Chemical Co., Inc., 40-40 Lawrence St., Flushing 54, N.Y.

Oleyl Oleate

Croda, Inc., 15 E. 26th St., New York 10, N.Y.

Oleyl Oleate (Cetiol V)

Fallek Products Co., Inc., 165 Broadway, New York 6, N.Y.

Olive Oil Fatty Acid Monoethanolamide

Dutton and Reinish, Ltd., London, England

Optical Dye

General Dyestuff Corp., 435 Hudson St., New York 14, N.Y.

Organic Chemicals

Carbide and Carbon Chemicals Corp., 30 E. 42nd St., New York 17, N.Y.

Oxidized Microcrystalline Wax

Bareco Wax Co., P.O. Box 2009, Tulsa, Oklahoma

Palatone

The Dow Chemical Co., Midland, Michigan

Pearl Essence

Argenta Products Co., Sea St., Eastport, Maine

Pectin, Powdered

Speas Company, Kansas City 1, Missouri

Pendit CA

Rayette, Inc., Chem. Division, 261 E. 5th St., St. Paul 1, Minn.

Petroleum Products

Atlantic Refining Co., Philadelphia 1, Pa.
L. Sonneborn & Sons, Inc., New York 10, N.Y.

Phantolid

Polak's Frutal Works, Middletown, N.Y.

Pharmaceuticals

Chas. L. Huisking & Co. Inc., 417 Fifth Ave., New York 16, N.Y.
Heyden Newport Chemical Corp., 342 Madison Ave., New York 17, N.Y.
Monsanto Chemical Co., 1700 S. Second St., St. Louis, Mo.

Phosphates

Victor Chemical Works, 155 N. Wacker Drive, Chicago 6, Illinois

Phosphates and Fluorides

Blockson Chemical Co., Joliet, Ill.
Victor Chemical Works, 155 N. Wacker Drive, Chicago 6, Ill.

Piperonyl Butoxide

Fairfield Chemical Division, 1701 Patapsco Ave., Baltimore, Md.

Polyethylene Glycol 4000

Carbide and Carbon Chemicals Co., 30 E. 42nd St., New York 17, N.Y.

Polyethylene Glycol 400 Distearate

Glyco Chemicals, Div. of Chas. L. Huisking & Co., Inc., 417 Fifth Ave., New York 16, N.Y.
Kessler Chemical Co., Inc., State Rd. & Gottman Ave., Philadelphia 35, Pa.

Polyoxyethylene Ester of Fatty and Resin Acids (Renex 20)

Atlas Powder Company, Wilmington 99, Delaware

Polyoxyethylene Lauryl Ether (Brij 35)

Atlas Powder Co., Wilmington 99, Delaware

Polyoxyethylene (40) Stearate

Atlas Powder Company, Wilmington 99, Delaware

Polyterge 102

Knapp Products, Inc., Lodi, N.J.

Polyvinylpyrrolidone (PVP) Iodine; PVP Type NP

General Aniline & Film Corp., 435 Hudson St., New York 14, N.Y.

Precipitated Chalk

H. J. Baker & Bros., 600 Fifth Ave., New York 20, N.Y.

Procaine Borate

Richmond Chemical Corp., 1741 Richmond Terrace, Staten Island 10, N.Y.

Propylene Glycol Monolaurate

Glyco Products Co., Inc., Empire State Bldg., New York 1, N.Y.

PVP-Vinyl Acetate

General Aniline and Film Corp., 230 Park Ave., New York City, N.Y.

Quaternary Ammonium Compound

Atlas Powder Company, Wilmington 99, Delaware

Renex 690

Atlas Powder Company, Wilmington 99, Delaware

Rotenone

S. B. Penick & Co., 100 Church St., New York 8, N.Y.

Sea Kem Irish Moss Extractive

Kem Products Co., Inc., 229 High St., Newark, N.J.

Seakem Type 104 Stabilizer

Seaplant Chem. Corp., 63 David St., New Bedford, Mass.

Shellac

The Montrose Corp., 138-A-41st St., Brooklyn 32, N.Y.

Silicates

Philadelphia Quartz Co., Philadelphia 6, Pa.

Silicone Fluid 555

Dow-Corning Corp., Midland, Michigan

Silicones

Dow-Corning Corp., Midland, Michigan
General Electric Company, Waterford, N.Y.

Sipon ES

American Alcolac Corp., 3440 Fairfield Rd., Baltimore 26, Md.

Soapmakers' Materials

Innis Speiden & Co., Inc., 120 Lexington Ave., New York 17, N.Y.
Philadelphia Quartz Co., Philadelphia 6, Pa.
Welch, Holme & Clarke Co., Inc., 439 West St., New York 14, N.Y.

Sodium Aluminum Chlorhydroxy Lactate Complex 40% Solution

Reheis Co., Inc., Berkeley Heights, New Jersey

Sodium Ethoxylated Lauryl Alcohol Sulfate Paste

American Alcolac Corporation, 3440 Fairfield Rd., Baltimore 26, Md.

Sodium Hexametaphosphate

Blockson Chemical Co., Joliet, Illinois

Sodium Lauryl Sulfate

Aceto Chemical Co., Inc., 40–40 Lawrence St., Flushing, N.Y.

Sodium Lauryl Sulfonate

Marchon Products Ltd., Whitehaven, England

Sodium or Potassium Zirconium Lactate

Titanium Alloy Mfg., Division of National Lead Co. and the Titanium Zirconium Co., 111 Broadway, New York 6, N.Y.

Sodium Stearate

Merck & Co., Inc., Rahway, N.J.

Solvents

Kessler Chemical Corp., 11th Ave and W. 26th St., New York, N.Y.

Sorbic Acid

Carbide and Carbon Chemicals Company, New York City, N.Y.

Sorbitan Monooleate (Span 80)

Atlas Powder Co., Wilmington, Delaware

Sorbitol

Merck & Co., Inc., Rahway, N.J.

"Sorbo"

Atlas Powder Co., Wilmington 99, Delaware

Stabilizers and Emulsifiers

Cherry-Burrell Corp., Cedar Rapids, Iowa

Stabilizer, Liquid

American Food Laboratories, 1000 Stanley Ave., Brooklyn 8, N.Y.

Stabilizer for Ice Cream

Stein-Hall, 285 Madison Ave., New York 17, N.Y.
Germantown Manufacturing Co., 5100 Lancaster Ave., Philadelphia 31, Pa.

Staley's Corn Syrup

A. E. Staley Manufacturing Co., Decatur, Illinois

Standard Vegetable Shortening

E. F. Drew & Co., 15 E. 26th St., New York, N.Y.

Stearic Acid

Atlas Powder Co., Wilmington 99, Delaware

Stearyl Alcohol U.S.P.

Aceto Chemical Co., Inc., 40–40 Lawrence St., Flushing 54, N.Y.

Sulfonated Oils

Jacques Wolf & Co., Passaic, N.J.

Sulfur, Colloidal

Mann Fine Chemicals, Inc., 136 Liberty St., New York 6, N.Y.

Super Hartolan

Croda Ltd., 15 East 26th St., New York 10, N.Y.

Talc, Powdered Minerals, Etc.

Charles B. Chrystal Co., Inc., 53 Park Pl., New York 7, N.Y.
Tamms Silica Co., 228 N. LaSalle St., Chicago 1, Ill.

Teepol

Shell Chemical Div. Shell Union Oil Corp., 100 Bush St., San Francisco, Calif.

Tegin (Glyceryl Monostearate, Self-Emulsifying)

Tegosept M & P

Goldschmidt Chemical Corp., 153 Waverly Place, New York 14, N.Y.

Tergitol Nonionic NPX

Carbide and Carbon Chemicals Co., 30 E. 42nd St., New York 17, N.Y.

Tetrahydronaphthalene

Baird Chemical Corporation, 10 West 33rd St., New York 1, N.Y.

Texapon BS
Texapon CS

Fallek Products Co., 165 Broadway, New York 6, N.Y.

Texofor A6

Clovers Ltd., Wortley Low Mills, Leeds 12, England

Triethanolamine

Carbide & Carbon Chemicals Corp., 30 E. 42nd St., New York, N.Y.
Dow Chemical Co., Midland, Mich.

Triethanolamine Lauryl Sulfate

American Alcolac Corporation, 3440 Fairfield Rd., Baltimore, Md.

Triethanolamine Ricinoleate

Philipp Brothers Chemicals, Inc., 37–39 Wall St., New York 5, N.Y.
The Baker Castor Oil Co., 118–122 Broadway, New York 5, N.Y.

Triton X–101

Rohm & Haas Company, Washington Square, Philadelphia 5, Pa.

Tuberose Extra Fine

Fritzsche Bros., Inc., 76 Ninth Ave., New York 11, N.Y.

Tuberyl Acetate

Verona Chemical Co., 26 Verona Ave., Newark 4, N.J.

Tween "20"

Atlas Powder Co., Wilmington 99, Delaware

Ultrapole S

Textilana Corporation, 12607 Cerise Ave., Hawthorne, Calif.

Undecylic Acid

The Baker Castor Oil Co., 40 Ave. A, Bayonne, N.J.

Vanillidine Acetone

F. Ritter & Company, 4001–4009 Goodwin Ave., Los Angeles 39, Calif.

Veegum H.V.

R. T. Vanderbilt Co., 230 Park Ave., New York 17, N.Y.

Vegetable Oils, Animal Fats, Fatty Acids, and Alkalies

Welch, Holme & Clark Co., Inc., 439 West St., New York 14, N.Y.

Veronol Aldehyde

Verona Chemical Co., 26 Verona Avenue, Newark, N.J.

Versalide

Givaudan-Delawanna, Inc., 321 W. 44th St., New York 36, N.Y.

Versene Na_4

The Dow Chemical Co., Midland, Michigan

Waxes BJ, F, O, OM, OP, S

Wax & Rosin Products, 42 Broadway, New York 4, N.Y.

Waxes (Carnauba, Ceresins, Ozokerites, Etc.)

E. A. Bromund Co., 256 Broadway, New York 13, N.Y.
Koster Kennan, Sayville, N.Y.
Will & Baumer Candle Co., Inc., Syracuse, N.Y.

Wecobee R & Hychol

Wecobee SS

E. F. Drew & Co., Inc., 15 E. 26th St., New York 10, N.Y.

Wood Flour

National Sawdust Co., 69 N. 6th St., Brooklyn, N.Y.

Ylang-Ylang Oil Bourbon

Fritzsche Bros. Inc., 76 Ninth Ave., New York 11, N.Y.

Zinc and Magnesium Stearates

M. W. Parsons-Plymouth, Inc., 59 Beekman St., New York, N.Y.

Zinc Oxide, U.S.P.

The New Jersey Zinc Co., 160 Front St., New York, N.Y.

Zinc Undecylenate

Baker Castor Oil Co., 118–122 Broadway, New York 5, N.Y.

Aerosol Valves

Oil Equipment Laboratories, Inc., 600 Pearl St., Elizabeth, N.J.
The Risdon Manufacturing Co., Naugatuck, Conn.

All Metal Circle Sifter

Allis-Chalmers, Industrial Equipment Division, Milwaukee 1, Wisc.

Autoclaves

Alco Product Div. of American Locomotive Co., Dunkirk, N.Y.

Aluminum Boxes

New Jersey Aluminum Co., Newark, N.J.

Bottles, Glass Jars, Etc.

Carr-Lowry Glass Co., Baltimore 3, Md.
Hazel Atlas Glass Co., Wheeling, W. Va.
Kimble Glass Co., Toledo 1, Ohio
Owens-Illinois Glass Co., Toledo 1, Ohio
Swindell Bros., Baltimore, Md.

Candy Cooker and Mixer

Savage Bros. Co., 2638 Gladys Ave., Chicago 12, Ill.

Cans and Tin Boxes

American Can Co., 100 Park Ave., New York, N.Y.
Continental Can Co., 633 Third Ave., New York 17, N.Y.
Crown Can Div. of Crown Cork & Seal Co., Erie Ave. and H St., Philadelphia, Pa.

Caps (Molded and Metal)

Armstrong Cork Co., Lancaster, Pa.

Collapsible Tubes

A. H. Wirz, Inc., 4th and Palmer Sts., Chester, Pa.
New England Collapsible Tube Co., 3132 S. Canal St., Chicago, Ill.

Colloid Mills

Chemicolloid Labs., 30 Church St., New York 7, N.Y.
Charles Ross & Son Co., 152 Classon Ave., Brooklyn 5, N.Y.

Driers

Witco Chemical Co., 122 East 42nd St., New York 17, N.Y.

Dustless Blenders

Sturtevant Mill Co., 106 Clayton St., Boston, Mass.

Filtering, Filling, Mixing Machinery

Alsop Engineering Corp., 305 Cass St., Milldale, Conn.
F. J. Stokes Machine Co., Philadelphia 20, Pa.
Karl Kiefer Machinery Co., Cincinnati, Ohio
The J. H. Day Co. Inc., 1149 Harrison Ave., Cincinnati, Ohio
The Hobart Manufacturing Co., Troy, Ohio
U. S. Bottlers Machinery, Chicago 18, Ill.

Filter Paper and Filtering Aids

August Giese & Son, 300 Fourth Ave., New York 16, N.Y.
Ertel Engineering Corp., Kingston 1, N.Y.
The Filter Paper Co., 2442 S. Michigan Ave., Chicago, Ill.

Glass-Lined Tanks

The Filter Paper Co., 2442 S. Michigan Ave., Chicago 16, Ill.
Pfaudler Co., 1000 West Ave., Rochester 3, N.Y.

Hand Refractometer

Bausch & Lomb Optical Co., Rochester 2, N.Y.

Homogenizer

Ultrasonic Company, 198 Pacific St., Newark, N.J.

Kettles & Vacuum Kettles

Hamilton Copper & Brass Works, Inc., Hamilton, Ohio

Laboratory Apparatus

Eimer & Amend, 633 Greenwich St., New York 14, N.Y.
Scientific Materials Co., Pittsburgh, Pa.

Laboratory Mills

American Pulverizer Co., 1131 Macklind Ave., St. Louis 10, Mo.

Lipstick Containers

The Plume & Atwood Mfg. Co., Waterbury, Conn.

Molds and Dies

Progressive Machinery Works, 137 W. 22nd St., New York 11, N.Y.
A. Cavalla, Inc., 163 W. 18th St., New York 11, N.Y.

Moulder & Filler

Excelsior Industrial Corporation, 611 W. 43rd St., New York 36, N.Y.

New Dial Type Candy Thermometer

Oringer Manufacturing Co., 154 State St., Boston, Mass.

New pH Meter

Dairyland Food Laboratories, Inc., Waukesha, Wisconsin

Paper Boxes

Hinde & Daugh, 4803 Decatur St., Sandusky, Ohio

Pocket pH *Meter*

Beckman Instruments Inc., Fullerton 1, California

Pocket Refractometer

National Instrument Co., 5005 Queensbury Ave., Baltimore 15, Md.

Portable Mixer

(3 Speed, No Clamping, 175, 325, 575 R.P.M.)

Consolidated Siphon Supply Co., Inc., 24 Wooster St., New York 13, N.Y.

Scales

The Exact Weight Scale Co., 935 W. 5th Ave., Columbus 8, Ohio

Soapmakers' Machinery

Houchin Machinery Co., Inc., Hawthorne, N.J.
Newman Tallow & Soap Machinery Co., Chicago 9, Ill.

Stainless Steel Kettles

B. H. Hubbert & Son, Inc., Baltimore 24, Md.
Lee Metal Products Co., Inc., 418 Pine St., Philipsburg, Pa.

Stainless Steel Tanks

Arthur Colton Co., 3400 E. Lafayette St., Detroit 7, Mich.
Metal Glass Products Co., Belding, Mich.
The Filter Paper Co., 2442 S. Michigan Ave., Chicago, Ill.

Starch Trays

Baywood Mfg. Co., Inc., 2757 Stillwell Ave., Brooklyn 24, N.Y.

Ultrasonic Emulsifier

Sonic Engineering Corp., 146 Selleck St., Stamford, Conn.

Vacuum Fruit Spread Cooker

Majonnier Bros. Co., 4601 West Ohio St., Chicago 44, Ill.

Vials and Miniatures

Glass Industries, Inc., 10 W. 33rd St., New York 1, N.Y.

Viscosity Cups

Eimer & Amend, 633 Greenwich St., New York 14, N.Y.

Weighing and Filling Machine

Wrights' Automatic Machinery Co., Durham, North Carolina

Index

O

P

T